Men's Issues and Men's Mental Health

Rob Whitley

Men's Issues and Men's Mental Health

An Introductory Primer

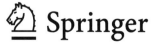

Rob Whitley
Douglas Research Centre
McGill University
Montreal, QC, Canada

ISBN 978-3-030-86319-7   ISBN 978-3-030-86320-3 (eBook)
https://doi.org/10.1007/978-3-030-86320-3

© Springer Nature Switzerland AG 2021

This work is subject to copyright. All rights are reserved by the Publisher, whether the whole or part of the material is concerned, specifically the rights of reprinting, reuse of illustrations, recitation, broadcasting, reproduction on microfilms or in any other physical way, and transmission or information storage and retrieval, electronic adaptation, computer software, or by similar or dissimilar methodology now known or hereafter developed.

The use of general descriptive names, registered names, trademarks, service marks, etc. in this publication does not imply, even in the absence of a specific statement, that such names are exempt from the relevant protective laws and regulations and therefore free for general use.

The publisher, the authors and the editors are safe to assume that the advice and information in this book are believed to be true and accurate at the date of publication. Neither the publisher nor the authors or the editors give a warranty, expressed or implied, with respect to the material contained herein or for any errors or omissions that may have been made. The publisher remains neutral with regard to jurisdictional claims in published maps and institutional affiliations.

This Springer imprint is published by the registered company Springer Nature Switzerland AG
The registered company address is: Gewerbestrasse 11, 6330 Cham, Switzerland

Preface

There is a growing interest in the field of men's mental health. This developing field is based on epidemiological findings that men experience elevated rates of certain mental health outcomes in comparison to women. For example, research consistently shows that men make up around 75% to 80% of all completed suicides in western countries. Likewise, rates of substance use disorder are significantly elevated in men, with around three out of four cases being male. Indeed, recent statistics indicate that males account for around 70% of overdose deaths related to the ongoing opioid crisis. Moreover, men still tend to under-utilize mental health services, with figures indicating that men account for around 30% of people who use mental health services. All this has led researchers, commentators, and journalists to describe men's mental health issues (and male suicide, in particular) in ominous terminology: a "silent epidemic," "an invisible crisis," "a quiet catastrophe," and "a gender gap that is a matter of life and death."

At the same time, there have been growing concerns about the general state and well-being of men and boys in western societies. These concerns are encapsulated in recent popular books on the topic, for example *Men on Strike* by Helen Smith, *The Boy Crisis* by Warren Farrell and John Gray, as well as *Man Interrupted* by Philip Zimbardo and Nikita Coulombe. In sum, these books argue that large numbers of men and boys are quietly suffering under the radar of society, with little response or empathy from official institutions or the general public. This has led to the formation of the term *Men's Issues*, an amorphous phrase referring to issues disproportionately experienced by males including homelessness, incarceration, and the aforementioned mental health issues. The examination of men's issues also involves shining a spotlight on patterns and trends within various sectors of society such as the educational system, the employment sector, and the family to assess the experience of men and boys therein.

This book attempts to merge these two emerging fields, through a rigorous and meticulous assessment of the scientific evidence related to men's mental health and men's issues. This involves the integration of findings from diverse fields including psychiatry, psychology, public health, epidemiology, and sociology. To my knowledge, this is the first book that attempts to rigorously synthesize scientific findings from these various disciplines to better understand men's issues and men's mental health. It is my intention to stretch and enrich existing work on the topic, avoiding a narrow focus on any one discipline or singular concept, instead examining the wider social context and broader cultural trends.

In pursuance of this aim, I was able to draw on my lengthy experience conducting research on women's mental health. Indeed, this was the focus of my research for many years, leading to research papers published in well-read journals including *Archives of Women's Mental Health, Social Science & Medicine,* and *Culture, Medicine & Psychiatry.* This research was conducted in diverse locations including immigrant neighbourhoods of Montreal (Québec), African-American neighbourhoods of Washington, DC, Kingston (Jamaica), and rural Ethiopia. While conducting such research, I was regularly accosted by female research participants making statements such as "What are you doing for our men?" and "We have forgotten about the boys around here." At the same time, a number of female students in my classes began making similar remarks, with one encouraging me to pursue my interest in men's mental health, writing an email to me stating that:

> I have an amazing father who worked extremely hard to give all of his children the same private education, regardless of their gender. I have a great boyfriend who does nothing but encourage me to succeed and throughout my education, I have had some great male teachers who have shared their knowledge and education with me, helping me to enhance my future. As someone who genuinely cares about men and their mental health, it was refreshing to hear something somewhat positive and from a different perspective in today's lecture…

More recently, I have been contacted by widows, mothers, wives, daughters, and other women with concerns about men's mental health, as well as by a variety of men across the world who have seen themselves or their loved ones struggle with mental health issues. Their collective concerns led me to refocus my scholarship onto men's mental health and helped spur the writing of this book, which attempts to fill a significant gap in the literature through a comprehensive overview of men's issues and men's mental health.

While this book is primarily intended for researchers, clinicians, academics, graduate students, and others working in fields related to men's mental health, much of the material can be easily read and understood by an intelligent lay reader. This means the book is accessible for men and women who may lack specialist knowledge in mental health sciences, but are motivated to inform themselves about core issues. This includes those working in the trenches to help men and boys such as teachers, social workers, religious ministers, sports coaches, and law enforcement. Indeed, it is my hope that the book will be useful to all who are interested in the topic.

Montreal, QC, Canada   Rob Whitley

Acknowledgments

In writing this book, I have been assisted by various research assistants, collaborators, and health advocates who have helped in various ways. This includes Lara Antebi, Victoria Carmichael, Sonora Grimsted, and Anne-Marie Saucier, whose assistance has been invaluable throughout the writing process. Thank you to one and all. I would also like to thank my employer, McGill University, who kindly granted me a leave of absence from teaching and administrative duties to write this book. Finally, I would like to thank Janet Kim of *Springer Nature* for her kind, helpful, and professional assistance in bringing this book to fruition.

Contents

1 An Introduction to Men's Issues and Men's Mental Health 1
   1.1 Beyond Masculinity 2
   1.2 Men's Issues and Men's Mental Health 3
   1.3 Common Issues 5
      1.3.1 Gender Stereotypes of Men 5
      1.3.2 Gender Empathy Gap 7
      1.3.3 Male Gender Blindness 9
   1.4 COVID-19 12
   1.5 Conclusion 13
   References 14

Part I Men's Mental Health

2 The Social Determinants of Male Suicide 23
   2.1 The Global Financial Crisis and Its Repercussions 23
   2.2 Which Men Are Killing Themselves? 24
      2.2.1 Middle-Aged Men 25
      2.2.2 Men in Rural and Remote Regions 25
      2.2.3 White Men 25
      2.2.4 Indigenous and Aboriginal Men 26
      2.2.5 Military Veterans 27
      2.2.6 Men Involved in the Criminal Justice System 27
   2.3 Social Context and Common Risk Factors 28
      2.3.1 Employment Issues 28
      2.3.2 Marital Status, Divorce and Family Issues 31
      2.3.3 Mental Disorders and Substance Use Issues 33
   2.4 Social Integration and Social Connection 35
   2.5 Conclusion 37
   References 37

3	**Wasted Lives: Substance Abuse, Substance Use Disorder and Addictions in Men**	45
	3.1 Addictions and Substance Abuse in DSM-5	46
	3.2 Alcohol-Related Disorders and Alcohol Use	47
	3.3 Cannabis-Related Disorders and Cannabis Use	48
	3.4 Opioid-Related Disorders and Opioid Use	49
	3.5 Gambling Disorder	51
	3.6 Internet Gaming Disorder	52
	3.7 Aetiology and Causation	53
	3.7.1 Educational Failure and Subsequent Failure to Launch	54
	3.7.2 Unemployment and Employment Issues	56
	3.7.3 Divorce, Separation and Loneliness	58
	3.8 The Consequences of SUD and Addictions	59
	3.9 Treatments	61
	3.10 Conclusion	62
	References	63
4	**Attention-Deficit/Hyperactivity Disorder in Young Males: The Medicalization of Boyhood?**	71
	4.1 What Is ADHD?	71
	4.2 The Epidemiology of ADHD	73
	4.3 US Studies on ADHD	75
	4.4 Risk Factors	77
	4.4.1 Middle-Childhood Years	77
	4.4.2 Childhood Maltreatment and Neglect	77
	4.4.3 Low Family Income	78
	4.4.4 Low Parental Education	78
	4.4.5 Single-Mother Families	78
	4.5 Educational Impact	80
	4.6 Impact into Adulthood	81
	4.7 Medication Issues	82
	4.7.1 Side Effects and Misuse	82
	4.7.2 Absolute Gender Differences in Medication Usage	83
	4.7.3 Relative Gender Differences in Medication Usage	84
	4.8 The Medicalization Hypothesis	85
	4.8.1 The Psychiatric Industry	88
	4.8.2 Big Pharma	89
	4.8.3 Mothers and Medicalization	90
	4.8.4 Schools and Education	92
	4.8.5 People with an ADHD Diagnosis	94
	4.9 Social Control	95
	4.10 Conclusion	96
	References	97

5	**Risk Factors and Rates of Depression in Men: Do Males Have Greater Resilience, or Is Male Depression Underrecognized and Underdiagnosed?**	105
	5.1 The Prevalence of Depression	106
	5.2 Gender Differentials in Prevalence and Treatment	107
	5.3 Male Resilience	108
	5.4 An Artefactual Difference?	110
	5.5 Bias in Diagnostic Criteria: A Male Depressive Syndrome?	111
	5.6 Risk Factors	113
	5.6.1 Low Educational Attainment	113
	5.6.2 Unemployment and Financial Strain	114
	5.6.3 Disability	115
	5.6.4 Homosexual Orientation	116
	5.6.5 Divorce	117
	5.6.6 Ethno-Racial Status	118
	5.7 Paternal Postpartum Depression	118
	5.8 Conclusion	120
	References	121
6	**Why Do Men Have Low Rates of Formal Mental Health Service Utilization? An Analysis of Social and Systemic Barriers to Care and Discussion of Promising Male-Friendly Practices**	127
	6.1 Masculinity and Men's Formal Service Use	129
	6.2 Stigma	130
	6.2.1 Stigma in the Media	131
	6.2.2 Stigma in the Workplace	132
	6.2.3 Stigma in the Family	133
	6.2.4 Stigma in Health Services	133
	6.3 Formal Mental Health Services: An Unwelcoming Environment?	134
	6.4 The Different Modalities of Healing	136
	6.5 Making Male-Friendly and Male-Sensitive Services	138
	6.6 Men's Sheds: An Innovative and Promising Practice	140
	6.7 Conclusion and Recommendations	142
	References	143

Part II Men's Issues and Their Relation to Men's Mental Health

7	**The Gender Gap in Education: Understanding Educational Underachievement in Young Males and Its Relationship to Adverse Mental Health**	153
	7.1 Background	153
	7.2 Low Educational Attainment: A Mental Health Risk Factor	155
	7.2.1 Suicide	155
	7.2.2 Substance Abuse	156

		7.2.3 Depression and Anxiety	157
	7.3	The Educational Gender Gap	158
		7.3.1 Primary Education	159
		7.3.2 Secondary Education	161
		7.3.3 Tertiary Education	164
	7.4	Failure to Launch and Male Loneliness	167
	7.5	Conclusion	168
	References		169
8	**Employment, Unemployment, and Workplace Issues in Relation to Men's Mental Health**		177
	8.1	Gender Differences in Paid Work	178
	8.2	Unemployment	179
	8.3	Employment, Unemployment, and Mental Health	179
		8.3.1 Suicide	181
		8.3.2 Substance Abuse	183
		8.3.3 Depression and Anxiety	185
	8.4	Employment Conditions and Workplace Environment	187
		8.4.1 Precarious Employment	187
		8.4.2 Job Stress and Job Strain	188
		8.4.3 Male-Dominated Occupations	190
		8.4.4 Occupational Health and Safety	191
		8.4.5 Workplace Stigma	193
	8.5	The Big Picture: Changing Economic Trends and Gender Differentials in Employment	194
	8.6	Conclusion	197
	References		198
9	**Family Ties: Marriage, Divorce, and the Mental Health of Men and Boys**		207
	9.1	Marital Status and Mental Health in Adults	208
		9.1.1 Depression	209
		9.1.2 Substance Abuse	210
		9.1.3 Suicide	211
		9.1.4 The Psychosocial Impact of Divorce for Men	212
		9.1.5 The Psychosocial Stress of Single Unmarried Men	214
		9.1.6 A Unifying Theory? Durkheim and Social Integration	216
		9.1.7 The Big Picture: A Worsening Situation?	217
		9.1.8 Implications of Trends for Mental Health	219
	9.2	The Effects of Divorce and Father Absence on Offspring Mental Health	220
		9.2.1 Single-Father Households	222
		9.2.2 Plausible Mechanisms and Pathways to Mental Health	223
		9.2.3 The Big Picture: Trends and Social Context	225
	9.3	Conclusion	227
	References		228

10 Men's Mental Health: Time for a Paradigm Shift 235
    10.1 Sociocultural Determinants of Mental Health 235
    10.2 Traditional Masculinity: Friend or Foe to Mental Health? 237
    10.3 A Strengths-Based Approach 239
    10.4 Stereotypes and Biases 240
    10.5 Male-Friendly Policies, Programs, and Procedures 242
    10.6 Conclusion 244
    References 244

Index 247

About the Author

Rob Whitley, PhD, is an associate professor in the Department of Psychiatry, McGill University (Montreal, Québec, Canada), and a research scientist at the Douglas Research Centre. He is also an Honorary Principal Fellow at the University of Melbourne, and has held honorary appointments at King's College London, Dartmouth Medical School (New Hampshire), and Howard University (Washington, DC). He has published over 150 academic papers in the field of social and cultural psychiatry, and has written over 100 mental health-related articles for lay audiences in diverse venues including *Psychology Today*, the *HuffPost*, the *Montreal Gazette*, the *Vancouver Sun*, and the *National Post*. Whitley is also a video-producer and film-maker, and has produced several documentaries and short fictional films related to men's mental health that have been featured in film festivals across North America. His research has been financially supported by a variety of public and private funding bodies including the Canadian Institutes of Health Research, the Social Sciences and Humanities Research Council of Canada, the Mental Health Commission of Canada, Veterans Affairs Canada, and Movember. He is currently a Fonds de recherche du Québec-Santé Senior Research Scholar.

Chapter 1
An Introduction to Men's Issues and Men's Mental Health

It's a man's world. Or is it? Recent statistics indicate that men are suffering numerous difficulties (or disparities) in modern western societies. There has been much media coverage of the gender pay gap – with men on average earning significantly more money than women – a complex issue revisited in the later chapter on employment issues (see Chap. 8). But what about the many other gender gaps where men are worse off than women? These are also complex issues that are discussed in the various chapters of this book, including:

 (i) The health gap, with men having an increased risk of various mental health issues including suicide, substance abuse and attention-deficit hyperactivity disorder, as well as lower rates of health service utilization.
 (ii) The education gap, with boys dropping out of high school at a much higher rate than girls, and also performing worse in exams at every level of education, with young men now making up a solid minority of postsecondary students.
 (iii) The justice gap, with men more likely to receive longer sentences than women for the same crime (even when controlling for prior criminal history), and less likely to obtain favourable outcomes from the family court system.

Many of these gender gaps are unknown to the general public, and some are quietly worsening under the radar of society, negatively affecting millions of males across the western world. The experience of these adverse outcomes is a tragedy for the males involved, and also a tragedy for their families, friends and society as a whole. As such, it is essential to document the facts and discuss underlying causes of the many psychosocial issues that are disproportionately affecting males. Therein lies the purpose of this book. The aim is to inform and educate the reader about these core issues, with a focus on men's mental health and well-being. Indeed, this book will give clinicians, social service practitioners, policy-makers, researchers, teachers, academics and others concrete, concise and up-to-date information that can be used to better address problems that affect males. Hopefully, the content of this book will inspire key stakeholders to take action to improve the lives of men and boys in the clinic, the classroom, the workplace or elsewhere.

In pursuance of this aim, this book moves beyond simplistic one-dimensional platitudes that glibly and wholly blame men for their existential woes; a phenomenon known in the social sciences as *victim blaming* (Crawford, 1977; Richards et al., 2003). This refers to a tendency to place sole responsibility for a physical or mental illness on the individual beliefs, behaviours, attitudes and lifestyle choices of the illness bearer: a common phenomenon in the literature on male psychology and in wider public discourse (Bilsker et al., 2018; Whitley, 2018; Essex, 1996).

Victim blaming typically involves a narrow deficit-based focus, and is inconsistent with an amassed body of public health research investigating social context, which indicates that health outcomes are determined by a constellation of supra-individual level factors (Krieger, 1994; Wilkinson, 1999; Marmot, 2005). An example of narrowly focused victim blaming is found in popular writing that blames men's mental health woes on stereotypical individual-level traits such as stubbornness and stoicism, without exercising any peripheral vision to examine social context and supra-individual level factors. Often, this involves the use of vague all-encompassing pseudo-intellectual terminology to describe the underlying causes of men's mental health issues, for example, 'male privilege' or 'toxic masculinity': unvalidated and unscientific terms that falsely paint a whole gender as poisonous or privileged.

Instead of taking a victim-blaming approach, this book focuses on the wider social determinants of men's mental health, with a focus on social context and cultural influences. This is consistent with the standard approach adopted in public health research, which uses a broad lens to examine the complex web of causation through holistic and multi-level analysis (Kawachi et al., 2020; Berkman et al., 2014; Krieger, 1994). This includes an intentional examination of distal upstream societal factors such as education (see Chap. 7) and employment (see Chap. 8), assessing their influence on proximal downstream individual outcomes such as suicide (see Chap. 2) and substance abuse (see Chap. 3). By definition, this wide-lensed public health approach avoids the aforementioned victim blaming frequently seen in discourse and scholarship that focuses on individual-level attributes. This public health approach is utilized throughout this book, which adopts a novel framework to men's issues and men's mental health through its focus on: (i) social determinants of mental health; (ii) upstream distal influences on psychosocial outcomes; and (iii) wider socio-cultural change that is affecting men.

1.1 Beyond Masculinity

As stated, this book attempts to overcome some of the limitations of a narrow approach to men's mental health, by deliberately examining social context and other upstream factors. This involves moving beyond a singular focus on the concept of masculinity, with a variety of scholars recently noting that this focus has tended to unduly dominate the conversation about men's mental health (Liddon & Barry, 2021; Seager & Barry, 2019; Whitley, 2018; Poole, 2016). This undue focus typically involves framing traditional masculinity in a negative manner. For example, a recent European Parliament report attributed mental health issues in men to "masculinity which may encourage suppression of emotions or resort to anger" (Committee on Women's Rights and Gender Equality, 2016). Other organizations have taken aim at masculinity, with the World Health Organization encouraging "programmes with men and boys that include deliberate discussions of gender and masculinity" as an answer to men's issues (Barker et al., 2007).

The limits of such an excessive concentration on the singular concept of masculinity are noted in a recent paper aptly titled "Men's Health: Beyond Masculinity", which notes that several men's health programs and policies "have located the problem as masculinity [and] suggested the problem is in men's heads" – further arguing for a better consideration of social determinants and social context (Elder & Griffith, 2016). Other researchers have come to a similar conclusion, with a report from the Men's Health Initiative of British Columbia noting that a singular focus on the supposed pathological role of masculinity risks "blaming the victim; undervaluing positive male traits; and alienating men in whom we seek to instil healthy behaviours" (Bilsker et al., 2010).

Such a singular focus on *masculinity* can propel a narrow research agenda, and can also lead to health promotion efforts which may be limited in their impact. For example, the US Agency for Healthcare Research and Quality ran a series of billboards with the slogan "this year thousands of men will die from stubbornness" (Elder & Griffith, 2016). Similarly, the website of Beyond Blue, an Australian mental health charity, states on its webpage devoted to male mental health that "men are known for bottling things up" (Whitley, 2018). Such campaigns have a subtext, namely, that men's mental health outcomes are principally determined by men's individual (and inherently self-defeating) beliefs and attitudes. But as this book will outline, this is a narrow one-dimensional framing of the issue that is not consistent with the wider public health and social science literature. Worse still, it can contribute to the aforementioned victim-blaming approach, which may exacerbate male mental health issues and deter mental health service utilization in men. Given this situation, the content of this book deliberately eschews an undue focus on the concept of masculinity, and instead represents a careful examination of social and cultural context.

1.2 Men's Issues and Men's Mental Health

The terms *men's mental health* and *men's issues* refer to two overlapping and intertwining fields, but as yet there are no commonly accepted consensual definitions of these two related terms. In this book, Chaps. 2, 3, 4, 5 and 6 deal with issues that would conventionally be characterized as men's mental health issues if adopting a traditional definition of that term. Chapter 2 deals with male suicide, Chap. 3 with substance abuse and addictions issues and Chap. 4 with attention-deficit hyperactivity disorder. These outcomes were chosen for in-depth analysis at the start of the book as considerable epidemiological research indicates that males experience these adverse mental health outcomes at a significantly higher rate than females. Thus, each of these chapters explores gender differences in prevalence, as well as underlying causes and possible explanations for elevated rates among males. Chapter 5 focuses on depression, which has traditionally been considered to affect women more than men at a rate of around 2:1. This chapter examines the literature suggesting that men may be more resilient to depression, as well as other research noting that the differences between men and women may be exaggerated due to measurement and reporting biases, entertaining the possibility that men actually have similar rates to women. Chapter 6 examines a growing corpus of research indicating that men tend to underutilize formal mental health services, but are more likely than women to engage with more informal mental health services. This includes an elucidation of differential patterns of service use by gender and an exploration of the underlying factors behind gender variations in service use.

In sum, Chaps. 2, 3, 4, 5 and 6 are devoted to topics that could be characterized as core men's mental health issues, if adopting a narrow definition of the term. Chapters 7, 8, 9 and 10 cast a broader net to discuss some of the wider factors that have been characterized as *men's issues*, linking these issues to the mental health outcomes described in earlier chapters. What are these purported men's issues? First, several scholars have argued that the educational system is failing boys and young men, with males experiencing elevated rates of high-school dropout, suspension and expulsion, as well as low rates of tertiary enrolment (Farrell & Gray, 2019; Sax, 2016; Hoff Sommers, 2013). This education gap is concerning, as low educational attainment has been linked to a variety of adverse mental health outcomes. All of this is discussed in Chap. 7. Second, a growing body of research indicates that many men are having difficulty adapting to broad changes in the world of work, particularly blue-collar men and men lacking a postsecondary education (Case & Deaton, 2020; Zimbardo & Coulombe, 2016; Baumeister, 2010). This is leading to high rates of unemployment and failure to launch among the affected men, which again has been linked to adverse mental health. All this is discussed in Chap. 8. Third, social trends indicate a massive change in typical family formation in recent decades, with an increase in divorce, the never-married, and single-person households, which can influence psychosocial well-being and wider ontological security (Bauman, 2003; Beck & Beck-Gernsheim, 1995; Giddens, 1992). For men, such changes often lead to separation from children, high rates of loneliness and social support deficits, which have been linked to adverse mental health. All this is discussed in Chap. 9. The final chapter brings all these separate strands together in a conclusion outlining ways to address the mental health and psychosocial issues plaguing a substantial portion of the male population.

1.3 Common Issues

Each chapter of this book is self-contained and discusses unique issues related to the central theme of the chapter in an in-depth and comprehensive manner. That said, there are a number of core concepts that transverse the various chapters of this book and are revisited frequently to illuminate points made. In particular, three overlapping and intertwining concepts underpin the central thesis of this book, namely, (i) gender stereotypes of men; (ii) the gender empathy gap; and (iii) male gender blindness. These three concepts are detailed and defined in turn in the next sub-section, with examples given to further understanding.

1.3.1 Gender Stereotypes of Men

Evidence from a variety of sources indicates the existence of enduring gender stereotypes across various sectors of society, with men sometimes stereotyped more negatively than women. One well-researched phenomenon is known as the women are wonderful effect (or *halo effect*); terms that were coined based on research indicating that people typically attribute significantly more positive and pleasant traits to women than to men (Krys et al., 2018; Rudman & Goodman, 2004; Eagly & Mladinic, 1994). Interestingly, both men and women tend to possess such biased stereotypes, with women typically stereotyped as warm and nurturing, while men are typically stereotyped as dominant and aggressive (Reynolds et al., 2020; Kite & Whitley, 2016).

One common manifestation of such biased gender stereotypes is the familiar *women as victim/men as villain* dichotomy, where men are sometimes framed as villainous threats to the social order and women as helpless passive victims, regardless of actual circumstances (Synnott, 2016; Reynolds et al., 2020; Baumeister, 2010). This stereotype contributes to wider public attitudes and beliefs about men and women, and can feed into policy emanating from governments as well as local institutions such as schools, healthcare providers and law enforcement. As will be noted throughout this book, this stereotype (and associated policies) can be harmful to men's mental health, as it can frame all men in a stereotypical manner (i.e. as villains or perpetrators), which can lead to the wider demonization of men in local settings. This demonization may be especially severe when intersecting with other harmful stereotypes. For example, black men (Oliver, 2003), military veterans (McCartney, 2011), single men (Morris et al., 2008) and men with mental illness (Whitley, 2013) may experience a harmful double stigma based on enduring stereotypes about their gender and demographic group, which can lead to emotional distress and social harm.

Numerous studies show that the media perpetuates the female victim/male villain dichotomy, regardless of actual circumstances. For example, one content analysis of Canadian newspaper articles found that the media more frequently described men with mental illness in stigmatizing and derogatory language, whereas women with mental illness were more often described with empathy and compassion (Whitley et al., 2015). A similar study found that the media tended to berate men for being silent about their depression and their reluctance to seek help, rather than encourage men to take action (Bengs et al., 2008). These findings overlap with stereotypes found in classical literature, where archetypal fictional characters such as Svengali, Don Juan, Lothario, Iago and Dracula are framed as a corruptive presence lurking in the shadows of polite society.

The presence of these stereotypes has led to the formulation of what is known as the chivalry hypothesis. This posits that the state and society act in a gallant and forgiving manner towards women, consistent with the passive victim stereotype; while acting in a more vindictive and suspicious manner towards men, consistent with the villainous perpetrator stereotype (Grabe et al., 2006). As said, this can manifest itself in various policy decisions. A notable example was the Canadian Government's decision to make single men (but not single women) a lower priority in its Syrian refugee resettlement program, concluding that single men are a potential threat to Canadian society (Houle, 2019). Another egregious example is a common airline policy that prohibits solo male passengers from sitting next to an unaccompanied minor, with such men being asked to swap seats with a female passenger, again implying that men are a potential threat and inherently prone to paedophilia (Dai, 2012). A further example could be seen in criminal court sentencing decisions, with one well-researched US study finding that men receive 63% longer sentences than women, even after controlling for the arrest offence and prior criminal history, with men also twice as likely to go to prison if convicted (Starr, 2012).

It has been argued that these negative stereotypes of men are perpetuated by all-encompassing buzzwords frequently seen in the media such as 'patriarchy', 'male privilege', 'rape culture' and 'toxic masculinity' which can shape wider attitudes and policies (Nuzzo, 2019; Barry et al., 2019). Such negative stereotypes may also have been fuelled by recent social movements including #MeToo and moral panics about male sexuality on campus and beyond (Liddon & Barry, 2021; Kipnis, 2017). In sum, the actions of a very small minority of men are often extrapolated to the whole population of men by various sectors of society, leading to the aforementioned negative stereotypes and associated policies which can discriminate against men. As will be argued throughout this book, such negative stereotypes can colour and shape the treatment of males by others, including treatment by: (i) health services; (ii) law enforcement; (iii) the legal system; (iv) employers; (v) teachers/professors; and (vi) the general public. This can affect mental health.

1.3.2 Gender Empathy Gap

The gender empathy gap is a relatively new phrase that refers to variations in public and private empathy towards men and women, with women typically receiving more empathy than men, even when controlling for situational factors (Collins, 2019; Seager, 2019). This gender empathy gap is influenced by the aforementioned stereotypes of men as villainous perpetrators and women as passive victims, and can also derive from chivalric notions that women are more worthy of care, forgiveness and attention than men (Grabe et al., 2006). According to growing research, this gender empathy gap is real, common and measurable.

Indeed, the gender empathy gap can be inferred from various statistics, which rarely raise more than a whimper of protest, and are largely unknown to the bulk of society. For example, men make up over 90% of the prison population, over 85% of the homeless population and are twice as likely than women to be a victim of crime (Brown et al., 2019; Wilkins, 2015). As detailed in Chap. 8, men account for around 90% of workplace deaths and injuries, with recently released figures indicating that male life expectancy is significantly lower than female life expectancy at 76 years on average for American men and 81 years for women (Arias & Xu, 2020). As further elucidated in Chap. 7, males are suffering multiple inequities in the school system, including higher rates of dropout, suspension and exclusion. However, there are very few public programs or interventions addressing these issues. On the contrary, the European Union, Germany, Japan, the United Kingdom, Canada and the World Bank recently announced an investment of nearly $4 billion for women's and girl's education across the world (Government of Canada, 2018). There was nothing for boys, who are often in dire need of help and assistance. All this could be related to variations in gender empathy, which have also been explored in several experimental studies comparing responses to men and women in distress.

For example, a recent paper describes a series of studies on gender-based moral typecasting, with over 3000 participants responding to a variety of vignettes detailing workplace harm involving men, women or characters of unspecified gender (Reynolds et al., 2020). This study found that participants generally:

(i) Assume a victim of workplace harm is female in vignettes where gender is unspecified
(ii) Felt less warmly towards a victim of workplace harm when they assumed that the victim was a male
(iii) Were more likely to perceive a fired male as less of a victim and experiencing less pain than a fired female
(iv) Perceived that males experienced less pain than females after hearing an ambiguous yet potentially offensive workplace joke
(v) Were more willing to punish and less willing to forgive male perpetrators of workplace harm than female perpetrators
(vi) Perceived managers as more intentionally harmful and immoral when they fired a group of women compared to firing a group of men.

In other words, this study demonstrates that men are less likely to be perceived as victims than women, that harm to men evokes less moral outrage than equivalent harm to women, and that people typically extend less empathy to men and are less sensitive to male suffering.

Of note, this study found that both male and female participants tended to show favouritism to women over men, indicating that differences in gender empathy are held by men and women alike. These findings are consistent with other research indicating that men are one of the few demographic groups who do not display in-group favouritism when making judgements and decisions, or when imparting empathy (Baumeister, 2010; Rudman & Goodman, 2004). This absence of in-group favouritism among males begins at an early age, with one study indicating that both adolescent boys and girls report more empathy to females in distress as compared to males in distress (Stuijfzand et al., 2016). This raises the question of whether the gender empathy gap has a biological basis, or is a product of wider socialization.

Interestingly, some studies indicate that biology can play a role in the gender empathy gap. For example, several studies indicate that the presence of neotenous features (known colloquially as 'cuteness') such as large eyes, small nose, flattened face, high-pitched voice and low muscle mass elicits more empathy, help, support and pity from third parties (Lishner et al., 2008; Keating et al., 2003; Dijker, 2001). Of note, such neotenous features are sexually dimorphic, thus being significantly more common in women than men, meaning that third parties may instinctively extend the same level of empathy and protection to women as they do to children (Cunningham et al., 1995; Barber, 1995; Gould, 1985). Indeed, a vignette-based study found that more muscular individuals receive less pity or attention for their suffering in comparison to leaner (i.e. more neotenous) individuals, with very muscular males receiving the least pity (Dijker, 2001). Like neotenous features per se, muscle mass is also sexually dimorphic, with men tending to have significantly more muscle mass than women (Lassek & Gaulin, 2009).

In other words, the possession of more childlike features in adolescence and adulthood can elicit more empathy and concern from others, but males tend to lose such features as they age, while females often maintain them into adulthood. Incidentally, neotenous features in females may also contribute to benevolent sexism, a paternalistic belief that adult women are like children and need care and protection (or 'safe spaces') from challenging environments and demanding situations.

Others have argued that the empathy gap may be due to evolutionary psychology. For example, men possess human sperm, while women possess human eggs. To put it crudely, human sperm is much more common than human eggs, meaning that sperm is less valuable and more disposable than human eggs. This means that (at a species level) women make a greater physiological contribution to reproduction, which may result in collective values that prioritize the protection of women from harm, while caring less about male suffering, as this ensures the reproductive vitality of a culture (Baumeister, 2010). This can be seen in social norms such as 'women and children first' in the face of disaster. For example, the survival of women was prioritized during the sinking of RMS Titanic, meaning 73% of women on board survived, compared to only 21% of men (Seager & Barry, 2019). Such phenomena led Farrell (1993) to write that "men are the disposable sex", while Baumeister (2010) argues that "men's lives are valued much less than women's...men are more expendable than women". To support such claims, both these authors argue that societies are often prepared to sacrifice men for the common good, whether this be in war, hazardous occupations, or other dangerous activities that protect and enhance civilization (and simultaneously lower the life expectancy of men). This occurs with little public outcry, again indicating a gender empathy gap between women and men.

However, it is commonly accepted that within a civilized society, evolutionary psychology or long-practiced social norms should not take precedence when making decisions about policy and practice, especially when this has public health consequences. In contrast, reason, science and ethics should combine to ensure equitable and evidence-based policy and decision-making. As will be detailed later in this book, such procedures are not always observed with regards to the mental health of men and boys, where services are underfunded and policies often punitive. The empathy gap is another real yet ignored phenomena that may be contributing to dysfunctional practices and policies regarding men and boys, and is thus revisited throughout this book.

1.3.3 *Male Gender Blindness*

A final concept reappearing regularly throughout this book is known as *male gender blindness*. This term was coined by psychologists Martin Seager and John Barry, and refers to the tendency to overlook or ignore issues, inequities and disparities disproportionately experienced by men and boys, perhaps fuelled by the gender empathy gap (Seager et al., 2014, 2016; Liddon et al., 2019). A cogent example of male gender blindness can be seen in a recent analysis of scientometric data comparing research on 'men's health' with research on 'women's health' (Nuzzo, 2019). This study found:

(i) Nearly a 10-fold difference in use of the term 'women's health' compared to 'men's health' in the title or abstract of scientific papers indexed in PubMed since 1970
(ii) 199 cases where the term 'men's health' was used in abstracts and titles of academic papers in 2018, compared to 900 cases for the term 'women's health'
(iii) Six specific scientific journals devoted to men's health, compared to 62 journals devoted to women's health.

This led the author to conclude that "men's health...has not been recognized and promoted in the same way as women's health...discussions on 'gender equity' in health tend to focus almost exclusively on women". This is a common conclusion from scholars working in the field of men's mental health. For example, Englar-Carlson (2019) writes that "for the most part, when scholars are writing about gender, they are often referring to women rather than the experiences of women and men", while Seager et al. (2016) state that "gender issues, however, have come almost exclusively to mean women's issues". This issue is dealt with in detail throughout this book, where it is often noted that reports, inquiries, action plans and interventions related to gender and mental health mainly focus on women and girls, and typically ignore men and boys.

For example, the European Parliament's Committee on Women's Rights and Gender Equality (2016) recently produced a report entitled "on promoting gender equality in mental health and clinical research", which was adopted by the Parliament in plenary session. However, the word *gender* is implicitly equated with *women* throughout the report, and only two paragraphs out of 163 are devoted to men's mental health. Likewise, a word count reveals that the words "women" and "girls" are mentioned 217 times, whereas "men" and "boys" are mentioned only 45 times; and when males are mentioned, it is mainly in a victim-blaming framework (Whitley, 2017).

Such blindness to male health is often seen in national action plans and health frameworks. For example, the US Department of Health and Human Services Office of Disease Prevention and Health Promotion (2020) created a set of "data-driven national objectives to improve health and well-being over the next decade" in a strategy entitled 'Healthy People 2030'. This strategy lists 35 specific objectives with the goal of promoting health and well-being for women, but only four objectives specific to men, again indicating a common blindness to men's issues.

Similarly, there are many publicly funded national bureaus and local clinics devoted to women's health, but very few devoted to men's health. For example, the US National Institute of Health contains a well-funded Office for Research on Women's Health, but there is as yet no analogous office for men's health research (Nuzzo, 2019). Similarly, one research study found that 49 out of 50 top US hospitals contain a women's health centre, but only 16 out of these 50 top hospitals contain an analogous men's health centre (Choy et al., 2015).

In Canada, the government contains a dedicated Minister for Women in charge of a government Department for Women and Gender Equality which (inter alia) funds projects in areas such as "ending violence against women and girls; improving the economic security and prosperity of women and girls; and encouraging women and girls in leadership roles" (Department for Women and Gender Equality, 2020). However, again there is no equivalent body devoted to furthering the welfare of men and boys, another example of male gender blindness at the governmental level. Also in Canada, the government recently concluded a lengthy *National Inquiry into Missing and Murdered Indigenous Women and Girls,* a worthy initiative that nevertheless failed to include any investigation of missing and murdered Indigenous men, even though figures indicate that Indigenous men are murdered and missing at a similar rate to Indigenous women (Jones, 2015).

1.3 Common Issues

Perhaps the most egregious case of male gender blindness relates to Intimate Partner Violence (IPV). The popular image of IPV is based on the aforementioned gender stereotype of a male villain and a female victim. But these hackneyed stereotypes paint a very incomplete picture, with recent research indicating a high number of male victims of domestic abuse. For example, a recent UK government survey indicated that 9% of males had experienced some form of partner abuse, which amounts to around 1.4 million British men (Office for National Statistics, 2018). This includes stalking, physical violence and sexual assault. Indeed, a seminal US research study found that male IPV victims are often slapped, kicked, punched, grabbed or choked (Hines et al., 2007). In Canada, a large survey concluded that "equal proportions of men and women (4%) reported being victims of spousal violence during the preceding 5 years" (Canadian Centre for Justice Statistics, 2016). However, this issue rarely receives public attention (let alone public services), with data indicating that there are over 600 shelters devoted to abused women in Canada, but zero shelters devoted to abused men (Roebuck et al., 2020; Beattie & Hutchins, 2015). This means that the 418,000 abused men across Canada typically lack services and support. For such men, there are no dedicated national inquiries, no government departments devoted to their welfare, and no specific official funding bureaus supporting research, interventions or programs.

This manifestation of male gender blindness in relation to IPV has real consequences for the affected men. Not only can it lead to a lack of services, but it can also inhibit male help-seeking behaviour. For example, the aforementioned surveys indicate that small proportions of men (less than 20% of victims) will tell the police or a health professional about their victimization. Evidence suggests that this may be due to well-grounded fears that they will be ridiculed, scorned or disbelieved by these authorities. In fact, a recent research paper found that the overarching experience of male IPV victims was that 'no one would ever believe me'. One victim noted 'I told friends, they laughed' while another stated '…the police, they laughed' (Bates, 2019). Indeed, Dutton (2012) found that over half of male victims who called the police reported being treated as the perpetrator, while several studies indicate that female perpetrators are much less likely to be arrested and charged than male perpetrators, even when injuries are sustained by the victim (Roebuck et al., 2020; Mahony, 2010; Millar & Brown, 2010).

In sum, the phenomena of IPV against men exemplifies the intersection of the three important concepts presented in this chapter: (i) stereotypes of men; (ii) the gender empathy gap; and (iii) male gender blindness. First, male victims are often considered perpetrators by the police and sometimes disbelieved by clinicians, suggesting that professionals' actions are coloured by negative stereotypes associated with the male villain/female victim Manichaean dichotomy. Second, male victims receive a lack of empathy for their plight, and are often met with laughter and ridicule from friends as well as law enforcement, suggesting differential levels of empathy for male and female victims of IPV. Third, there appears to be a wilful blindness to male victims of IPV, as evidenced by the lack of official services and support for this population, as well as governmental inertia to address this issue.

1.4 COVID-19

Another example that can be used to illustrate male gender blindness and the gender empathy gap is related to COVID-19. This book was written during the COVID-19 pandemic in 2020–2021. Undoubtedly, this pandemic and its associated lockdowns have had a powerful effect on the mental health of men and women alike, but at the time of writing hard data on mental health is lacking. In contrast, there is a growing corpus of research on physical health and COVID-19, pointing to gender differentials in: (i) mortality; (ii) severity; and (iii) rates of testing and vaccination.

With regards to mortality, a variety of studies indicate that men are significantly more likely to die from COVID-19 than women, even though incidence rates of COVID-19 are similar (Stokes et al., 2020). For example, an analysis of data from eight developed countries found a M:F rate ratio of 1.4 (confidence interval not presented), with men in the 40- to 60-year-old age category experiencing over double the rates of their female peers (Bhopal & Bhopal, 2020). A similar US study found a M:F rate ratio of 1.4 (95% CI 1.2–1.6) among White Americans and 1.5 (95% CI 1.3–1.7) among Black Americans (Rushovich et al., 2021). Data from the US Centers for Disease Control and Prevention (CDC) (2021b) indicates that 54% of COVID-19-related deaths have been male, with 46% female.

With regards to severity, evidence suggests that men typically experience more severe symptoms of COVID-19 than women. For example, one study from the CDC analysed outcomes from over 1.3 million confirmed cases in the USA, finding a preponderance of severe outcomes in males (Stokes et al., 2020) such as:

 (i) 16% of males with COVID-19 were hospitalized, compared to 12% of females
 (ii) 2.8% of males with COVID-19 were admitted to the ICU, compared to 1.7% of females
(iii) 6% of males with COVID-19 died, compared to 4.8% of females

These findings overlap with a study of 29 countries finding men accounted for a higher proportion of deaths, ICU admissions and hospitalizations (Global Health 5050, 2021).

With regard to rates of testing and vaccination, research indicates that men are significantly less likely to be tested or vaccinated than women. For example, the aforementioned study of 29 countries found that the average vaccination coverage across these countries was 14% of women and 10% of men (March 2021), with women accounting for 60% of people who have received two vaccination doses (Global Health 5050, 2021). Data from the CDC in mid-April 2021 indicates that 35 million females had been vaccinated, compared to 27 million males, meaning that men accounted for only 43% of vaccinations at that time (CDC, 2021a).

However, these differentials are largely unknown to the general public and are rarely discussed by the media, policy-makers, researchers or other key societal stakeholders. In contrast, much media attention has focused on the deleterious impact of COVID-19 on women (e.g. Henriques, 2020; Madgavkar et al., 2020; Topping, 2020), with one representative BBC article entitled 'How COVID-19 is changing women's lives' (Savage, 2020). Similarly, health researchers have tended to focus on women, with a recent emblematic article (in the prestigious journal *Nature*) entitled 'women are most affected by pandemics', concluding that 'addressing some of the issues that women face in outbreaks highlights a broader landscape of inequalities' (Wenham et al., 2020).

A core theme of this book is that men's health and women's health is not a zero-sum game, and that a gendered approach to mental health should be a hallmark of a caring and inclusive society. This must include a careful consideration of the impact of wider social context on the mental health of both males and females, as well as tailored policy and service responses that account for gender differentials and preferences. As such, it is very important to assess the impact of COVID-19 on women and girls, and there are various socio-economic domains where women appear to be experiencing a higher rate of inequities compared to men, which demand a tailored policy response (Wenham et al., 2020).

However, there has been little analogous discussion of the impact of COVID-19 on men and boys, and little policy or service response taking a targeted approach to reducing COVID-19-related inequities in males. In fact, one recent article aptly notes that the focus is rarely on men in discussions of gender and COVID-19, even though COVID-19-related morbidity and mortality is higher in men than women (Ellison et al., 2021). This absence of attention to the impact of COVID-19 on men could be due to the aforementioned *gender empathy gap* as well as male gender blindness. Moreover, *gender stereotypes* can also play a role, with women more easily framed as victims of COVID-19 than men by the media, policy-makers and the public at large. A core thesis of this book is that these three phenomena also limit and constrain thinking and action about men's mental health, which is harmful to the affected men, their families, and society as a whole.

1.5 Conclusion

A definable scientific field of men's mental health has only recently emerged, and even then this has been a quiet emergence. Similarly, there has been little academic interest in what have been termed *men's issues*. In contrast, there has been considerable popular writing and discourse about men's mental health, both in the legacy media and social media. This has tended to engage in scientifically illiterate victim blaming of men experiencing psychosocial distress, with little acknowledgement of the complex web of causation. This book attempts to rectify this situation, through a comprehensive public health-inspired multi-level analysis of men's mental health and men's issues with a focus on social context. This involves documenting and analysing distal and proximal social determinants of mental health, as well as a critical examination of the nature and configuration of mental health services. So far, many discussions about men's mental health have led to a singular message: that individual men need to change. But an essential thesis of this book is that society, its institutions, and health services in particular need to change in order to successfully address the many psychosocial issues plaguing men.

References

Arias, E., & Xu, J. (2020). United States life tables, 2018. *National Vital Statistics Reports, 69*(12), 1–44.

Barber, N. (1995). The evolutionary psychology of physical attractiveness: Sexual selection and human morphology. *Ethology & Sociobiology, 16*(5), 395–424. https://doi.org/10.1016/0162-3095(95)00068-2

Barker, G., Ricardo, C., & Nascimento, M. (2007). *Engaging men and boys in changing gender-based inequity in health: Evidence from programme interventions*. World Health Organization. Retrieved May 10, 2021 from https://www.who.int/gender/documents/Engaging_men_boys.pdf

Barry, J., Kingerlee, R., Seager, M., & Sullivan, L. (Eds.). (2019). *The Palgrave handbook of male psychology and mental health*. Palgrave Macmillan.

Bates, E. (2019). "No one would ever believe me": An exploration of the impact of intimate partner violence victimization on men. *Psychology of Men and Masculinities, 21*(4), 497–507. https://doi.org/10.1037/men0000206

Bauman, Z. (2003). *Liquid love: On the frailty of human bonds*. Polity Press.

Baumeister, R. F. (2010). *Is there anything good about men?: How cultures flourish by exploiting men*. Oxford University Press.

Beattie, S., & Hutchins, H. (2015). *Shelters for abused women in Canada, 2014*. In *Statistics Canada*. Retrieved May 6, 2021, from https://www150.statcan.gc.ca/n1/en/pub/85-002-x/2015001/article/14207-eng.pdf?st=bySNKZoM

Beck, U., & Beck-Gernsheim, E. (1995). *The normal chaos of love*. Polity Press.

Bengs, C., Johansson, E., Danielsson, U., Lehti, A., & Hammarström, A. (2008). Gendered portraits of depression in Swedish newspapers. *Qualitative Health Research, 18*(7), 962–973. https://doi.org/10.1177/1049732308319825

Berkman, L. F., Kawachi, I., & Glymour, M. M. (Eds.). (2014). *Social epidemiology* (2nd ed.). Oxford University Press. http://ndl.ethernet.edu.et/bitstream/123456789/31016/1/Lisa%20F.%20Berkman.pdf

Bhopal, S. S., & Bhopal, R. (2020). Sex differential in COVID-19 mortality varies markedly by age. *The Lancet, 396*(10250), 532–533. https://doi.org/10.1016/S0140-6736(20)31748-7

Bilsker, D., Fogarty, A. S., & Wakefield, M. A. (2018). Critical issues in men's mental health. *Canadian Journal of Psychiatry. Revue Canadienne de Psychiatrie, 63*(9), 590–596. https://doi.org/10.1177/0706743718766052

References

Bilsker, D., Goldenberg, L., & Davison, J. A. (2010). *A roadmap to men's health: Current status, research, policy & practice*. University of Alberta. Retrieved May 10, 2021, from https://www.ualberta.ca/anesthesiology-pain-medicine/media-library/eliassons-wellness-docs/mens-mental-health/a-roadmap-to-mens-health.pdf

Brown, J. S. L., Sagar-Ouriaghli, I., & Sullivan, L. (2019). Help-seeking among men for mental health problems. In J. A. Barry, R. Kingerlee, M. Seager, & L. Sullivan (Eds.), *The Palgrave handbook of male psychology and mental health* (pp. 397–415). Palgrave Macmillan.

Canadian Centre for Justice Statistics. (2016, January 21). *Family violence in Canada: A statistical profile, 2014*. Statistics Canada. Retrieved May 6, 2021, from https://www150.statcan.gc.ca/n1/pub/85-002-x/2016001/article/14303-eng.pdf

Case, A., & Deaton, A. (2020). *Deaths of despair and the future of capitalism*. Princeton University Press.

Centers for Disease Control and Prevention (CDC). (2021a). *Demographic characteristics of people receiving COVID-19 vaccinations in the United States*. Centers for Disease Control and Prevention. Retrieved May 6, 2021, from https://covid.cdc.gov/covid-data-tracker/#vaccination-demographic

Centers for Disease Control and Prevention (CDC). (2021b). *Demographic trends of COVID-19 cases and deaths in the US reported to CDC*. Centers for Disease Control and Prevention. Retrieved May 6, 2021, from https://covid.cdc.gov/covid-data-tracker/#demographics

Choy, J., Kashanian, J. A., Sharma, V., Masson, P., Dupree, J., Le, B., & Brannigan, R. E. (2015). The men's health center: Disparities in gender specific health services among the top 50 "best hospitals" in America. *Asian Journal of Urology, 2*(3), 170–174. https://doi.org/10.1016/j.ajur.2015.06.005

Collins, W. (2019). *The empathy gap: Male disadvantages and the mechanisms of their neglect*. LPS Publishing.

Committee on Women's Rights and Gender Equality. (2016, December 12). *On promoting gender equality in mental health and clinical research (2016/2096(INI))*. European Parliament. Retrieved May 10, 2021, from https://www.europarl.europa.eu/doceo/document/A-8-2016-0380_EN.html

Crawford, R. (1977). You are dangerous to your health: The ideology and politics of victim blaming. *International Journal of Health Services, 7*(4), 663–680. https://doi.org/10.2190/YU77-T7B1-EN9X-G0PN

Cunningham, M. R., Roberts, A. R., Barbee, A. P., Druen, P. B., & Wu, C.-H. (1995). "Their ideas of beauty are, on the whole, the same as ours": Consistency and variability in the cross-cultural perception of female physical attractiveness. *Journal of Personality and Social Psychology, 68*(2), 261–279. https://doi.org/10.1037/0022-3514.68.2.261

Dai, S. (2012, August 13). All men are potential pedophiles in the eyes of Australian Airlines. *The Atlantic*. https://www.theatlantic.com/international/archive/2012/08/all-men-are-potential-pedophiles-eyes-australian-airlines/324776/

Department for Women and Gender Equality. (2020, November 26). *Department for women and gender equality – Women's program*. Government of Canada. Retrieved May 6, 2021, from https://www.canada.ca/en/women-gender-equality/news/2019/03/department-for-women-and-gender-equality%2D%2Dwomens-program.html

Dijker, A. J. (2001). The influence of perceived suffering and vulnerability on the experience of pity. *European Journal of Social Psychology, 31*(6), 659–676. https://doi.org/10.1002/ejsp.54

Dutton, D. G. (2012). The case against the role of gender in intimate partner violence. *Aggression & Violent Behavior, 17*(1), 99–104. https://doi.org/10.1016/j.avb.2011.09.002

Eagly, A. H., & Mladinic, A. (1994). Are people prejudiced against women? Some answers from research on attitudes, gender stereotypes, and judgments of competence. *European Review of Social Psychology, 5*(1), 1–35. https://doi.org/10.1080/14792779543000002

Elder, K., & Griffith, D. M. (2016). Men's health: Beyond masculinity. *American Journal of Public Health, 106*(7), 1157. https://doi.org/10.2105/AJPH.2016.303237

Ellison, J. M., Semlow, A. R., Jaeger, E. C., Bergner, E. M., Stewart, E. C., & Griffith, D. M. (2021, March 26). *Why COVID-19 policy should explicitly consider men's health*. Medical News Today. Retrieved May 6, 2021, from https://www.medicalnewstoday.com/articles/why-covid-19-policy-should-explicitly-consider-mens-health

Englar-Carlson, M. (2019). Forward. In J. A. Barry, R. Kingerlee, M. Seager, & L. Sullivan (Eds.), *The Palgrave handbook of male psychology and mental health* (pp. vii–xiv). Palgrave Macmillan.

Essex, C. (1996). Men's health: Don't blame the victims. *British Medical Journal, 312*(7037), 1040. https://doi.org/10.1136/bmj.312.7037.1040a

Farrell, W. (1993). *The myth of male power*. Berkley Books.

Farrell, W., & Gray, J. (2019). *The boy crisis: Why our boys are struggling and what we can do about it*. BenBella Books.

Giddens, A. (1992). *The transformation of intimacy: Sexuality, love, and eroticism in modern societies*. Stanford University Press.

Global Health 5050. (2021, March). *The COVID-19 sex-disaggregated data tracker: March update report*. Global Health 5050. Retrieved May 6, 2021, from https://globalhealth5050.org/wp-content/uploads/March-2021-data-tracker-update.pdf

Gould, S. J. (1985). *Ontogeny and phylogeny*. Harvard University Press.

Government of Canada. (2018, June 10). *Advancing gender equality and women's empowerment*. Government of Canada. Retrieved May 10, 2021, from https://pm.gc.ca/en/news/backgrounders/2018/06/10/advancing-gender-equality-and-womens-empowerment

Grabe, M. E., Trager, K. D., Lear, M., & Rauch, J. (2006). Gender in crime news: A case study test of the chivalry hypothesis. *Mass Communication and Society, 9*(2), 137–163. https://doi.org/10.1207/s15327825mcs0902_2

Henriques, M. (2020, April 12). Why Covid-19 is different for men and women. *British Broadcasting Corporation (BBC)*. https://www.bbc.com/future/article/20200409-why-covid-19-is-different-for-men-and-women

Hines, D. A., Brown, J., & Dunning, E. (2007). Characteristics of callers to the domestic abuse helpline for men. *Journal of Family Violence, 22*, 63–72. https://doi.org/10.1007/s10896-006-9052-0

Hoff Sommers, C. (2013). *The war against boys: How misguided policies are harming our young men* (Reissue ed.). Simon & Schuster.

Houle, R. (2019, February 12). *Results from the 2016 Census: Syrian refugees who resettled in Canada in 2015 and 2016*. Statistics Canada. Retrieved May 10, 2021, from https://www150.statcan.gc.ca/n1/pub/75-006-x/2019001/article/00001-eng.htm

Jones, A. (2015). Adam Jones: Aboriginal men are murdered and missing far more than aboriginal women. A proper inquiry would explore both. *National Post*. https://nationalpost.com/opinion/adam-jones-aboriginal-men-are-murdered-and-missing-far-more-than-aboriginal-women-a-proper-inquiry-would-explore-both

Kawachi, I., Lang, I., & Ricciardi, W. (Eds.). (2020). *Oxford handbook of public health practice 4e*. Oxford University Press.

Keating, C., Randall, D. W., Kendrick, T., & Gutshall, K. A. (2003). Do babyfaced adults receive more help? The (cross-cultural) case of the lost resume. *Journal of Nonverbal Behavior, 27*(2), 89–109. https://doi.org/10.1023/A:1023962425692

Kipnis, L. (2017). *Unwanted advances: Sexual paranoia comes to campus*. Harper Collins.

Kite, M. E., & Whitley, B. E., Jr. (2016). *Psychology of prejudice and discrimination* (3rd ed.). Routledge.

Krieger, N. (1994). Epidemiology and the web of causation: Has anyone seen the spider? *Social Science & Medicine, 39*(7), 887–903. https://doi.org/10.1016/0277-9536(94)90202-X

Krys, K., Capaldi, C. A., van Tilburg, W., Lipp, O. V., Bond, M. H., Vauclair, C.-M., Manickam, L. S. S., Domínguez-Espinosa, A., Torres, C., Lun, V. M.-C., Teyssier, J., Miles, L. K., Hansen, K., Park, J., Wagner, W., Arriola Yu, A., Xing, C., Wise, R., Sun, C.-R., & Ahmed, R. A. (2018). Catching up with wonderful women: The women-are-wonderful effect is smaller in more

References

gender egalitarian societies. *International Journal of Psychology, 53*(1), 21–26. https://doi.org/10.1002/ijop.12420

Lassek, W. D., & Gaulin, S. J. C. (2009). Costs and benefits of fat-free muscle mass in men: Relationship to mating success, dietary requirements, and native immunity. *Evolution and Human Behavior, 30*(5), 322–328. https://doi.org/10.1016/j.evolhumbehav.2009.04.002

Liddon, L., & Barry, J. (Eds.). (2021). *Perspectives in male psychology: An introduction*. Wiley-Blackwell.

Liddon, L., Kingerlee, R., Seager, M., & Barry, J. A. (2019). What are the factors that make a male-friendly therapy? In J. Barry, R. Kingerlee, M. Seager, & L. Sullivan (Eds.), *The Palgrave handbook of male psychology and mental health*. Palgrave Macmillan.

Lishner, D., Oceja, L. V., Stocks, E., & Zaspel, K. (2008). The effect of infant-like characteristics on empathic concern for adults in need. *Motivation and Emotion, 32*(4), 270–277. https://doi.org/10.1007/s11031-008-9101-5

Madgavkar, A., White, O., Krishnan, M., Mahajan, D., & Azcue, X. (2020, July 15). *COVID-19 and gender equality: Countering the regressive effects*. McKinsey Global Institute. Retrieved May 6, 2021, from https://www.mckinsey.com/featured-insights/future-of-work/covid-19-and-gender-equality-countering-the-regressive-effects

Mahony, T. H. (2010). *Police-reported dating violence in Canada, 2008*. Statistics Canada. Retrieved May 10, 2021, from https://www150.statcan.gc.ca/n1/pub/85-002-x/2010002/article/11242-eng.htm

Marmot, M. (2005). Social determinants of health inequalities. *The Lancet, 365*(9464), 1099–1104. https://doi.org/10.1016/S0140-6736(05)71146-6

McCartney, H. (2011). Hero, victim or villain? The public image of the British Soldier and its implications for defense policy. *Defense & Security Analysis, 27*(1), 43–54. https://doi.org/10.1080/14751798.2011.557213

Millar, P., & Brown, G. (2010). Explaining gender differences in police arresting and charging behavior in cases of spousal violence. *Partner Abuse, 1*(3), 314–331. https://doi.org/10.1891/1946-6560.1.3.314

Morris, W. L., DePaulo, B. M., Hertel, J., & Taylor, L. C. (2008). Singlism—Another problem that has no name: Prejudice, stereotypes and discrimination against singles. In M. A. Morrison & T. G. Morrison (Eds.), *The psychology of modern prejudice* (pp. 165–194). Nova Science Publishers.

Nuzzo, J. L. (2019). Men's health in the United States: A national health paradox. *The Aging Male, 23*(1), 42–52. https://doi.org/10.1080/13685538.2019.1645109

Office for National Statistics. (2018). *Domestic abuse: Findings from the Crime Survey for England and Wales – Appendix tables*. Office for National Statistics. Retrieved May 6, 2021, from https://www.ons.gov.uk/peoplepopulationandcommunity/crimeandjustice/datasets/domesticabusefindingsfromthecrimesurveyforenglandandwalesappendixtables

Office of Disease Prevention and Health Promotion. (2020). *Healthy people 2030*. U.S. Department of Health and Human Services. Retrieved May 6, 2021, from https://health.gov/healthypeople/objectives-and-data/browse-objectives

Oliver, M. B. (2003). African American men as "criminal and dangerous": Implications of media portrayals of crime on the "criminalization" of African American men. *Journal of African American Studies, 7*(2), 3–18. https://doi.org/10.1007/s12111-003-1006-5

Poole, G. (2016, November). *The need for male-friendly approaches to suicide prevention in Australia*. Mengage. Retrieved May 10, 2021, from https://www.mengage.org.au/images/Preventing-Male-Suicide-AMHF-desktop.pdf

Reynolds, T., Howard, C., Sjåstad, H., Zhu, L., Okimoto, T. G., Baumeister, R. F., Aquino, K., & Kim, J. (2020). Man up and take it: Gender bias in moral typecasting. *Organizational Behavior and Human Decision Processes, 161*, 120–141. https://doi.org/10.1016/j.obhdp.2020.05.002

Richards, H., Reid, M., & Watt, G. (2003). Victim-blaming revisited: A qualitative study of beliefs about illness causation, and responses to chest pain. *Family Practice, 20*(6), 711–716. https://doi.org/10.1093/fampra/cmg615

Roebuck, B., McGlinchey, D., Hastie, K., Taylor, M., Roebuck, M., Bhele, S., Hudson, E., & Grace Xavier, R. (2020, August 14). *Male survivors of intimate partner violence in Canada*. Office of the Federal Ombudsman for Victims of Crime (OFOVC). Retrieved May 10, 2021, from https://www.victimsfirst.gc.ca/res/cor/IPV-IPV/Male%20Survivors%20of%20IPV%20in%20Canada,%202020.pdf

Rudman, L. A., & Goodman, S. A. (2004). Gender differences in automatic in-group bias: Why do women like women more than men like men? *Journal of Personality and Social Psychology, 87*(4), 494–509. https://doi.org/10.1037/0022-3514.87.4.494

Rushovich, T., Boulicault, M., Chen, J. T., Danielsen, A. C., Tarrant, A., Richardson, S. S., & Shattuck-Heidorn, H. (2021). Sex disparities in COVID-19 mortality vary across US racial groups. *Journal of General Internal Medicine*. https://doi.org/10.1007/s11606-021-06699-4

Savage, M. (2020, June 30). How Covid-19 is changing women's lives. *British Broadcasting Corporation*. https://www.bbc.com/worklife/article/20200630-how-covid-19-is-changing-womens-lives

Sax, L. (2016). *Boys adrift: The five factors driving the growing epidemic of unmotivated boys and underachieving young men* (Revised and Updated ed.). Basic Books.

Seager, M. (2019). From stereotypes to archetypes: An evolutionary perspective on male help-seeking and suicide. In J. A. Barry, R. Kingerlee, M. Seager, & L. Sullivan (Eds.), *The Palgrave handbook of male psychology and mental health* (pp. 227–248). Palgrave Macmillan.

Seager, M., & Barry, J. A. (2019). Positive masculinity: Including masculinity as a valued aspect of humanity. In J. A. Barry, R. Kingerlee, M. Seager, & L. Sullivan (Eds.), *The Palgrave handbook of male psychology and mental health* (pp. 105–122). Palgrave Macmillan.

Seager, M., Barry, J. A., & Sullivan, L. (2016). Challenging male gender blindness: Why psychologists should be leading the way. *Clinical Psychology Forum, 285*, 35–40.

Seager, M., Sullivan, L., & Barry, J. (2014). The male psychology conference, University College London, June 2014. *New Male Studies: An International Journal, 3*(2), 41–68.

Starr, S. (2012). Estimating gender disparities in federal criminal cases. *American Law and Economics Review, 17*(1), 127–159. https://doi.org/10.2139/ssrn.2144002

Stokes, E. K., Zambrano, L. D., Anderson, K. N., Marder, E. P., Raz, K. M., El Burai Felix, S., Tie, Y., & Fullerton, K. E. (2020). Coronavirus disease 2019 case surveillance – United States, January 22–May 30, 2020. *MMWR Morbidity and Mortality Weekly Report, 69*, 759–765. https://doi.org/10.15585/mmwr.mm6924e2

Stuijfzand, S., De Wied, M., Kempes, M., Van de Graaff, J., Branje, S., & Meeus, W. (2016). Gender differences in empathic sadness towards persons of the same- versus other-sex during adolescence. *Sex Roles, 75*(9), 434–446. https://doi.org/10.1007/s11199-016-0649-3

Synnott, A. (2016). *Re-thinking men: Heroes, villains and victims*. Routledge. https://www.taylorfrancis.com/books/mono/10.4324/9781315606132/re-thinking-men-anthony-synnott

Topping, A. (2020, March 27). Mothers say they are being kept at work in UK as fathers stay home. *The Guardian*. https://www.theguardian.com/world/2020/mar/27/mothers-say-they-being-kept-at-work-uk-as-fathers-stay-home?CMP=share_btn_tw

Wenham, C., Smith, J., Davies, S. E. Feng, H., Grépin, K. A., Harman, S., Herten-Crabb, A., & Morgan, R. (2020, July 8). Women are most affected by pandemics – Lessons from past outbreaks. *Nature*. Retrieved May 6, 2021, from https://www.nature.com/articles/d41586-020-02006-z

Whitley, R. (2013). Fear and loathing in New England: examining the health-care perspectives of homeless people in rural areas. *Anthropology & Medicine, 20*(3), 232–243. https://doi.org/10.1080/13648470.2013.853597

Whitley, R. (2017, May 12). Gender and mental health: Do men matter too? *Psychology Today*. Retrieved May 10, 2021, from https://www.psychologytoday.com/ca/blog/talking-about-men/201705/gender-and-mental-health-do-men-matter-too

Whitley, R. (2018). Men's mental health: Beyond victim-blaming. *The Canadian Journal of Psychiatry, 63*(9), 577–580. https://doi.org/10.1177/0706743718758041

References

Whitley, R., Adeponle, A., & Miller, A. R. (2015). Comparing gendered and generic representations of mental illness in Canadian newspapers: An exploration of the chivalry hypothesis. *Social Psychiatry and Psychiatric Epidemiology, 50*(2), 325–333. https://doi.org/10.1007/s00127-014-0902-4

Wilkins, D. (2015). *How to make mental health services work for men.* Men's Health Forum. Retrieved May 10, 2021, from https://www.menshealthforum.org.uk/sites/default/files/pdf/how_to_mh_v4.1_lrweb_0.pdf

Wilkinson, R. G. (1999). Health, hierarchy, and social anxiety. *Annals of the New York Academy of Sciences, 896*(1), 48–63. https://doi.org/10.1111/j.1749-6632.1999.tb08104.x

Zimbardo, P. G., & Coulombe, N. (2016). *Man, interrupted: Why young men are struggling what we can do about it.* Red Wheel.

Part I
Men's Mental Health

Chapter 2
The Social Determinants of Male Suicide

There is one undeniable fact regarding suicide and gender – men make up the vast majority of completed suicides across the world. Indeed, the World Health Organization reports that around two out of three suicides across the globe are male (WHO, 2018). These global figures signify an alarming suicide rate among men per se. However, a more granular analysis indicates certain regions have even higher proportions of male suicide. In Europe, men make up around 80% of completed suicides, while in the Americas men make up around 75% of completed suicides.

In Canada, approximately 3000 men die by suicide per year, which translates to over 50 deaths per week. In the USA, around 35,000 men die by suicide every year, which translates to around 1 every 15 minutes. This has led Professor Dan Bilsker of Simon Fraser University to declare that we are in the midst of a "silent epidemic of male suicide" (Bilsker & White, 2011).

Worryingly, rates of male suicide appear to be rising, after a period of declining rates. For example, a US Centers for Disease Control and Prevention (CDC) report noted that age-adjusted male suicide rates in the USA showed a period of slight decline from the mid-1980s to 2006. But this same report notes that male suicide increased by around 2% per year from 2006 to 2017, reflecting a 26% increase in male suicides since 1999 (Hedegaard et al., 2018).

2.1 The Global Financial Crisis and Its Repercussions

Several studies have linked this rise in male suicides to the 2007–2008 Global Financial Crisis (GFC) and its repercussions, especially the subsequent Great Recession, which negatively affected aspects of the economy dominated by men (Case & Deaton, 2020). One study indicated a significant rise in US suicides from

2007–2010, resulting in around 5000 excess suicide deaths (Reeves et al., 2012). The authors attributed around a quarter of these suicides to rising rates of unemployment – an issue discussed later in this chapter, as well as in much more detail in Chap. 8, which is devoted to issues surrounding employment and men's mental health.

Similar trends have been observed in other parts of the world. For example, a steady downward trend in male suicides was witnessed in most Western European countries in the years before the Global Financial Crisis (Stuckler et al., 2011). However, a comprehensive cross-national study found a significant increase in male suicide in 2009 across the world. This was especially marked in Europe – a 4% increase (95% CI: 3.4–5.1); and the Americas – a 6% increase (95% CI: 5.4–7.5) (Chang et al., 2013). In contrast, this study found that rates of female suicide remained stable in Europe, with a less marked 2% increase (95% CI: 1.1–3.5) in the Americas.

Other research has examined suicide rates within specific European nations, pointing to a similar rise in male suicide, often ascribed to financial and employment issues arising from the GFC. For example, a time trend analysis compared actual suicides with expected suicides in 2008–2010 in the UK, finding a significant rise in suicides, with 846 excess male suicides (95% CI: 818–877) compared to 155 excess female suicides (95% CI: 121–189). Interestingly, this study found that regions with higher rates of unemployment had higher rates of male suicide (Barr et al., 2012). Similar increases in male suicide after the Global Financial Crisis have been observed in Greece (Kentikelenis et al., 2011), Italy (De Vogli et al., 2013), and several other European countries (Stuckler et al., 2011).

Interestingly, the male suicide rate has continued to rise in the Americas and Europe in more recent years, even though the most severe consequences of the Global Financial Crisis have passed. For example, a recent report noted that the unadjusted suicide rate (for both males and females) in the USA has risen from 15 suicide deaths per 100,000 in 2005 to 18 suicide deaths per 100,000 in 2017 (US Department of Veterans Affairs, 2019). Male suicides rates are even higher, with the CDC noting 22 suicides per 100,000 in 2017 – a 30 year high.

2.2 Which Men Are Killing Themselves?

It is important to state that suicide can affect all demographics, and that no group of men are immune from risk of suicide. It is also important to state that suicide also remains a rare event, even in high-risk populations. That said, the amassed research indicates that certain groups of men are at a higher risk of suicide. These include: (i) middle-aged men; (ii) men living in rural and remote regions; (iii) White men; (iv) Indigenous men; (v) military veterans; and (vi) men involved in the criminal justice system. All of these groups are dealt with in detail next.

2.2.1 Middle-Aged Men

In terms of age, suicides in western countries are particularly pronounced among men ages 40–60 years. In general, these men have higher rates than older and younger men, though men over 75 years old tend to have high rates, with young men having the lowest rates (WHO, 2018). As discussed later in this chapter, these elevated rates have been linked to the experience of severe life events that often occur in the middle-years of life, including divorce (see Chap. 9), job loss (see Chap. 8), foreclosure and bankruptcy.

2.2.2 Men in Rural and Remote Regions

In terms of region, men living in small towns, rural regions and sparsely populated areas have particularly high rates of suicide (Hirsch, 2007). In the USA, flyover states such as Wyoming, Montana, New Mexico and Utah have the highest rates of male suicide. Alaska also has high rates. Indeed, a recent CDC report indicates that the most rural US counties have a suicide rate 1.8 times higher than the most urban counties (Hedegaard et al., 2018). There are similarly high rates in rural and remote regions of Canada (Burrows et al., 2013), Australia (Alston, 2012) and the UK (Levin & Leyland, 2005). This has been linked to a variety of employment and socio-economic factors, namely, declines in traditional industries and decreasing economic opportunity for blue-collar men lacking postsecondary education, discussed later in this chapter, and in much more detail in a devoted chapter later in this book (see Chap. 8). It should also be noted that Aboriginal and Indigenous men often live in these regions (see Sect. 2.2.4).

2.2.3 White Men

In terms of ethnicity, ethnic minority men within western countries tend to have lower rates of suicide than Whites of European ancestry, as well as lower rate of mental illness per se. For example, African-Americans, Hispanics and Asian Americans within the USA tend to have significantly lower rates of suicide than White men of European ancestry (Sullivan et al., 2013). Similarly, White men of European ancestry in Canada and Australia tend to have higher rates than both non-European immigrants, as well as Canadian-born ethnic minorities (Malenfant, 2004; Ide et al., 2012). This has been attributed to various factors. On the one hand, ethnic minority men may live in subcultures that tend to have higher rates of religiosity, more inter-generational bonding, and greater social support from extended family and friends (Whitley et al., 2017; Lawrence et al., 2016; Sax, 2016). On the other hand, White men may live in subcultures characterized by high levels of individualism, which can lead to isolation and a lack of social support (Bellah et al., 1996; Putnam 2001). This thesis is considered in more detail in Sect. 2.4, where social integration and connection are discussed.

2.2.4 Indigenous and Aboriginal Men

The only ethnic group in the USA that has similar rates to Whites are American Indians. One recent study found that American Indians had slightly lower rates than Whites, but higher rates than Blacks, Hispanics and Asian Americans (Sullivan et al., 2013). Another recent study found that American Indians had a 50% higher rate of suicide than Whites in the USA, with especially high rates in Alaska and the Northern Plains (Herne et al., 2014).

In contrast, studies consistently and unequivocally indicate that Indigenous Canadian men and Aboriginal Australian men have considerably higher rates than all other ethnic groups in their respective nations (Pollock et al., 2018). Indeed, evidence suggests that some remote Inuit communities in Northern Quebec have a youth suicide rate over 10 times higher than the Quebec average, with most suicides being single young men (Boothroyd et al., 2001; Kral, 2012). Again, higher rates are seen in rural, remote and sparsely populated areas, linked to factors such as unemployment, lack of opportunity, poor living conditions, and lack of hope (Hicks, 2007, Kral, 2012; O'Keefe & Wingate, 2013).

Importantly, tens of thousands of Canadian Indigenous males (and females) experienced a unique, lengthy and incomparable stressor during their youth. This stressor was their forced separation from their families and communities to attend government-sponsored residential schools located outside their home communities, the last of which closed in 1996. These residential schools were part of Canada's long-term assimilationist policy vis-à-vis Aboriginal people. Evidence suggests that many of these institutions enacted a strict regime, and that mental, physical and sexual abuse (and neglect) were common (Royal Commission on Aboriginal Peoples, 1996). Unsurprisingly, a large corpus of research has linked such adverse childhood experience to suicide, substance use and other mental health issues in later adulthood (Brodsky & Stanley, 2008; Elias et al., 2012).

Evidence suggests that these negative sequalae have had a cumulative and collective effect within Aboriginal communities, leading to some level of intergenerational traumas (Bombay et al., 2014). A similar phenomenon occurred in Australia with the stolen generation, where mixed-race Indigenous children were systematically removed from their families and relocated to governmental institutions. Again, this traumatic experience has been linked to high rates of suicide in Indigenous and Aboriginal populations therein (Hunter & Harvey, 2002).

2.2.5 Military Veterans

Another group of men with a higher risk of suicide are military veterans. Indeed, a recent report from the US Department of Veterans Affairs (2019) noted that the rate of suicide among US male veterans was 30% higher than other adult men, with the highest rates in young veterans ages 18–34 years. This report notes that the current age-adjusted suicide rate among male veterans is 39 per 100,000, meaning around 13 male veterans per day die by suicide in the USA. Similar findings were contained in two recent reports from Veterans Affairs Canada, which found that male veterans had a 36% higher risk of suicide than other adult men (VanTil et al., 2018; Simkus et al., 2017). Similar to the US data, these Canadian reports found that young male veterans were most at risk, with an age-adjusted rate of 28 male suicides per 100,000 in the first 10 years after discharge – the most vulnerable period for veterans. Importantly, the preponderance of suicides among recently discharged and younger US and Canadian veterans will include large numbers of men who served in recent conflicts such as Afghanistan and Iraq.

Again, these suicides have been linked to unique stressors experienced by military personnel, especially for those involved in frontline combat. By definition, such personnel have faced immense dangers to life and limb, and may have witnessed close-quarter death and destruction. This can increase risk of PTSD, which is significantly higher in veterans as compared to the general population (Thompson et al., 2015). Moreover, the transition to civilian life can be challenging for veterans, with around 50% reporting difficulties in adjustment after discharge (Rose et al., 2018), and only 29% of veterans reporting high levels of social support, which can lead to loneliness, alienation and social isolation (Ketcheson et al., 2018). Again, this is considered in more detail in Sect. 2.4, where social integration and connection are discussed.

2.2.6 Men Involved in the Criminal Justice System

Men involved in the justice system also have an elevated rate of suicide. One study found that 11.5% of male suicides in the 40- to 64-year old age category were involved in the criminal justice system, compared to 3.8% of female suicides (Hempstead & Phillips, 2015). Moreover, men in prison have a higher rate of suicide. One cross-national study found that 93% of prison suicides are male, and that men in prison were three times (RR => 3.0) more likely to kill themselves than men in the general population (Fazel et al., 2017). Similarly, a report from the US Suicide Prevention Resource Center (2016) found that men "die by suicide in jails at a rate 1.5 times that of women".

2.3 Social Context and Common Risk Factors

It is important to state that the reasons for suicide are complex, and suicide is rarely the result of a single factor. Instead, a combination of proximal and distal risk factors tend to interact over time to increase suicide risk (Player et al., 2015; Joiner, 2007). Some of these proximal risk factors are more chronic and ongoing, for example, loneliness and isolation; while some can be more acute, for example, the sudden loss of employment or an unexpected divorce (Affleck et al., 2018). These can be compounded by distal upstream factors such as adverse childhood experiences (e.g. experience within a residential school), as well as proximal downstream issues such as lack of appropriate local health services. Evidence suggests that some individual-level risk factors may be more prevalent and experienced more intensely in men compared to women. In particular, the research literature indicates that three strong risk factors may be contributing to higher rates of suicide in men, namely: (i) employment issues; (ii) marital status, divorce and family issues; and (iii) mental disorders and substance use issues. These are discussed next.

2.3.1 Employment Issues

An amassed corpus of research indicates that several individual-level employment issues are risk factors for male suicide. The literature indicates that these employment issues can be divided into two forms: (i) job loss: an acute event that can be sudden and unexpected; and (ii) unemployment: a more chronic experience describing a period without work. Importantly, the impact of both job loss and unemployment on suicide appears to be greater for men than women.

Indeed, the aforementioned GFC led to an observed and dramatic increase in unexpected and sudden male job loss, which also led to a rise in male unemployment in the following years (Stuckler et al., 2011). Evidence suggests that this significantly contributed to the rise in male suicides during and after the GFC, which (as previously mentioned) occurred at a much greater rate than female suicides (Chang et al., 2013; Hedegaard et al., 2018).

Other research unrelated to the GFC indicates that unemployed men have a significantly higher rate of suicide than other men and unemployed women (Payne et al., 2008). For example, Milner et al. (2014) conducted a meta-analysis of five high-quality population-based cohort studies, finding that unemployment was a risk factor for suicide, with a relative risk of 1.58 (95% CI 1.33–1.83) compared to employment. The pooled risk ratios indicated that relative risk was much higher in unemployed men (RR 1.51: 95% CI 1.19–1.83) compared to unemployed women (RR 1.15: 95% CI 0.85–1.45). These results are consistent with an earlier systematic review and meta-analysis of population-based case-control and cohort studies, finding that unemployed men had a relative risk of suicide of 1.68 (95% CI: 1.11–2.54), compared to employed men (Li et al., 2011).

2.3 Social Context and Common Risk Factors

These findings have been confirmed by a variety of single-jurisdiction studies. For example, one seminal case-control study in Denmark found that unemployment was a significant risk factor for male suicides, but not for female suicides (Qin et al., 2000). This study found that unemployed men were over twice as likely to kill themselves as compared to employed men (OR = 2.21; 95% CI: 1.69–2.88), and also significantly more likely to kill themselves as compared to unemployed women. In contrast, unemployed females were not significantly more likely to kill themselves compared to employed females (OR = 1.37; 95% CI: 0.86–2.19). Such results have been replicated in more recent studies examining gender, employment and suicide (Gunnell & Chang, 2016).

Relatedly, unemployment has also been associated with high rates of suicide among the above-described vulnerable male subgroups. For example, high unemployment levels in certain Canadian and Australian Aboriginal communities have been linked to their high rates of suicide (Kumar & Tjepkema, 2019; Penney et al., 2009; De Leo et al., 2011). Likewise, elevated rates of suicide among veterans has been linked to difficulties finding employment after release from the services, which may be particularly difficult for infantrymen and others without specialist skills that are valued in civilian life (Kline et al., 2011). This increased risk of suicide among men experiencing job loss and unemployment has been explained by a variety of factors.

A core factor relates to financial impact. Men are typically still the primary family breadwinner, and their income is often necessary to pay for food, housing and other costs associated with supporting a household (Klesment & Van Bavel, 2017). The loss of income can lead to severe financial difficulties including household austerity, bankruptcy and foreclosure. Indeed, the loss of a family home can have a particularly negative impact, with several studies associating the rising rate of white middle-aged male suicide with the experience of foreclosure (Houle & Light, 2017; Kerr et al., 2017). Similarly, other studies have found an association between bankruptcy and suicide (Komoto, 2014; Kidger et al., 2011). In other words, unemployment and job loss can lead to severe financial consequences which can have a devasting impact on family well-being and quality of life. This financial loss can interact with other factors to increase suicide risk for men. One way this can occur is through downward social mobility and a subsequent reduction of socio-economic status.

Indeed, several studies have noted that men of lower socio-economic status have a particularly high risk of suicide, higher than comparable women, as well as men of a higher socio-economic status (Classen & Dunn, 2012). For example, a stratified sub-analysis within the aforementioned Li et al. (2011) review found that men in low status occupations (defined as manual/non-skilled/blue-collar workers) were more likely to kill themselves than men in high-status occupations (RR = 2.67; 95% CI 1.53–4.68). In contrast, this review found that women in low status occupations were not significantly more likely to kill themselves compared to women in high-status occupations (RR-1.27: 95% CI 0.54–2.94). Moreover, this review found that the population attributable fraction for suicide associated with low occupational status was 33% (range: 18.5%–46.5%) for men, but only 7% (range: −14.2%–34.4%) for women.

Of note, socio-economic status is typically defined as a combination of educational achievement and current occupational status meaning that men of low socio-economic status can experience a double jeopardy as they tend to: (i) lack higher education, which may limit current employment opportunities and has been independently identified as a risk factor for suicide (see Chap. 7); and (ii) be unemployed or working in insecure low-paid jobs. The influence of the wider socio-economic macro-environment vis-à-vis employment and men's mental health is discussed in more detail in Chap. 8, but a focused overview is given below.

In sum, wider upstream socio-economic change may result in an increased downstream risk of suicide and other mental health issues for men of low socio-economic status. For example, nations such as the USA, Australia and the UK have witnessed a massive decline in traditional industries that have typically employed large portions of local men giving such men financial security, as well as pride, purpose and meaning (Case & Deaton, 2020). This includes industries such as manufacturing, mining, fisheries, forestry and oil/gas – some of which have been closed down, or outsourced to other locations such as China. These declines are sometimes concentrated in discrete geographical areas, where a single industry (e.g. coal mining, shipbuilding, or car production) has typically employed large numbers of local men, giving many opportunities to both high-skilled and low-skilled men. The loss of these industries has been linked to increases in male suicide (as well as substance misuse – see Chap. 3) in such areas, and may explain the aforementioned higher rates of male suicide seen in smaller towns and rural regions, where the decline or loss of a dominant employer/industry can hit the local male population hard (Rivera et al., 2017; Browning & Heinesen, 2012; Myles et al., 2017; Alston 2012; Crawford & Prince, 1999).

To close this section, it is worth noting that men make up the overwhelming proportion of people working in the most dirty, dangerous and demanding industries – as witnessed by the fact that over 90% of workplace fatalities are male, and 75% of serious workplace injuries are male (US Bureau of Labor Statistics, 2020; Myers et al., 1998). In fact, the male-dominated professions of farming, fishing, law enforcement, military, construction, forestry, mining and transport services have been identified as the professions with the highest rates of suicide (Milner et al., 2013; Tiesman et al., 2014; Kposowa, 1999). In contrast, clerical and office workers had the lowest rates. These phenomena led Farrell (1993) to dub these male-dominated occupations as the death professions, due to the increased risk of both suicide and occupational deaths occurring therein.

The higher rates of suicide in such professions has been linked to various factors. First, the very nature of these jobs can expose workers to accident and injury, and sometimes to assault and violence – all of which can contribute to an increased risk of mental disorders such as PTSD and Substance Use Disorder, both of which are risk factors for suicide (see Sect. 2.3.3). Second, these jobs tend not to follow a 9–5 schedule, but often involve long hours, shift work, and considerable time away from friends and family. This can contribute to loneliness, isolation and lack of social support, again consistently identified as risk factors for suicide (Kleiman & Liu, 2013; Monk, 2000). Third, industries such as fishing, farming and forestry are subject to the whims of the seasonal and economic cycle, with periods of intense work often punctuated by periods of inertia and unemployment (Alston, 2012). This may be especially so in remote and rural Aboriginal communities, where work can also be conducted under harsh environmental conditions (Condon et al., 1995).

Of note, professions such as law enforcement and farming tend to offer ready access to lethal means for suicide such as firearms or poison, meaning that at-risk suicidal individuals in these professions do not have to overcome the same barriers in planning and performing a suicide as other men and women experiencing suicidal ideation. Such factors can also contribute to higher rates of suicide in some of these male-dominated professions.

2.3.2 Marital Status, Divorce and Family Issues

The category of *single men* is an umbrella term including men who are never married, widowed, separated or divorced. The literature indicates that all these groups have higher risk of suicide than married men, but that divorced and separated men are at highest risk. Moreover, a robust finding across the suicide literature is that never-married, separated and divorced men have a greater risk of suicide compared with never-married, separated and divorced women (Evans et al., 2014; Payne et al., 2008).

For example, a recent study of data from the large-scale US National Longitudinal Mortality Study consisting of 1.38 million people examined the relationship between suicide and marital status (Kposowa et al., 2020). This study stratified results by gender, finding that divorced and separated men had a twofold relative risk (adjusted RR 2.01: 95% CI 1.73–2.38) of suicide compared to married men, while divorced and separated women had a less marked adjusted relative risk of 1.46 (95% CI 1.10–1.95).

These findings are consistent with previous analyses from earlier waves of this longitudinal survey. For example, Kposowa (2000) found that divorced men were over two times more likely to die by suicide in comparison to married men (RR = 2.08; 95% CI: 1.58–2.72), with divorced men also having significantly higher rates than widowed and never-married men. In this study, rates of suicide in widowed and never-married men were much lower than divorced men, and were not significantly different from the rates for married men. In another analysis, Kposowa (2003) directly compared rates between divorced men and divorced women, finding that divorced men had a relative risk of killing themselves that was over 8 times higher than divorced women (RR = 8.36; 95% CI: 4.24–16.38). In other words, this series of analyses from a large-scale US longitudinal study found that divorce and separation are risk factors for suicide for both males and females, but risk was dramatically higher amongst divorced men.

These results converge with other findings from elsewhere. For example, a large-scale national cohort study of completed suicides in Sweden found that unmarried men were almost twice as likely to kill themselves when compared to married men (HR = 1.97; 95% CI: 1.85–2.10); and significantly more likely to kill themselves when compared to unmarried women, with the highest rates among divorced men (Crump et al., 2014). Interestingly, European countries with higher rates of divorce tend to have higher rates of male suicide. For example, Lithuania has the highest suicide mortality rate of all EU countries, with males dying by suicide at nearly six times the rate of women in that country (Eurostat, 2020a). It also has one of the highest divorce rates, again indicating a correlation between divorce and male suicide (Eurostat, 2020b).

Other studies have made broad comparisons between married and unmarried men, indicating that unmarried men per se are at greater risk of suicide compared to married men. For example, the aforementioned large-scale Danish case-control study found that the age-adjusted relative risk of suicide in single men was over double that of married or cohabiting men (OR = 2.59; 95% CI: 2.18–3.09), and significantly higher than the suicide rate for single women (Qin et al., 2000). Likewise, a large-scale US study using data from the National Center for Health Statistics notes that unmarried men ages 40–60 years were 3.5 times more likely to die by suicide compared to married men of the same age, with markedly higher rates for unmarried men compared to unmarried women (Phillips et al., 2010). Similarly, another large-scale US study showed hazard ratios demonstrating that unmarried men ages 40–75 years had a twofold risk of suicide compared to married men of the same age group (Tsai et al., 2014).

In sum, data from various surveys and various countries using various methodologies indicate that unmarried men per se have an elevated risk of suicide compared to married men, and this is more pronounced among men who are divorced and (to a slightly lesser extent) separated. This implies that the psychosocial experience of divorce can be particularly painful for men, and that it can be an acute stressor with chronic consequences. This could be related to several factors.

First, data indicates that around 70% of divorces are initiated by the wife, meaning that divorce can be a shocking and unwanted transition for the husband (Rosenfield, 2018). This means the husband often has to scramble to mobilize his psychological, social and financial resources to deal with a sudden and unplanned transformation. Many men, particularly low-income men, may lack these resources, which can lead to confusion and distress (McManus & DiPrete, 2001).

Second, women are more likely to maintain larger friendship and extended family networks when married, whereas men tend to rely on their partner and children for social interaction and social support (Kalmijn, 2003; Alexander et al., 2001). This means that men tend to experience a more intense fall in social support and interaction after a divorce, due to a lack of a social safety net. This can leave them lonely and isolated precisely when they need social support the most (Rotermann, 2007; Wyllie et al., 2012; Houle et al., 2008).

Third, fathers are typically separated from their children after a divorce, with studies from a variety of western jurisdictions indicating that the mother has sole or majority responsibility in over 80% of divorces (Grall, 2016; US Census Bureau, 2016; Kaspiew et al., 2015; Department of Justice Canada, 2000). In a review of the literature, Payne et al. (2008, p. 30) note that "divorce may be particularly devastating for men because they are mainly the ones who lose their home, children and family". This separation from children can be particularly painful, leading to a massive void and sense of loss, which can breed shame, guilt, alcohol abuse, a sense of failure and psychological distress (Wallerstein & Blakeslee, 2004; Bartlett, 2004; Stack, 2000). This experience can be a living bereavement for the men involved, which again can contribute towards suicidal tendencies.

Relatedly, many men report a negative and highly stressful experience within the family court system, with a common perception being that these courts marginalize father involvement in child-rearing responsibilities and fail to recognize the value of father–child relationships (Felix et al., 2013). This experience can lead to a loss of faith in society as a whole, especially when such courts demand weighty support payments but give minimal access, which can lead to psychological distress and a serious decline in quality of life (Shiner et al., 2009; McManus & DiPrete, 2001). Indeed, one scoping review found that separation from children is often cited as a primary cause of male suicide in many coroner's inquests (Struszczyk et al., 2019). All this led Kposowa (2003, p. 993) to note that 'in the end, the father loses not only his marriage but his children…it may well be that the observed association between divorce and suicide in men is the impact of post-divorce (court sanctioned) "arrangements"'.

Of note, there have been increases in rates of divorce, separation and the number of people living alone in recent decades. At the same time, people have been having fewer children, and when they do it is typically at a later age in life, transforming the nature of the typical family and the traditional life trajectory. All this is discussed in much greater detail in Chap. 9, where social and cultural trends related to marital status and the family are discussed in relation to mental health.

2.3.3 *Mental Disorders and Substance Use Issues*

One of the most prominent risk factors for male suicide is the presence of a mental disorder. For example, a systematic review of the suicide literature found that the relative risk of suicide for men with any mental disorder was 7.5 (Li et al., 2011). Interestingly, this study found higher rates in men with schizophrenia (RR = 11.9; 95% CI: 10.93–12.83) and men with affective disorders such as depression (RR = 11; 95% CI: 7.71–15.68), as compared to men with substance use disorders (RR = 6.9; 95% CI: 4.51–10.50) and men with personality disorders (RR = 4.1; 95% CI: 2.95–5.80). A more recent Swedish cohort study of over 3 million people found that PTSD was a significant risk factor for suicide, finding that men with PTSD were almost four times (HR: 3.96: 95% CI 3.12–5.03) more likely to kill themselves than men without PTSD (Fox et al., 2021).

Similar findings were found in some of the aforementioned large-scale studies. For example, a Swedish national cohort study found that the presence of any mental disorder was a strong risk factor, with a diagnosed mental disorder found in 39% of male suicides (Crump et al., 2014). Over half of these had a substance use disorder, while just under half had depression. Importantly, these figures may be underestimations, as the method of case ascertainment was based on medical records of diagnosed mental disorders, thus excluding undiagnosed disorders. Indeed, psychological autopsy studies suggest that up to 90% of suicide decedents had a mental disorder, often undiagnosed and untreated (Arsenault-Lapierre et al., 2004).

Of note, multi-variate analysis in this Swedish study indicated that the presence of any mental disorder produced a 12-fold risk for suicide in men (95% CI: 11.31–13.13), relative to men never diagnosed with a mental disorder. Depression had a 15-fold risk for men (95% CI: 14.37–21.47), the highest risk of all mental disorders, whereas schizophrenia (95% CI: 3.39–4.70) and substance use disorders (95% CI: 3.79–4.95) had a fourfold risk. Interestingly, these authors also conducted a time series analysis, indicating a 25-fold risk (95% CI: 22.25–29.14) for men during the three months following a diagnosis of depression – suggesting that this is a critical period when suicide risk increases (Crump et al., 2014).

These findings are consistent with results from a variety of studies indicating that suicide risk increases dramatically in the immediate months following psychiatric hospitalization, again suggesting the existence of a critical time period (Qin & Nordentoft, 2005). For example, the aforementioned Danish case-control study found that recent psychiatric hospitalization was the strongest predictor of male suicide, with men discharged in the previous year being 20 times more likely to die by suicide than men never admitted (Qin et al., 2000). In this study, men discharged in the previous month were at particular risk, and over 100 times more likely to die by suicide (OR = 154.2; 95% CI: 89.55–265.55) than men never admitted to a psychiatric hospital.

These findings also indicate that large proportions of men who die by suicide have had recent contact with the official healthcare system, indicating that suicidal men are in fact willing to seek help and talk about their issues (contrary to popular belief). Indeed, a seminal review of the suicide literature found that 78% of men had contact with a primary healthcare provider in the year before suicide, while 35% had contact with a specialized mental health provider (Luoma et al., 2002). Another study found that 30% of male suicides were receiving mental health treatment at the time of their death (Hempstead & Phillips, 2015). This belies the victim-blaming myth that the high rate of male suicide is due to men obstinately avoiding health services because of 'toxic masculinity' or pathological stubbornness (Whitley, 2018). It also implies that health services may not be adequately responding to men's needs and preferences, a phenomena discussed in greater detail in Chap. 6.

An overarching explanation of the high rate of male suicide is that a constellation of chronic, acute, proximal and distal risk factors interact to increase risk of suicide. These can typically include sudden and unexpected transitions, such as job loss and relationship breakdown, which tend to affect male suicidality much more intensely than female suicidality. Such acute stressors can worsen existing mental health issues, or precipitate new mental health issues, which can further increase suicide risk for men. These men often seek help from official health services, but may find such services unappealing, with some evidence suggesting that men perceive mental health services to be 'inherently feminized' (see Chap. 6) and unsuited to their needs (Morison et al., 2014; Bilsker et al., 2010; Ogrodniczuk et al., 2016). This may lead vulnerable men to avoid or disengage from health services and struggle in silence alone, which can sometimes involve attempts to self-medicate distress through substance abuse (see Chap. 3).

Indeed, one large-scale US study found that around 35% of men (ages 40–64 years) who died by suicide had either alcohol dependence or other substance abuse problems (Hempstead & Phillips, 2015), with similar statistics witnessed in other studies of male suicide (e.g. Suominen et al., 2004; Marzuk & Mann, 1988). This overlaps with findings from the aforementioned Swedish cohort study indicating that men with a substance use disorder have a fourfold risk of suicide compared to men with no psychiatric disorder (Crump et al., 2014). Importantly, such substance abuse issues can arise due to life course insult including adverse childhood experience (such as forced attendance at residential schools for Aboriginal Canadians), or early adult hardship such as participation in war (Kuh et al., 2003). It can also be an acute issue, with at-risk individuals attempting to self-medicate due to increasing stress and distress brought about by psychosocial issues such as job loss, divorce and dealing with a mental illness (Brownhill et al., 2002). In other words, both chronic and acute substance misuse can contribute to suicide risk.

2.4 Social Integration and Social Connection

In sum, the research literature indicates that certain subgroups of men are at increased risk of suicide. This includes Aboriginal men, military veterans, divorced men, unemployed men, and men with mental illness. Each of these separate groups face unique and sometimes incomparable stressors, which can contribute to the high rates of observed suicide in the said group. But are there any common underlying psychosocial experiences that can contribute to the higher rates of suicide in these groups? The short answer to this question is yes, as explained in detail next.

To a greater or lesser extent, men in these groups frequently face high levels of isolation, social stigma and financial strain. They may also be stereotyped on account of their demographic status as well as their gender, and there may be a lack of public empathy for their plight (see Chap. 1). Indeed, a common factor among men in these groups may be real or perceived rejection from mainstream society, leading to ongoing feelings of disaffection and estrangement. In short, an underlying factor explaining high rates of suicide in such disparate groups may be a strong sense of social alienation, characterized by a diminished sense of meaning and purpose in life, which in turn can weaken primary reasons for living (Kleiman & Beaver, 2013; Rodgers, 2011; Stack, 2000). Research on this topic has tended to centre upon the related sociological concepts of *social integration* and *social disintegration*.

Importantly, the social integration of adult men in western countries is typically provided by meaningful participation in: (i) a nuclear family and (ii) the workforce. As such disintegration of a nuclear family and disintegration of employment can have a particularly pernicious effect on men. Likewise, stigmatizing stereotypes targeted at groups such as people with mental illness and Aboriginal people may impede entry into the workforce in the first place, thus contributing to social alienation, lack of social integration and ongoing marginalization.

Indeed, the key conclusion of Durkheim's famous tome 'Suicide: A Study in Sociology' was that social integration (and lack thereof) was the core underlying factor explaining differential rates of suicide in nineteenth century Europe. Durkheim noted that groups such as childless women and unmarried men had higher rates of suicide, which were imputed to lack of social integration. Similarly, he noted that Roman Catholics and Jews had lower suicide rates than Protestants, arguing that this was due to Protestantism evolving into a more individualistic and less socially cohesive worldview than Catholicism or Judaism (Durkheim, 1897). This led him to coin terms such as egoistic suicide, referring to suicides by people lacking meaningful social connections and social integration, and anomic suicide, referring to suicides by people discombobulated by dramatic social, economic or political upheaval.

Durkheim's conceptualizations have been used by many contemporary researchers. For example, the theory of anomic suicide has been used to help explain higher rates of suicide after the GFC (Hodwitz & Frey, 2016) and in the former Soviet Republics (Värnik & Wasserman, 1992). Likewise, the theory of egoistic suicide has been used to explain higher rates of suicide in divorced men (Rossow, 1993) and unemployed men (DeFina & Hannon, 2014). Central to these Durkheimian understandings of suicide is the role of meaning and purpose. For example, considerable research indicates that men tend to draw significant amount of existential meaning from their protector and provider family breadwinner roles (Alston, 2012; Oliffe et al., 2011; Dyke & Murphy, 2006). This can be a powerful source of pride and purpose, and failure to fulfil these roles can leave men shamed and stigmatized in the eyes of themselves, their family and wider society – thus weakening intrapsychic, social and familial integrity (Affleck et al., 2018). Indeed, considerable research indicates that a real or perceived lack of supportive relationships is a risk factor for suicide (Centers for Disease Control and Prevention, 2008), with suicidal individuals consistently reporting lower levels of social support than non-suicidal individuals (O'Connor, 2003). An absence or failure of social support at critical social junctures, including both individual-level transitions such as losing a job or getting a divorce, or macro-level socio-economic upheaval such as the GFC or the COVID-19 pandemic may signify a failure of social integration, which in turn can increase risk of suicide for men.

2.5 Conclusion

Men die by suicide at a considerably higher rate than women, with some groups of men having particularly high rates of suicide such as Aboriginal men, military veterans, middle-aged men, men in rural and remote areas and men with mental illness. Worryingly, rates of male suicide have increased steadily since 1999. Evidence suggests that some risk factors pose substantially greater risks for males than females, particularly unemployment and divorce. Such factors can combine and interact, leading to a weakening of social integration and social connection, while also diminishing sense of meaning and purpose for the men involved. Importantly, all of these risk factors are affected by the wider cultural context, including macro-level socio-economic trends that are discussed in much greater detail in Part II of this book.

References

Affleck, W., Carmichael, V., & Whitley, R. (2018). Men's mental health: Social determinants and implications for services. *Canadian Journal of Psychiatry, 63*(9), 581–589. https://doi.org/10.1177/0706743718762388

Affleck, W., Thamotharampillai, U., Jeyakumar, J., & Whitley, R. (2018). "If one does not fulfill his duties, he must not be a man": Masculinity, mental health and resilience amongst Sri Lankan Tamil refugee men in Canada. *Culture, Medicine, and Psychiatry, 42*, 840–861. https://doi.org/10.1007/s11013-018-9592-9

Alexander, R., Feeney, J., Hohaus, L., & Noller, P. (2001). Attachment style and coping resources as predictors of coping strategies in the transition to parenthood. *Personal Relationships, 8*(2), 137–152. https://doi.org/10.1111/j.1475-6811.2001.tb00032.x

Alston, M. (2012). Rural male suicide in Australia. *Social Science & Medicine, 74*(4), 515–522. https://doi.org/10.1016/j.socscimed.2010.04.036

Arsenault-Lapierre, G., Kim, C., & Turecki, G. (2004). Psychiatric diagnoses in 3275 suicides: A meta-analysis. *BMC Psychiatry, 4*, 37. https://doi.org/10.1186/1471-244X-4-37

Barr, B., Taylor-Robinson, D., Scott-Samuel, A., McKee, M., & Stuckler, D. (2012). Suicides associated with the 2008-10 economic recession in England: Time trend analysis. *BMJ, 345*, e5142. https://doi.org/10.1136/bmj.e5142

Bartlett, E. E. (2004). The effects of fatherhood on the health of men: A review of the literature. *Journal of Men's Health and Gender, 1*(2-3), 159–169. https://doi.org/10.1016/j.jmhg.2004.06.004

Bellah, R. N., Madsen, R., Sullivan, W. M., Swidler, A., & Tipton, S. M. (1996). *Habits of the heart: Individualism and commitment in American life: updated edition with a new introduction.* University of California Press.

Bilsker, D., Goldenberg, L., & Davison, J. (2010). *A roadmap to men's health: Current status, research, policy and practice.* Men's Health Initiative of British Columbia, UBC and Centre for Applied Research in Mental Health and Addiction. Retrieved May 22, 2020, from https://www.sfu.ca/carmha/publications/roadmap-to-mens-health.html

Bilsker, D., & White, J. (2011). The silent epidemic of male suicide. *British Columbia Medical Journal, 53*(10), 529–534.

Bombay, A., Matheson, K., & Anisman, H. (2014). The intergenerational effects of Indian Residential Schools: Implications for the concept of historical trauma. *Transcultural Psychiatry, 51*(3), 320–338. https://doi.org/10.1177/1363461513503380

Boothroyd, L. J., Kirmayer, L. J., Spreng, S., Malus, M., & Hodgins, S. (2001). Completed suicides among the Inuit of northern Quebec, 1982–1996: A case-control study. *CMAJ, 165*(6), 749–755.

Brodsky, B. S., & Stanley, B. (2008). Adverse childhood experiences and suicidal behavior. *Psychiatric Clinics of North America, 31*(2), 223–235. https://doi.org/10.1016/j.psc.2008.02.002

Brownhill, S., Wilhelm, K., Barclay, L., & Parker, G. (2002). Detecting depression in men: A matter of guesswork. *International Journal of Men's Health, 1*(3), 259–280. https://doi.org/10.3149/jmh.0103.259

Browning, M., & Heinesen, E. (2012). Effect of job loss due to plant closure on mortality and hospitalization. *Journal of Health Economics, 31*(4), 599–616. https://doi.org/10.1016/j.jhealeco.2012.03.001

Burrows, S., Auger, N., Tamambang, L., & Barry, A. D. (2013). Suicide mortality gap between Francophones and Anglophones of Quebec, Canada. *Social Psychiatry and Psychiatric Epidemiology, 48,* 1125–1132. https://doi.org/10.1007/s00127-012-0637-z

Case, A., & Deaton, A. (2020). *Deaths of despair and the future of capitalism.* Princeton University Press.

Centers for Disease Control and Prevention (CDC). (2008). *Strategic direction for the prevention of suicidal behavior: Promoting individual, family, and community connectedness to prevent suicidal behavior.* Centers for Disease Control and Prevention. Retrieved May 22, 2020, from http://www.cdc.gov/ViolencePrevention/pdf/Suicide_Strategic_Direction_Full_Version-a.pdf

Chang, S. S., Stuckler, D., Yip, P., & Gunnell, D. (2013). Impact of 2008 global economic crisis on suicide: Time trend study in 54 countries. *BMJ, 347,* f5239. https://doi.org/10.1136/bmj.f5239

Classen, T. J., & Dunn, R. A. (2012). The effect of job loss and unemployment duration on suicide risk in the United States: A new look using mass-layoffs and unemployment duration. *Health Economics, 21*(3), 338–350. https://doi.org/10.1002/hec.1719

Condon, R. G., Collings, P., & Wenzel, G. (1995). The best part of life: Subsistence hunting, ethnicity, and economic adaptation among young adult Inuit males. *Arctic Institute of North America, 48*(1), 31–46. https://doi.org/10.14430/arctic1222

Crawford, M. J., & Prince, M. (1999). Increasing rates of suicide in young men in England during the 1980s: The importance of social context. *Social Science & Medicine, 49*(10), 1419–1423. https://doi.org/10.1016/S0277-9536(99)00213-0

Crump, C., Sundquist, K., Sundquist, J., & Winkleby, M. A. (2014). Sociodemographic, psychiatric and somatic risk factors for suicide: A Swedish national cohort study. *Psychological Medicine, 44*(2), 279–289. https://doi.org/10.1017/S0033291713000810

De Leo, D., Sveticic, J., Milner, A., & McKay, K. (2011). *Suicide in indigenous populations of Queensland.* Australian Academic Press.

De Vogli, R., Marmot, M., & Stuckler, D. (2013). Excess suicides and attempted suicides in Italy attributable to the great recession. *Journal of Epidemiology & Community Health, 67,* 378–379. https://doi.org/10.1136/jech-2012-201607

DeFina, R., & Hannon, L. (2014). The changing relationship between unemployment and suicide. *Suicide and Life-Threatening Behavior, 45*(2), 217–229. https://doi.org/10.1111/sltb.12116

Department of Justice Canada, Family, Children and Youth Section. (2000). *Selected statistics on Canadian families and family law: Second edition.* Department of Justice Canada. Retrieved May 22, 2020, from https://www.justice.gc.ca/eng/rp-pr/fl-lf/famil/stat2000/index.html#a01

Durkheim, E. (1897). *Suicide: A study in sociology* (J. A. Spaulding & G. Simpson, Trans.). The Free Press.

Dyke, L. S., & Murphy, S. A. (2006). How we define success: A qualitative study of what matters most to women and men. *Sex Roles, 55,* 357–371. https://doi.org/10.1007/s11199-006-9091-2

References

Elias, B., Mignone, J., Hall, M., Hong, S. P., Hart, L., & Sareen, J. (2012). Trauma and suicide behaviour histories among a Canadian indigenous population: An empirical exploration of the potential role of Canada's residential school system. *Social Science & Medicine, 74*(10), 1560–1569. https://doi.org/10.1016/j.socscimed.2012.01.026

Eurostat. (2020a, June). *Causes of death statistics*. Eurostat. Retrieved April 20, 2021, from https://ec.europa.eu/eurostat/statistics-explained/index.php/Causes_of_death_statistics#Causes_of_death_by_sex

Eurostat. (2020b, October 6). *Marriage and divorce statistics*. Eurostat. Retrieved April 20, 2021, from https://ec.europa.eu/eurostat/statistics-explained/pdfscache/6790.pdf

Evans, R., Scourfield, J., & Moore, G. (2014). Gender, relationship breakdown, and suicide risk: A review of research in Western countries. *Journal of Family Issues, 37*(16), 2239–2264. https://doi.org/10.1177/0192513X14562608

Farrell, W. (1993). *The myth of male power*. Berkley Books.

Fazel, S., Ramesh, T., & Hawton, K. (2017). Suicide in prisons: An international study of prevalence and contributory factors. *Lancet Psychiatry, 4*(12), 946–952. https://doi.org/10.1016/S2215-0366(17)30430-3

Felix, D. S., Robinson, W. D., & Jarzynka, K. J. (2013). The influence of divorce on men's health. *Journal of Men's Health, 10*(1), 3–7. https://doi.org/10.1016/j.jomh.2012.09.002

Fox, V., Dalman, C., Dal, H., Hollander, A. C., Kirkbride, J. B., & Pitman, A. (2021). Suicide risk in people with post-traumatic stress disorder: A cohort study of 3.1 million people in Sweden. *Journal of Affective Disorders, 279*, 609–616. https://doi.org/10.1016/j.jad.2020.10.009

Grall, T. (2016, January). *Custodial mothers and fathers and their child support: 2013*. US Census Bureau. Retrieved May 22, 2020, from https://www.census.gov/content/dam/Census/library/publications/2016/demo/P60-255.pdf

Gunnell, D., & Chang, S. S. (2016). Economic recession, unemployment, and suicide. In R. C. O'Connor & J. Pirkis (Eds.), *The international handbook of suicide prevention* (2nd ed., pp. 284–300). Whitley Blackwell.

Hedegaard, H., Curtin, S. C., & Warner, M. (2018, November). *Suicide mortality in the United States, 1999–2017*. National Center for Health Statistics. Retrieved May 22, 2020, from https://www.cdc.gov/nchs/products/databriefs/db330.htm#:~:text=occurring%20after%202006.-,From%201999%20through%202017%2C%20the%20age%2Dadjusted%20suicide%20rate%20increased,1999%20to%2022.4%20in%202017

Hempstead, K. A., & Phillips, J. A. (2015). Rising suicide among adults aged 40-64 years: The role of job and financial circumstances. *American Journal of Preventive Medicine, 48*(5), 491–500. https://doi.org/10.1016/j.amepre.2014.11.006

Herne, M. A., Bartholomew, M. L., & Weahkee, R. L. (2014). Suicide mortality among American Indians and Alaska Natives, 1999–2009. *American Journal of Public Health, 104*, S336–S342. https://doi.org/10.2105/AJPH.2014.301929

Hicks, J. (2007). The social determinants of elevated rates of suicide among Inuit youth. *Indigenous Affairs, 4*, 30–37.

Hirsch, J. K. (2007). A review of the literature on rural suicide. *Crisis, 27*, 189–199. https://doi.org/10.1027/0227-5910.27.4.189

Hodwitz, O., & Frey, K. (2016). Anomic suicide: A Durkheimian analysis of European normlessness. *Sociological Spectrum, 36*(4), 236–254. https://doi.org/10.1080/02732173.2016.1148652

Houle, J., Mishara, B. L., & Chagnon, F. (2008). An empirical test of a mediation model of the impact of the traditional male gender role on suicidal behavior in men. *Journal of Affective Disorders, 107*(1-3), 37–43. https://doi.org/10.1016/j.jad.2007.07.016

Houle, J. N., & Light, M. T. (2017). The harder they fall? Sex and race/ethnic specific suicide rates in the U.S. foreclosure crisis. *Social Science & Medicine, 180*, 114–124. https://doi.org/10.1016/j.socscimed.2017.03.033

Hunter, E., & Harvey, D. (2002). Indigenous suicide in Australia, New Zealand, Canada and the United States. *Emergency Medicine, 14*(1), 14–23. https://doi.org/10.1046/j.1442-2026.2002.00281.x

Ide, N., Kõlves, L., Cassaniti, M., & De Leo, D. (2012). Suicide of first-generation immigrants in Australia, 1974–2006. *Social Psychiatry and Psychiatric Epidemiology, 47*, 1917–1927. https://doi.org/10.1007/s00127-012-0499-4

Joiner, T. (2007). *Why people die by suicide*. Harvard University Press.

Kalmijn, M. (2003). Shared friendship networks and the life course: An analysis of survey data on married and cohabiting couples. *Social Networks, 25*(3), 231–249. https://doi.org/10.1016/S0378-8733(03)00010-8

Kaspiew, R., Carson, R., Qu, L., Horsfall, B., Tayton, S., Moore, S., Coulson, M., & Dunstan, J. (2015, October). *Court Outcomes Project (Evaluation of the 2012 Family Violence Amendments)*. Australian Institute of Family Studies. Retrieved April 15, 2021, from www.aifs.gov.au/publications/court-outcomes-project

Kentikelenis, A., Karanikolos, M., Papanicolas, I., Basu, S., McKee, M., & Stuckler, D. (2011). Health effects of financial crisis: omens of a Greek tragedy. *The Lancet, 378*(9801), 1457–1458. https://doi.org/10.1016/S0140-6736(11)61556-0

Kerr, W. C., Kaplan, M. S., Huguet, N., Caetano, R., Giesbrecht, N., & McFarland, H. (2017). Economic recession, alcohol, and suicide rates: Comparative effects of poverty, foreclosure, and job loss. *American Journal of Preventive Medicine, 52*(4), 469–475. https://doi.org/10.1016/j.amepre.2016.09.021

Ketcheson, F., King, L., & Richardson, J. D. (2018). Association between social support and mental health conditions in treatment-seeking Veterans and Canadian Armed Forces personnel. *Journal of Military, Veteran and Family Health, 4*(1), 20–32. https://doi.org/10.3138/jmvfh.2017-0001

Kidger, J. K., Gunnell, D., Jarvik, J. G., Overstreet, K. A., & Hollingworth, W. (2011). The association between bankruptcy and hospital-presenting attempted suicide: A record linkage study. *Suicide and Life-Threatening Behavior, 41*(6), 676–684. https://doi.org/10.1111/j.1943-278X.2011.00063.x

Kleiman, E. M., & Beaver, J. K. (2013). A meaningful life is worth living: Meaning in life as a suicide resiliency factor. *Psychiatry Research, 210*(3), 934–939. https://doi.org/10.1016/j.psychres.2013.08.002

Kleiman, E. M., & Liu, R. T. (2013). Social support as a protective factor in suicide: Findings from two nationally representative samples. *Journal of Affective Disorders, 150*(2), 540–545. https://doi.org/10.1016/j.jad.2013.01.033

Klesment, M., & Van Bavel, J. (2017). The reversal of the gender gap in education, motherhood, and women as main earners in Europe. *European Sociological Review, 33*(3), 465–481. https://doi.org/10.1093/esr/jcw063

Kline, A., Ciccone, D. S., Falca-Dodson, M., Black, C. M., & Losonczy, M. (2011). Suicidal ideation among National Guard troops deployed to Iraq: The association with postdeployment readjustment problems. *Journal of Nervous and Mental Disease, 199*(12), 914–920. https://doi.org/10.1097/NMD.0b013e3182392917

Komoto, Y. (2014). Factors associated with suicide and bankruptcy in Japanese pathological gamblers. *International Journal of Mental Health and Addiction, 12*, 600–606. https://doi.org/10.1007/s11469-014-9492-3

Kposowa, A. J. (1999). Suicide mortality in the United States: Differentials by industrial and occupational groups. *American Journal of Industrial Medicine, 36*(6), 645–652. https://doi.org/10.1002/(SICI)1097-0274(199912)36:6<645::AID-AJIM7>3.0.CO;2-T

Kposowa, A. J. (2000). Marital status and suicide in the National Longitudinal Mortality Study. *Journal of Epidemiology & Community Health, 54*(4), 254–261. https://doi.org/10.1136/jech.54.4.254

Kposowa, A. J. (2003). Divorce and suicide risk. *Journal of Epidemiology and Community Health, 57*(12), 993. https://doi.org/10.1136/jech.57.12.993

Kposowa, A. J., Ezzat, D. A., & Breault, K. D. (2020). Marital status, sex, and suicide: New longitudinal findings and Durkheim's marital status propositions. *Sociological Spectrum, 40*(2), 81–98. https://doi.org/10.1080/02732173.2020.1758261

References

Kral, M. J. (2012). Postcolonial suicide among Inuit in Arctic Canada. *Culture, Medicine, and Psychiatry, 36*, 306–325. https://doi.org/10.1007/s11013-012-9260-4

Kuh, D., Ben-Shlomo, Y., Lynch, J., Hallqvist, J., & Power, C. (2003). Life course epidemiology. *Journal of Epidemiology & Community Health, 57*, 778–783. https://doi.org/10.1136/jech.57.10.778

Kumar, M. B., & Tjepkema, M. (2019, June 28). *Suicide among First Nations people, Métis and Inuit (2011–2016): Findings from the 2011 Canadian Census Health and Environment Cohort (CanCHEC)*. Statistics Canada. Retrieved March 18, 2021, from https://www150.statcan.gc.ca/n1/pub/99-011-x/99-011-x2019001-eng.htm

Lawrence, R. E., Oquendo, M. A., & Stanley, B. (2016). Religion and suicide risk: A systematic review. *Archives of Suicide Research, 20*(1), 1–21. https://doi.org/10.1080/13811118.2015.1004494

Levin, K. A., & Leyland, A. H. (2005). Urban/rural inequalities in suicide in Scotland, 1981–1999. *Social Science & Medicine, 60*(12), 2877–2890. https://doi.org/10.1016/j.socscimed.2004.11.025

Li, Z., Page, A., Martin, G., & Taylor, R. (2011). Attributable risk of psychiatric and socio-economic factors for suicide from individual-level, population-based studies: A systematic review. *Social Science & Medicine, 72*(4), 608–616. https://doi.org/10.1016/j.socscimed.2010.11.008

Luoma, J. B., Martin, C. E., & Pearson, J. L. (2002). Contact with mental health and primary care providers before suicide: A review of the evidence. *American Journal of Psychiatry, 159*(6), 909–916. https://doi.org/10.1176/appi.ajp.159.6.909

Malenfant, E. C. (2004). Suicide in Canada's immigrant population. *Health Reports, 15*(2), 9–17.

Marzuk, P. M., & Mann, J. J. (1988). Suicide and substance abuse. *Psychiatric Annals, 18*(11), 639–645. https://doi.org/10.3928/0048-5713-19881101-07

McManus, P. A., & DiPrete, T. A. (2001). Losers and winners: The financial consequences of separation and divorce for men. *American Sociological Review, 66*(2), 246–268. https://doi.org/10.2307/2657417

Milner, A., Page, A., & LaMontagne, A. D. (2014). Cause and effect in studies on unemployment, mental health and suicide: A meta-analytic and conceptual review. *Psychological Medicine, 44*(5), 909–917. https://doi.org/10.1017/S0033291713001621

Milner, A., Spittal, M. J., Pirkis, J., & LaMontagne, A. D. (2013). Suicide by occupation: Systematic review and meta-analysis. *British Journal of Psychiatry, 203*(6), 409–416. https://doi.org/10.1192/bjp.bp.113.128405

Monk, A. (2000). The influence of isolation on stress and suicide in rural areas: An international comparison. *Rural Society, 10*(3), 393–403. https://doi.org/10.5172/rsj.10.3.393

Morison, L., Trigeorgis, C., & John, M. (2014). Are mental health services inherently feminised? *The Psychologist, 27*(6), 414–416.

Myers, J. R., Kisner, S. M., & Fosbroke, D. E. (1998). Lifetime risk of fatal occupational injuries within industries, by occupation, gender, and race. *Human and Ecological Risk Assessment: An International Journal, 4*(6), 1291–1307. https://doi.org/10.1080/10807039891284677

Myles, N., Large, M., Myles, H., Adams, R., Liu, D., & Galletly, C. (2017). Australia's economic transition, unemployment, suicide and mental health needs. *Australian & New Zealand Journal of Psychiatry, 51*(2), 119–123. https://doi.org/10.1177/0004867416675035

O'Connor, R. C. (2003). Suicidal Behaviour as a cry of pain: Test of a psychological model. *Archives of Suicide Research, 7*, 297–308. https://doi.org/10.1080/713848941

O'Keefe, V. M., & Wingate, L. R. (2013). The role of hope and optimism in suicide risk for American Indians/Alaska Natives. *Suicide and Life-Threatening Behavior, 43*(6), 621–633. https://doi.org/10.1111/sltb.12044

Ogrodniczuk, J., Oliffe, J., Kuhl, D., & Gross, P. A. (2016). Men's mental health: Spaces and places that work for men. *Canadian Family Physician, 62*(6), 463–464.

Oliffe, J. L., Han, C. S. E., Ogrodniczuk, J. S., Phillips, J. C., & Roy, P. (2011). Suicide from the perspectives of older men who experience depression: A gender analysis. *American Journal of Men's Health*, 444–454. https://doi.org/10.1177/1557988311408410

Payne, S., Swami, V., & Stanistreet, D. L. (2008). The social construction of gender and its influence on suicide: A review of the literature. *Journal of Men's Health, 5*(1), 23–35. https://doi.org/10.1016/j.jomh.2007.11.002

Penney, C., Senécal, S., & Bobet, E. (2009). Mortalité par suicide dans les collectivités inuites au Canada: taux et effets des caractéristiques des collectivités/Suicide mortality in Inuit communities in Canada: Rates and effects of community characteristics. *Cahiers Québécois de Démographie, 38*(2), 311–343. https://doi.org/10.7202/044818ar

Phillips, J. A., Robin, A. V., Nugent, C. N., & Idler, E. L. (2010). Understanding recent changes in suicide rates among the middle-aged: Period or cohort effects? *Public Health Reports, 125*(5), 680–688. https://doi.org/10.1177/003335491012500510

Player, M. J., Proudfoot, J., Fogarty, A., Whittle, E., Spurrier, M., Shand, F., Christensen, H., Hadzi-Pavlovic, D., & Wilhelm, K. (2015). What interrupts suicide attempts in men: A qualitative study. *PLoS One, 10*(6), e0128180. https://doi.org/10.1371/journal.pone.0128180

Pollock, N. J., Naicker, K., Loro, A., Mulay, S., & Coleman, I. (2018). Global incidence of suicide among Indigenous peoples: A systematic review. *BMC Medicine, 16*, 145. https://doi.org/10.1186/s12916-018-1115-6

Putnam, R. D. (2001). *Bowling alone*. Routledge.

Qin, P., Agerbo, E., Westergård-Nielsen, N., Eriksson, T., & Mortensen, P. B. (2000). Gender differences in risk factors for suicide in Denmark. *British Journal of Psychiatry, 177*(6), 546–550. https://doi.org/10.1192/bjp.177.6.546

Qin, P., & Nordentoft, M. (2005). Suicide risk in relation to psychiatric hospitalization: Evidence based on longitudinal registers. *Archives of General Psychiatry, 62*(4), 427–432. https://doi.org/10.1001/archpsyc.62.4.427

Reeves, A., Stuckler, D., McKee, M., Gunnell, D., Chang, S. S., & Basu, S. (2012). Increase in state suicide rates in the USA during economic recession. *The Lancet, 380*(9856), 1813–1814. https://doi.org/10.1016/S0140-6736(12)61910-2

Rivera, B., Casal, B., & Currais, L. (2017). Crisis, suicide and labour productivity losses in Spain. *European Journal of Health Economics, 18*, 83–96. https://doi.org/10.1007/s10198-015-0760-3

Rodgers, P. (2011). *Understanding risk and protective factors for suicide: A primer for preventing suicide*. Suicide Prevention Resource Center. Retrieved May 22, 2020, from https://rhyclearinghouse.acf.hhs.gov/sites/default/files/docs/21124-Understanding_Risk_and_Protective.pdf

Rose, S., VanDenKerkhof, E., & Schaub, M. (2018). Determinants of successful transition literature review. *Journal of Military, Veteran and Family Health, 4*(1), 90–99. https://doi.org/10.3138/jmvfh.4313

Rosenfield, M. J. (2018). Who wants the breakup? Gender and breakup in heterosexual couples. In D. Alwin, D. Felmlee, & D. Kreager (Eds.), *Social networks and the life course: Integrating the development of human lives and social relational networks* (pp. 221–243). Springer.

Rossow, I. (1993). Suicide, alcohol, and divorce; Aspects of gender and family integration. *Addiction, 88*(12), 1659–1665. https://doi.org/10.1111/j.1360-0443.1993.tb02041.x

Rotermann, M. (2007). Marital breakdown and subsequent depression. *Health Reports, 18*(2), 33–44.

Royal Commission on Aboriginal Peoples. (1996, October). *Report on the Royal Commission on Aboriginal Peoples*. Public Works and Government Services Canada. Retrieved May 22, 2020, from https://www.bac-lac.gc.ca/eng/discover/aboriginal-heritage/royal-commission-aboriginal-peoples/Pages/final-report.aspx

Sax, L. (2016). *Boys Adrift*. Basic Books.

Shiner, M., Scourfield, J., Fincham, B., & Langer, S. (2009). When things fall apart: Gender and suicide across the life-course. *Social Science & Medicine, 69*(5), 738–746. https://doi.org/10.1016/j.socscimed.2009.06.014

Simkus, K., VanTil, L., & Pedlar, D. (2017, November 13). *2017 veteran suicide mortality study (1976 to 2012)*. Veterans Affairs Canada, Research Directorate. Retrieved May 22, 2020, from https://www.veterans.gc.ca/eng/about-vac/research/research-directorate/publications/reports/vsms-2017

Stack, S. (2000). Suicide: A 15-year review of the sociological literature Part I: Cultural and economic factors. *Suicide and Life-Threatening Behavior, 30*(2), 145–162. https://doi.org/10.1111/j.1943-278X.2000.tb01073.x

References

Struszczyk, S., Galdas, P. M., & Tiffin, P. A. (2019). Men and suicide prevention: A scoping review. *Journal of Mental Health, 28*(1), 80–88. https://doi.org/10.1080/09638237.2017.1370638

Stuckler, D., Basu, S., Suhrcke, M., Coutts, A., & McKee, M. (2011). Effects of the 2008 recession on health: A first look at European data. *The Lancet, 378*(9786), 124–125. https://doi.org/10.1016/S0140-6736(11)61079-9

Suicide Prevention Resource Center (SPRC). (2016). *Preventing suicide among men in the middle years: Recommendations for suicide prevention programs*. Suicide Prevention Resource Center. Retrieved May 22, 2020, from http://www.sprc.org/sites/default/files/resource-program/SPRC_MiMYReportFinal_0.pdf

Sullivan, E. M., Annest, J. L., & Luo, F. (2013). Suicide among adults aged 35–64 years–United States, 1999–2010. *Morbidity and Mortality Weekly Report, 62*(17), 321–325. https://doi.org/10.15585/mmwr.mm6430a6

Suominen, K., Isometsä, E., Haukka, J., & Lönnqvist, J. (2004). Substance use and male gender as risk factors for deaths and suicide. *Social Psychiatry and Psychiatric Epidemiology, 39*, 720–724. https://doi.org/10.1007/s00127-004-0796-7

Thompson, J. M., MacLean, M. B., Van Til, L., Sudom, K., Sweet, J., Poirier, A., McKinnon, K., Dursun, S., Sudom, K., Zamorski, M., Sareen, J., Ross, D., Hoskins, C., & Pedlar, D. (2015, May 15). *Canadian armed forces veterans: Mental health findings from the 2013 Life After Service Survey*. Veterans Affairs Canada, Research Directorate. Retrieved May 22, 2020, from http://publications.gc.ca/collections/collection_2016/acc-vac/V32-260-2016-eng.pdf

Tiesman, H. M., Konda, S., Hartley, D., Menendez, C. C., Ridenour, M., & Hendricks, S. (2014). Suicides in U.S. workplaces, 2003–2010: A comparison with non-workplace suicides. *American Journal of Preventive Medicine, 48*(6), 674–682. https://doi.org/10.1016/j.amepre.2014.12.011

Tsai, A. C., Lucas, M., Sania, A., Kim, D., & Kawachi, I. (2014). Social integration and suicide mortality among men: 24-year cohort study of U.S. health professionals. *Annals of Internal Medicine, 161*(2), 85–95. https://doi.org/10.7326/M13-1291

US Bureau of Labor Statistics. (2020, December 16). Table 1. Fatal occupational injuries by selected demographic characteristics, 2015–19. Retrieved March 12, 2021, from https://www.bls.gov/news.release/cfoi.t01.htm

US Census Bureau (2016, November 17). *The majority of children live with two parents, Census Bureau reports*. U.S. Census Bureau. Retrieved April 21, 2021, from https://www.census.gov/newsroom/press-releases/2016/cb16-192.html

US Department of Veterans Affairs. (2019). *2019 national veteran suicide prevention annual report*. US Department of Veterans Affairs. Retrieved March 26, 2020, from https://www.mentalhealth.va.gov/docs/data-sheets/2019/2019_National_Veteran_Suicide_Prevention_Annual_Report_508.pdf

VanTil, L. D., Simkus, K., Rolland-Harris, E., & Pedlar, D. J. (2018). Veteran suicide mortality in Canada from 1976 to 2012. *Journal of Military, Veteran and Family Health, 4*(2), 110–116. https://doi.org/10.3138/jmvfh.2017-0045

Värnik, A., & Wasserman, D. (1992). Suicides in the former Soviet republics. *Acta Psychiatrica Scandinavica, 86*(1), 76–78. https://doi.org/10.1111/j.1600-0447.1992.tb03230.x

Wallerstein, J. S., & Blakeslee, S. (2004). *Second chances: Men, women, and children a decade after divorce*. Houghton Mifflin Harcourt.

Whitley, R. (2018). Men's mental health: Beyond victim-blaming. *Canadian Journal of Psychiatry, 63*(9), 577–580. https://doi.org/10.1177/0706743718758041

Whitley, R., Wang, J., Fleury, M. J., Liu, A., & Caron, J. (2017). Mental health status, health care utilisation, and service satisfaction among immigrants in Montreal: An epidemiological comparison. *The Canadian Journal of Psychiatry, 62*(8), 570–579. https://doi.org/10.1177/0706743716677724

World Health Organization (WHO). (2018). *Mental health atlas 2017*. World Health Organization.

Wyllie, C., Platt, S., Brownlie, J., Chandler, A., Connolly, S., Evans, R., Kennelly, B., Kirtley, O., Moore, G., O'Connor, R., & Scourfield, J. (2012). *Men, suicide and society: Why disadvantaged men in mid-life die by suicide*. Samaritans. Retrieved May 22, 2020, from https://media.samaritans.org/documents/Samaritans_MenSuicideSociety_ResearchReport2012.pdf

Chapter 3
Wasted Lives: Substance Abuse, Substance Use Disorder and Addictions in Men

The concept of *addiction* is an important part of psychiatric discourse and popular discourse. In psychiatry, the concept of addiction is typically used in relation to psychoactive substances such as alcohol, cannabis and opioids. However, it is also used in relation to behaviours unrelated to substances such as pathological gambling and Internet gaming, which are sometimes the target of psychiatric treatment. In popular discourse, the concept of addiction is used in relation to a range of other behaviours that are not typically targeted by psychiatry – and can include smartphone addiction, sex addiction and 'shopaholics'. In the 1990s, Dr. Aviel Goodman posited a definition of addiction with two core characteristics that allows for a broad understanding, and has been highly utilized in the scientific literature. Goodman (1990) describes addiction as:

> A behaviour, that can function both to produce pleasure and to provide escape from internal discomfort, is employed in a pattern characterized by (1) recurrent failure to control the behaviour (powerlessness) and (2) continuation of the behaviour despite significant negative consequences (unmanageability).

This broad definition centres on the related concepts of *powerlessness* and *unmanageability*. Other definitions of addiction typically include these two concepts, sometimes building on them by defining other core elements of addiction including *preoccupation, compulsion* and *impulsiveness* (Sussman & Sussman, 2011; Hesse, 2006).

A related concept is that of *abuse* (or its cognate term *misuse*), which is often used in popular discourse as synonym for addiction. However, the terms *abuse* and *misuse* are typically used in the psychiatric literature to refer to a less extreme and intense version of addiction, including drug abuse and alcohol abuse. For example, people who use drugs excessively may not become addicted to them, but may still regularly abuse them, which can lead to functional impairment and negative biopsychosocial sequalae. In psychiatry, abuse and misuse are typically considered pathological behaviours per se, and are often considered as precursors to more serious forms of addiction. In sum, there is a nuanced difference between the terms *addiction* and *abuse/misuse*, but all three terms are considered pathological behaviours in need of clinical action.

Common across all understandings and definitions of addiction and abuse is the emphasis on negative consequences: an essential element of Goodman's (1990) definition. This typically involves negative biological, psychological and social consequences. As detailed later in this chapter, addictions and abuse have been linked to an increased risk of injuries, poisoning and overdoses, and can contribute towards harmful health behaviours such as a poor diet, lack of exercise and sleep difficulties. Moreover, addictions can also lead to negative psychosocial consequences interfering with factors such as education, employment, and family/ friendship relations. In short, addictions and abuse are serious public health and mental health issues, with negative consequences for individuals, families and society as a whole. As such, organizations such as the American Psychiatric Association (APA) and the World Health Organization (WHO) have officially categorized certain addictions and abusive behaviours as mental disorders.

3.1 Addictions and Substance Abuse in DSM-5

Mental illnesses are officially classified in a large manual published by the APA known as the Diagnostic and Statistical Manual of Mental Disorders, Fifth Edition (DSM-5). This book contains 947 pages and lists hundreds of mental disorders in a variety of thematized chapters, with each chapter having various sections and subsections. One chapter is specifically entitled *Substance-Related and Addictive Disorders*. The beginning of this chapter outlines the core concept of *Substance Use Disorder* (SUD), which is the official umbrella term given to a variety of more specific disorders that are described in subsections in the rest of the chapter. These specific disorders are diagnosed using 11 overarching criteria including preoccupation with the substance, heavy usage and functional impairment. These are rated on a continuum from mild to severe. The three most prominent and potentially severe SUDs in this chapter of DSM-5 are: (i) Alcohol-Related Disorders; (ii) Cannabis-Related Disorders; and (iii) Opioid-Related Disorders. Additionally, the chapter lists *Gambling Disorder* as a *Non-Substance-Related Mental Disorder,* the only addiction in DSM which is not related to a psychoactive substance. Other concepts that are popularly considered addictions such as *sex addiction* or *smartphone addiction* are not listed in DSM-5, and thus are not officially categorized as mental disorders (as yet).

Large-scale surveys indicate that lifetime prevalence of SUDs is high, with a 2012 Statistics Canada report indicating that around 22% of Canadians (over six million people) met the criteria for a SUD during their lifetime (Pearson et al., 2013). Similar results have been seen elsewhere. For example, the large-scale and rigorous US Substance Abuse and Mental Health Services Administration (SAMHSA) National Survey on Drug Use and Health (NSDUH) indicates that 19.3 million people in the USA have had a SUD in the past year (SAMHSA, 2019). Of note, these and other surveys indicate that the prevalence of alcohol-related, cannabis-related, opioid-related and gambling disorders is much higher in men than in women; indicating that men account for around 75% of all SUD cases (Polak et al., 2015; Greenfield et al., 2010; Compton et al., 2007; Hasin et al., 2007). This means that around 15 million men in the USA alone were affected by these disorders in the past year, which amounts to over 10% of the US adult male population.

Focused epidemiological studies have given precise estimates by gender, consistently finding significantly higher rates in men compared to women. A landmark large-scale epidemiological study found that 12-month population prevalence of SUD was 16.1% in men and 6.6% in women (Kessler et al., 1994). This more than twofold differential was confirmed in another rigorous study finding that men were over twice as likely (OR 2.6: 99% CI: 2.0-3.3) to have a SUD during a 12-month period than women (Compton et al., 2007). More recently, a 2012 Statistics Canada survey indicated that 6.4% of Canadian men met the threshold for at least one reported SUD compared to 2.5% of women (Pearson et al., 2013). Analogous figures are seen in studies in other English-speaking countries, with the Australian National Survey of Mental Health and Well-Being finding that 3.2% of males and 1.3% of females met criteria for non-alcohol drug use disorder in the past 12 months (Hall et al., 2002). This male preponderance at a M:F rate of around 2.5:1 is largely unknown by the public, and generally operates under the radar of society.

Moreover, much evidence suggests that men initiate substance use at an earlier age than women (Marsh et al., 2018; Greenfield et al., 2010), with onset often occurring in late adolescence or early adulthood. Of note, this is a vital period of biopsychosocial development that lays a foundation for later life, meaning that the negative impact of substance use can be amplified in men. For example, late adolescence and early adulthood entail intense brain development, and are times when young adults are launching into the world as independent citizens by entering the workforce and/or beginning postsecondary education. This can be interrupted or curtailed by substance abuse – perhaps contributing to lower youth employment (see Chap. 8) and university graduation rates (see Chap. 7) in men compared to women (Kleinfeld, 2009; Marshall, 2012).

As can be seen above, there are many commonalities across the different substance use disorders. These commonalities are revisited later in this chapter in separate sections devoted to discussion of aetiology, impact and treatment. That said, there are variations in terms of prevalence, gender ratios and time trends. As such, a brief description of the major substance use disorders is given in turn below, along with important statistics relevant to each disorder discussed.

3.2 Alcohol-Related Disorders and Alcohol Use

National and international surveys indicate that alcohol is by far the most abused substance. This may be due to its legality, affordability and social acceptability. These surveys also indicate that men are much more likely to experience an alcohol-related disorder than women. For example, the 2018 US National Survey on Drug Use and Health indicated that 14.4 million adults had an alcohol-related disorder in the past year, which is 5.8% of the adult population (SAMHSA, 2019). Just over nine million of these cases were men (7.6% of adult men), and just over five million were women (4.1% of adult women). This survey also indicates that men are much more likely to drink alcohol per se as compared to women.

Surveys elsewhere indicate a similar gender difference in alcohol-related disorders of around 2.5:1. For example, a large-scale Canadian survey found that 4.7% of men met the criteria for alcohol-related disorders in the past year, compared to 1.7% of women in the previous year (Pearson et al., 2013). Likewise, the Australian National Survey of Mental Health and Well-Being found that 9.5% of males and 3.6% of females met the criteria for an alcohol use disorder in the past year (Hall et al., 2002). In sum, this male preponderance is seen across jurisdictions.

Similarly, men are considerably more likely to engage in chronic or acute alcohol abuse, which may not reach the threshold for a SUD diagnosis, but can impair functioning and have negative biopsychosocial sequelae. For example, Canadian national guidelines recommend that men consume no more than 15 drinks a week (defined as *chronic risk*), with no more than three drinks a day most days (defined as *acute risk*) (Canadian Centre on Substance Use and Addiction, 2019). The chronic-risk guidelines were exceeded by 22% (2.5 million) of males who drank alcohol, while the acute-risk guidelines were exceeded by 17% (1.9 million) of males who drank (Tanner et al., 2014). These figures are considerably higher than analogous figures for women.

Similarly, the 2018 US National Survey on Drug Use and Health (NSDUH) indicates that 31% of adult males had reported binge drinking (acute risk) in the last month, compared to 22% of adult females. In this survey, binge drinking was defined as five or more drinks on one occasion for males, and four or more on one occasion for females. Of note, binge drinking and alcohol use disorder tends to occur in younger age groups for both men and women, with 18–25-year-olds having higher rates than people aged 25+ years (SAMHSA, 2019).

3.3 Cannabis-Related Disorders and Cannabis Use

Research indicates that men tend to consume more cannabis than women. For example, the 2018 NSDUH indicates that 23 million US adult men had used cannabis in the past year, in contrast to 17.3 million women, with the rate of use slowly increasing from 2015 to 2018. Of note, 24% of young adult men had used cannabis in the last month, compared to 20% of young adult women. Similar figures are seen in the Canadian Tobacco, Alcohol and Drugs Survey (Government of Canada, 2019), indicating that 15% of adult Canadians had used cannabis in the last year, with prevalence significantly higher among men (19%: 2.7 million men) than women (11%: 1.7 million). The 19% rate of usage in men is a significant increase from the 2015 figure of 15%.

Additionally, surveys indicate that men experience cannabis use disorders at a rate considerably higher than women. For example, a Canadian survey indicates that men have over double the rate of cannabis-related disorders, with 12-month prevalence of 1.9% for men and 0.7% for women (Pearson et al., 2013). This survey also indicates that lifetime prevalence is over double the rate in men than women. In the USA, the 2018 NSDUH indicates that 7.4 million US adults had a cannabis-use disorder, including 5.9% of young adults, though figures are not broken down by sex (SAMHSA, 2019). However, other US studies indicate a rate over double in men compared to women, with a large nationally representative sample indicating that 12% of men and 5% of women met criteria for lifetime prevalence of cannabis-related disorders (Stinson et al., 2006).

Importantly, evidence suggests that experience of cannabis-related disorders is generally longer and more severe in men than women. For example, data from the US National Epidemiologic Survey on Alcohol and Related Conditions indicates that men with cannabis-related disorders had: (i) more symptoms; (ii) longer episodes; (iii) higher consumption of joints; (iv) slower recovery rates; and (v) an older age at remission, as compared to women (Khan et al., 2013). For example, the average duration of the disorder was 40 months in men and 31 months in women.

Furthermore, young men appeared at particular risk, with higher rates in men ages 18–25 years.

Of note, rates of treatment seeking are very low for both men and women, but are lower for men (see Chap. 6 for greater discussion). This may be due to the lack of specific treatment for cannabis-related disorders. Moreover, some research indicates that people with such disorders do not want to attend generic substance misuse treatments, due to an unwillingness to mix with people with more severe alcohol and 'hard drug' issues (Khan et al., 2013).

Importantly, changes in the law may affect rates of cannabis use disorder; however, sufficient data is not yet available to examine the impact of recent changes. For example, Canada became the first English-speaking nation to legalize cannabis in 2018, and some US states have legalized or decriminalized the possession of cannabis for medicinal and recreational use. This provides the conditions for a natural experiment on the relationship between legalization, cannabis use and onset of cannabis use disorder, but comprehensive data on these impacts is not yet available.

3.4 Opioid-Related Disorders and Opioid Use

The word *opioid* is an umbrella term referring to a class of psychoactive drugs (natural or synthetic) with analgesic properties that can also create euphoric side effects. The word *opiates* refers to naturally occurring opioids deriving from the opium poppy. *Morphine* and *codeine* are perhaps the best-known opiates with a legitimate medical use, often prescribed by physicians as a painkiller. Heroin is made from morphine through chemical processing, meaning it is a semi-synthetic opiate. In some jurisdictions such as the USA and Australia, heroin is deemed to have no medical use, and is thus an illicitly produced street drug available illegally on the black market.

Other subtypes of opioids include synthetic man-made substances such as *methadone, fentanyl, hydrocodone* and *oxycodone*, which are prescription painkillers with legitimate medical uses. These prescription opioids are generally prescribed by physicians as a painkiller for people experiencing chronic or acute pain deriving from a variety of sources. This can include pain from accidents, injuries, military service and post-operative pain, as well as palliative care for illnesses such as terminal cancer. These synthetic opioids tend to be much stronger than opiates, with the Centers for Disease Control and Prevention stating that fentanyl is "50-100 times more potent than morphine" (CDC, 2020). Of note, opioids such as fentanyl can be illicitly manufactured for sale on the black market. This is a common practice, which is partly fuelling fentanyl misuse.

The term *opioid misuse* is an overarching term that can refer to: (i) heroin misuse; (ii) the use of illicitly manufactured opioids such as fentanyl; and (iii) prescription opioid misuse (sometimes known as *non-medical prescription opioid use*). The latter term refers to a phenomenon whereby prescription opioids become available on the black market and used by people without a valid prescription. Similarly, some people misuse the medical system to obtain opioid prescriptions, or alternatively obtain opioids from family and friends who possess a valid prescription.

This difference between these three types of opioid misuse is important, with a leading research team stating that 'the opioid crisis is increasingly characterized as two epidemics intertwined: the heroin epidemic and the non-medical use of prescription opioids epidemic' (Marsh et al., 2018). The use of illicitly manufactured fentanyl could be considered a third epidemic of increasing prominence. Importantly, opioid misuse can be extremely dangerous, with a high risk of drug-related deaths, overdose and addiction. Indeed, the CDC (2020) reports that opioids were implicated in 446,000 deaths in the USA between 1999 and 2018. Moreover, usage can lead to severe functional impairment, which can negatively affect work, education and social relationships.

The 2018 NSDUH indicates that 10.3 million Americans (3.7% of the adult population) misuse opioids, with over 97% of these misusing prescription opioids, with the rest abusing heroin (SAMHSA, 2019). Importantly, both heroin abuse and prescription opioid misuse are significantly higher in men than women (Tetrault et al., 2008; Marsh et al., 2018). For example, NSDUH data indicates that past year prescription opioid misuse is 4.5% for men and 3.7% for women, while lifetime prevalence is 11.9% for men and 9.2% for women (Silver & Hur, 2020).

Similar figures are seen in the 2017 Canadian Tobacco, Alcohol and Drugs Survey, indicating that around 5% of men and 2% of women had engaged in non-cannabis illegal drug abuse in the last year (Government of Canada, 2019). Indeed, this same survey indicates that 11% of Canadian males (1.6 million people) had used opioid pain relievers, though precise breakdowns for opioid misuse are not given (Government of Canada, 2019). Unsurprisingly, men are significantly more likely to meet criteria for opioid-related disorders than women, with the 2017

NSDUH data showing 12-month rates of 1.9% for men and 1.2% for women (Silver & Hur, 2020).

With regard to heroin use, the 2018 NSDUH found that just over 800,000 Americans had used heroin in the last 12 months. A study of data from 2007 to 2014 found that the prevalence of past-year heroin use was over double the rate in men compared to women (Marsh et al., 2018). This same study also found that the prevalence rate for men had more than doubled between 2007 and 2014. This is consistent with another study, which found that heroin use in men had increased by 50% between 2002 and 2013 (Jones et al., 2015).

Again, evidence suggests that opioid misuse and heroin use can affect men more severely. For example, research indicates that men are more likely to inject heroin, as well as use greater amounts of heroin for a longer time (Kelly et al., 2009). Moreover, men comprised around 70% of opioid deaths by overdose in the USA in 2018, a total of 32,078 male deaths, compared to 14,724 female deaths. Around 70% of these deaths were due to prescription opioids and fentanyl (Silver & Hur, 2020; Wilson et al., 2020). Similar percentages are seen in Canada, with the British Columbia Coroners Service (2020) reporting that over 75% of opioid-related overdose deaths are male. Worryingly, one study found that overdose deaths from prescription opioids have increased 3.6 times for men between 1999 and 2010 (Marsh et al., 2018). Of note, Silver & Hur (2020) state that "the majority of research on gender and the opioid epidemic focuses on women", indicating that the scientific literature on this topic is characterized by the male gender blindness discussed in Chap. 1.

Some positive news is that opioid misuse may be declining in the USA over the last few years. The 2018 NSDUH notes a reduction from 12.6 million opioid misusers in 2015 to 10.3 million in 2018, despite population growth. Heroin use has also declined from 2016 to 2018. Moreover, a recent CDC study indicated a 2% decline in opioid-related overdoses between 2017 and 2018, including reduction in both heroin-related overdoses and prescription-opioid-related overdoses (Wilson et al., 2020). This may be due to ongoing efforts to reduce high-dose opioid prescribing by family physicians. That said, this CDC study notes a 10% increase in overdoses due to illicitly manufactured fentanyl, indicating that opioid misuse remains a massive social and health issue in North America, particularly for men. Worryingly, over 75% of people with opioid-related disorders do not get treatment, with service utilization rates higher in women than men, a fact discussed later in Sect. 3.9.

3.5 Gambling Disorder

Gambling disorder (sometimes known as *pathological gambling* or *gambling addiction*) is the only non-substance-based disorder in the addictions subsection of DSM-5. This disorder is characterized by symptoms, including preoccupation with gambling, using increasing amounts of money, and unsuccessful efforts to control gambling. Like other addictive disorders, it can have severe psychosocial consequences leading to financial, relationship and employment problems.

Research consistently indicates that gambling disorder has a higher prevalence in men compared to women. For example, data from the large-scale US National Epidemiologic Survey on Alcohol and Related Conditions (NESARC) indicates that the lifetime prevalence rate for men is 0.64%, while for women it is 0.23% – a ratio of roughly 3:1 (Blanco et al., 2006). While these rates are very low, rates of sub-clinical pathological gambling (sometimes known as *at-risk gambling* or *problem gambling*) are considerably higher in men and again marked by a significant gender differential (Merkouris et al., 2016). Indeed, the NESARC data indicates a 6.8% prevalence of pathological gambling for men, and 3.3% for women (Blanco et al., 2006).

Men are also significantly more likely to have an earlier age of onset and a longer average duration than women, with most cases concentrated in the 18- to 35-year-old age group, and a higher rate among single men (Merkouris et al., 2016). Likewise, several studies have found that the negative psychosocial sequalae of gambling such as financial and employment issues are more severe for men than for women (Gonzalez-Ortega et al., 2013; Rodda et al., 2014). Such a negative impact can be especially harmful for men on low incomes and with limited potential for future earnings, such as low-skilled or older men (Subramaniam et al., 2015) Worryingly, only 7% of men with pathological gambling had sought treatment for a gambling disorder, in comparison to 16% of women, meaning that few men are receiving help or support (Blanco et al., 2006).

3.6 Internet Gaming Disorder

Some forms of addiction are not included in the DSM-5 main classification system but are listed in a separate section of DSM-5 as 'conditions for future research'. One of these conditions is known as *Internet Gaming Disorder* (IGD) – characterized by the excessive use of online games. The APA states that 'this proposed condition is limited to gaming and does not include problems with general use of the internet, online gambling, or use of social media or smartphones', and lists nine proposed symptoms including 'preoccupation with gaming', 'withdrawal symptoms', and 'inability to reduce playing'. These are based on the generic overarching criteria relevant to all the substance use disorders described at the start of this chapter.

However other respected organizations beyond the APA have officially declared that Internet gaming disorder is a real mental illness. Most notably, 'gaming disorder' is listed as a mental illness in the 11th edition of the International Classification of Disease (ICD-11), released by the World Health Organization in 2018 (WHO, 2018). ICD-11 is used by clinicians outside the USA to diagnose conditions, and by researchers to categorize and investigate these conditions. As such, inclusion in ICD-11 gives a mental condition an officially endorsed status as a mental disorder, and can have real consequences in clinics across the world. The symptoms of 'gaming disorder' listed in ICD-11 overlap with the proposed symptoms in DSM-5 focusing on lack of control, preoccupation and consequences "of sufficient severity to result in significant impairment in personal, family, social, educational, occupational or other important areas of functioning".

Given both the relative newness of the phenomena and the above-described disagreements regarding its status as a mental condition, there is a lack of research on gaming disorder in comparison to other addictive disorders, especially in North America and Western Europe. In fact, the centre of gravity for gaming disorder research and treatment is East Asia, with the most rigorous research studies occurring in countries such as Singapore, Hong Kong, Taiwan, Korea and China (Petry & O'Brien, 2013). These countries have reported high rates of Internet gaming disorder, and consider it to be a serious public health issue (Bass, 2015). As such, they have taken a lead in establishing research programs and associated treatments (Fam, 2018; King et al., 2017).

The research literature indicates that males are more likely to play video games compared to females, with males accounting for around 80% of gamers (Dong et al., 2019; Chen et al., 2018). Just like other addictive disorders, studies consistently indicate that males have a higher rate of IGD compared to females. For example, a recent meta-analysis found that the pooled prevalence of IGD was 4.6% (95% CI: 3.4-6.0) in adolescents, with a prevalence of 6.8% (95% CI: 4.3%-9.7%) in adolescent males, and 1.3% (95% CI: 0.6-2.2) in adolescent females (Fam, 2018).

Internet gaming conjures up images of a stereotypical male 'nerd' – a young man holed up in his parent's basement playing video games all day long. These gendered stereotypes are often the butt of humour, jokes and ridicule, displaying the lack of empathy for men with mental health issues discussed in Chap. 1. But these stereotypes can mask a serious problem, common to other addiction-related disorders. For example, gaming disorder is associated with a number of psychosocial issues such as social deficits, poor academic performance and unemployment – all of which can contribute to *failure to launch* in young adults (Petry et al., 2014), discussed in detail in Chap. 7. Moreover, excessive gaming can lead to other adverse outcomes including visual impairments, back pain, sleep deprivation and poor nutrition (Zimbardo & Coulombe, 2016). In sum, Internet gaming is a public health issue with a range of negative physical, mental and psychosocial consequences, which should not be ignored, regardless of its DSM-5 status.

3.7 Aetiology and Causation

As detailed above, men have higher rates of substance misuse, addictions and substance use disorder than women. The reasons behind these gender differentials are complex, and should not be ascribed to a single cause. Indeed, a review of the relevant literature indicates broad multi-factorial patterns that point to a number of common risk factors and social determinants which can explain elevated rates of addictions and substance misuse in men.

One of the most insightful surveys contributing to the literature on causation was conducted by William Compton and colleagues at the US National Institute on Drug

Abuse (Compton et al., 2007). In this study, data from over 40,000 US adults was analysed to assess alcohol and drug abuse. Though this data is relatively old (and predates the rise in opioid use), it is still one of the most rigorous and comprehensive surveys, and its results are aligned with more recent research.

This study found that certain subgroups of men had lower or higher risk of both alcohol and drug abuse. Interestingly, low rates were observed in Asian and Hispanic men, as well as in men aged 65+. Other groups of men had much higher rates, including: (i) men of lower socioeconomic status, as marked by lower education and income levels; (ii) single, widowed, separated, and divorced men; and (iii) Native American men. More recent research indicates that these three groups remain at risk in the present, though newer research on opioid misuse indicate that white men of low socio-economic status have particularly elevated rates of both prescription opioid/fentanyl misuse and heroin use (Marsh et al., 2018; Pouget et al., 2018). This may be especially pronounced in small towns and rural areas where there are less employment and educational opportunities (see Sect. 3.7.2).

Interestingly, other surveys have asked men directly why they misuse substances. Silver & Hur, (2020) found that 45% of men state that they use opioids for pain relief, while 23% use it to 'get high'. Similarly, Nolen-Hoeksema (2004) reports that 'men consistently report stronger motives to drink to escape from or cope with distress than women, and these motives are more strongly associated with alcohol-related problems'. Indeed, many other studies indicate that: (i) escapism; (ii) coping with distress; and (iii) self-medication are common reasons for substance abuse, including studies of alcohol use, cannabis use, drug use, Internet gaming disorder and gambling disorder (Chen et al., 2018; Merkouris et al., 2016).

Interestingly, the nature of the 'pain' or 'distress' in need of relief is not always specified in these studies, and has surprisingly not been the topic of purpose-built research on substance use disorders in men, perhaps displaying the male gender blindness discussed in Chap. 1. However, some literature, including the aforementioned Compton et al., (2007) study, indicates that this pain, distress and escapism could be related to a variety of factors that disproportionately affect men including: (i) educational failure and subsequent failure to launch; (ii) unemployment and employment issues; and (iii) divorce, separation and loneliness, all discussed separately in the following subsections.

3.7.1 Educational Failure and Subsequent Failure to Launch

As discussed in greater detail in Chap. 7, males are experiencing significantly higher rates of educational failure than females, including higher rates of high school dropout, lower rates of postsecondary enrollment, and worse performance on exams. This phenomenon is known as *low educational attainment*. A growing body of research indicates that low educational attainment is correlated with a variety of substance use disorders (SUDs). For example, the aforementioned Compton et al., (2007) study found that those with lower educational attainment (defined as less than high school graduation) had elevated rates of SUDs, with an odds ratio of 1.4 (99% CI: 1.0-2.1) as compared to those with more than a high school education.

Such findings have been replicated by more recent studies. For example, a longitudinal analysis of data from the National Epidemiologic Survey on Alcohol and Related Conditions (NESARC) (N = 34,653; 87% response rate) found a negative association between education and any SUD or substance use dependence, with the lowest rates of dependence/disorder among people with a graduate or professional degree (12.3%), and the highest rates among those with a high school diploma (24.2%) or less than high school education (22.7%). Indeed, those with less than high school education were over twice as likely (OR: 2.55: 99% CI: 2.01-3.23) to have any SUD or substance dependence than those with a graduate or professional degree (Erickson et al., 2016). Neither the NESARC study nor the Compton study stratified educational attainment by gender.

Another US study of over 1000 individuals found that the risk of developing a substance use disorder was significantly higher among high school dropouts compared to those with a college degree, with an adjusted OR = 3.5 (95% CI:1.71-7.17) (Fothergill et al., 2008). Similarly, a Mexican study found an elevated risk of substance use disorder among high school dropouts, with an OR = 2.16 (95% CI: 1.49-3.13) compared to current students (Benjet et al., 2009). But again, the odds ratios were not differentially specified by gender in these two studies.

One study that intentionally investigated gender differences in SUDs examined alcohol-use disorders (AUD) in a longitudinal analysis of over 1000 Americans (Crum et al., 2006). This study found that adult men who were high school dropouts had an adjusted OR of 3.37 (95% CI: 1.36–8.34) for AUD, compared to adult men with a college degree or higher. In contrast, adult women who were high school dropouts had an adjusted OR of 2.37 (95% CI: 0.79-7.10) for AUD compared to adult women with a college degree or higher. In other words, this study finds that low educational attainment is a more powerful risk factor for men compared to women, and the longitudinal nature of this (and other) studies accounts for reverse causation.

Many of these findings were summarized in a recent systematic review, with a preponderance of studies finding that secondary school dropout increased risk of a SUD, as well as risk of opioid use, cannabis use and injecting drug use (Esch et al., 2014). As previously mentioned, opioid misuse is an issue of growing societal concern, prompting several recent research studies on the topic. One cross-sectional analysis of young adults participating in the 2015 National Survey on Drug Use and Health found that opioid misuse and related SUD symptoms were significantly higher among high school dropouts, compared to those in tertiary education or employment (Schepis et al., 2018). In this study, 11.4% of high school dropouts had misused opioids in the last year, compared to 6.1% of those in college. Similarly, youth who had dropped out of high school had misused tranquilizers or sedatives at a rate of around 3:1 compared to those still in high school (6.7% vs. 2.7%). The authors did not stratify their results by gender, but a variety of other studies indicate that less educated men have particularly high rates of both heroin misuse and prescription opioid/fentanyl misuse (e.g., Marsh et al., 2018; Pouget et al., 2018).

As discussed in Chap. 7, successful participation in education can impart a strong sense of here-and-now meaning, purpose and routine to adolescents and young adults. Moreover, a successful educational experience can set a firm foundation for life, opening up doors to employment, social integration and financial success. Contrariwise, a lack of education can increase the risk of unemployment, subsequent financial strain, loneliness and alienation from mainstream society. This can create considerable mental pain and psychosocial distress, which in turn can lead to a lack of hope and existential despair (Case & Deaton, 2020). In this rendering of the situation, substance misuse could be considered a dysfunctional response to a dysfunctional situation.

3.7.2 Unemployment and Employment Issues

As discussed in greater detail in Chap. 8, men still derive much purpose and meaning in life from their work and associated workplace activities. But some groups of men (especially blue-collar and working-class men) are experiencing high rates of unemployment in the new service-based economy. This is partly due to a decline in manufacturing and other traditional industries, especially in small towns and rural/remote areas, where opportunities can be particularly scarce.

Evidence suggests that unemployment is a risk factor for substance abuse, substance dependence and substance use disorder. For example, Henkel (2011) conducted a review of the literature examining over 130 relevant studies, finding that the unemployed are around two to three times more likely to engage in problematic substance use. A sub-analysis of longitudinal data in this review indicates that the unemployed have a higher probability of developing a SUD compared to the employed, thus ruling out reverse causation. This includes higher rates of cannabis abuse, alcohol abuse and injecting drug abuse. This review notes that only a few studies give prevalence rates by gender, but those that do reveal a clear pattern: unemployed men have significantly higher rates of substance abuse and SUD than employed men and unemployed women. In contrast, differences between unemployed and employed women were less marked and less consistent. These findings align with a variety of different studies across different western jurisdictions that have focused on specific substances and specific substance use disorders.

In terms of alcohol abuse, a Finnish study of over 1000 young adults found that 20.1% of unemployed males engaged in hazardous drinking, compared to 7.1% of employed males (Kestilä et al., 2008). These figures were higher than the analogous figures for women, which were 14.7% for unemployed women and 4.5% for employed women. In other words, the unemployed were around three times more likely to engage in alcohol abuse compared to the employed, with unemployed men having the highest prevalence.

In terms of cannabis abuse, a French study of over 3000 young adults revealed that 19.3% of unemployed males used cannabis at least 10 times per month, compared to 12.4% of employed males (Legleye et al., 2008). Again, analogous figures for females were lower, with only 4.4.% of unemployed females and 4.3% of employed females engaging in similar levels of cannabis use. This study also found that unemployed males were significantly more likely to use other illegal drugs such as cocaine, heroin and ecstasy in comparison to employed males and unemployed females. In terms of past year use, 10.4% of unemployed males had used these drugs, compared to 5.2% of employed males, and 3.4% of unemployed females.

These results are consistent with an Australian study of over 10,000 adults which found that 19% of unemployed men engage in harmful use of alcohol, cannabis, opioids, sedatives or stimulants, compared to 9% of employed men (Andrews et al., 2001). Again, these rates were higher than analogous figures for unemployed women (11%) and employed women (4%). In sum, this literature indicates a two to threefold increased risk for substance abuse in unemployed men compared to employed men, and unemployed men have higher rates than unemployed women.

In terms of SUD, the landmark large-scale US Epidemiological Catchment Area study indicates that job loss can increase the risk of alcohol use disorder more than sixfold, though these studies did not report differential prevalence by gender (Dooley et al., 1992; Catalano et al., 1993). But the aforementioned Henkel (2011) review of the literature assessed a variety of studies including longitudinal research (thus accounting for reverse causation) concluding that men are at greater risk of SUD than women after a job loss and a period of unemployment. This is consistent with earlier reviews, which found that unemployed men had higher rates of alcohol use disorder than unemployed women and employed men, especially after job loss (Hammarström, 1994).

Indeed, rates of substance use disorder and associated fentanyl and opioid misuse appear to be higher in certain geographical areas, including areas with high rates of male unemployment and declining industries (Case & Deaton, 2020). This association implies a causal link between small-area deprivation, economic opportunity and substance abuse. It may also help explain high rates of substance use among Native Americans, Indigenous Canadians and Aboriginal Australians, who sometimes live in remote and isolated regions with little work or meaningful occupation. This may contribute towards a wider lack of purpose and meaning, leading some men to misuse substances in a drastic attempt to escape the associated pain and numb their psychological distress, while simultaneously filling a temporal and existential vacuum in their lives.

Moreover, it should be noted that men make up the overwhelming majority of people working in high-risk dangerous occupations including law enforcement, military personal, manufacturing, oil/gas workers, construction workers, fisheries, forestry and other manual labour (see Chap. 8). Given this situation, it is unsurprising that statistics indicate that men make up over 90% of workplace fatalities and over 75% of serious workplace injuries, including police and soldiers wounded in the line of duty (US Bureau of Labor Statistics, 2020a, 2020b; Myers et al., 1998).

It may be that men are disproportionately driven to substance misuse to control physical pain and mental distress incurred in these dangerous and demanding workplaces, where men make up the bulk of the workforce. Such substance misuse can begin mildly to control pain associated with occupational injuries, but can spiral into a more serious issue as individual men desperately attempt to grapple with ongoing (and sometimes worsening) pain. Such a hypothesis is supported by the research. For example, some studies indicate that a common clinical trajectory for the self-management of chronic pain is the use of alcohol or cannabis, followed by the legitimate use of prescription opioids, followed by the nonmedical use of opioids, followed by the use of heroin (Marsh et al., 2018). In some cases, this can be an effort to control physical or mental pain related to the workplace, which may be much more common in male-dominated professions compared to female-dominated ones. This hypothesis is discussed in more detail in Chap. 8.

3.7.3 Divorce, Separation and Loneliness

A growing body of research has examined the relationship between marital status and substance use. This research indicates higher rates of substance use among unmarried men, particularly among divorced men. For example, Edwards et al., (2018) conducted a longitudinal analysis of over 650,000 Swedes finding high rates of drug abuse onset in both sexes after a divorce with a summary hazard ratio of 7.31 (95% CI 6.91-7.74). For women, the hazards ratio was 6.80 (95% CI 6.25-7.39), while for men the hazards ratio was 8.29 (95% CI 7.65-8.97), indicating that divorce may have a greater mental health impact on men than women. Interestingly, this study also assessed the association between drug abuse onset and widowhood, finding a hazards ratio of 5.27 (95% CI 3.42-8.14) for women and 4.22 (95% CI 2.10-8.46) for men, implying that widowhood is a potent risk factor for drug abuse, but is weaker than divorce, and affects men less than women.

These results overlap with a similar Swedish study of over 900,000 individuals which examined alcohol use disorder onset after a divorce, which found a hazards ratio of 5.98 (95% CI: 5.65-6.33) for men after a divorce, while widowhood in men incurred a hazards ratio of 3.85 (95% CI: 2.81-5.28) (Kendler et al., 2017). Taken in the round, the combined results from these two studies suggest that the loss of a spouse through divorce or widowhood is detrimental to the mental health of both men and women; but divorce is a more powerful risk factor than widowhood, with divorce being particularly egregious for substance abuse in men. Moreover, the longitudinal nature of these two (and other) studies accounts for issues of reverse causation.

The previously described findings are consistent with studies elsewhere. For example, the aforementioned Compton et al., (2007) study found that the never married had an odds ratio of 2.0 (99% CI: 1.5-2.7) compared to the married for past year alcohol or drug use disorder; while the widowed, separated and divorced had an odds ratio of 2.6 (99% CI: 1.8-3.7) compared to the married. This suggests that the unmarried per se are at greater risk of substance use disorder than the married, with widowed, separated, and divorced men at particular risk. Similarly, another US study of over 8000 people examined past year alcohol use disorder, finding that all divorced and separated individuals had an adjusted odds ratio of 1.7 (95% CI

0.89-3.28) compared to all married, while men per se had an adjusted odds ratio of 5.86 (95% CI 3.50-9.82) compared to women per se, again signifying that divorced and separated men may be at greater risk than other demographics (Lin et al., 2011).

As discussed in much greater detail in Chap. 9, divorce and separation can have a variety of negative sequalae for men and women, but some factors may disproportionately impact men. For example, many men report negative experience in family courts, with data suggesting that only about one in six men have primary or sole custody of their children, often with minimal visitation rights (Beaupré et al., 2014). This separation from children can be soul-destroying and a living bereavement for the affected men, leaving them isolated and alienated from mainstream society.

Moreover, divorced men (along with single men per se) by definition lack the support and social integration of a nuclear family, which can contribute towards chronic loneliness. Indeed, surveys regularly indicate higher rates of loneliness in men compared to women (Cigna, 2020; YouGov, 2019). This male loneliness may be related to the 'stigma of singlehood' that can be especially severe for male singletons, who may be negatively stereotyped as potential perpetrators or villains (see Chap. 1), making them an object of suspicion and concern in a variety of social contexts (Byrne & Carr, 2005; DePaulo 2007). This may deter divorced and unmarried men from making pro-social efforts to address loneliness, with research indicating that young men are less likely to volunteer, participate in associations or clubs, or engage in political or charitable organizations compared to young women (Marcelo et al., 2007).

Instead, some men may be driven to engage in communities of substance abuse, in order to make social connections and reduce loneliness. Indeed, research indicates that men often become entangled in substance use networks to form social connections and be part of a community (Tanner et al., 2014; Chen et al., 2018). This can help achieve the desired escapism, as well as reducing the pain and distress associated with loneliness. In other words, the social needs of divorced and unmarried men may be impeded due to wider stigmas, stereotypes and suspicions (discussed in Chap. 1) targeted at single men, leading some to engage in pathological behaviours and communities centred upon substance abuse to better meet their social needs.

3.8 The Consequences of SUD and Addictions

Research studies indicate that adverse consequences associated with substance use disorder, addictions and substance misuse are higher among men than women. For example, the 2017 Canadian Tobacco, Alcohol and Drugs Survey reports that the prevalence of reported harms due to illegal drug use was 6% among men (518,000 people) and 3% among women (302,000 people), that is, double the rate in males compared to females (Government of Canada, 2019).

Importantly, the research literature indicates a bidirectional relationship between education/employment and SUD and addictions. As previously stated, low educational attainment and unemployment have been shown to be strong risk factors for a variety of adverse substance use outcomes in several longitudinal studies that rule out reverse causation. However, evidence also suggests that SUD and addictions issues are risk factors for adverse employment and educational outcomes. Indeed, several research studies suggest that SUD and addictions issues can contribute towards the much higher rate of educational dropout in men as compared to women (Vaughn et al., 2014; Maynard et al., 2015; Gonzales et al., 2016). These substance use issues can also prevent men from successfully entering the workforce, and can also result in unemployment, stagnation and dismissal for poor performance or flouting codes-of-conduct (Romelsjo et al., 2004; Brady & Randall, 1999). In other words, the bi-directional relationship between SUD and education/employment can create a vicious circle (or spiral) contributing to long-term issues.

Substance misuse and addictions can also have a deleterious impact on family and social relations. For example, gambling, Internet gaming and substance use can all result in an individual spending time and financial resources away from the family unit (Marsh et al., 2018). This can have a negative impact on parent-child and spousal relations, which can adversely affect the mental and physical health of the individual and their family (Khan et al., 2013).

Importantly, substance misuse by definition can have a detrimental effect on physical health. For example, prolonged alcohol use can lead to liver cirrhosis, which kills twice as many men as women. Similarly, opioid use and binge drinking can lead to accidents, injuries and overdoses – all of which are significantly more prevalent in men than women (Compton et al., 2007). Indeed, it has been noted that 77,000 people in 2015–2016 were hospitalized for alcohol use in Canada, most of whom were men (Smith, 2019). Relatedly, statistics from the World Health Organization indicate that around 13% of deaths worldwide can be attributed to alcohol, drugs or tobacco use. This may contribute towards the significantly lower life expectancy observed in men compared to women, as well as the lower life expectancy in men with SUD (Plunk et al., 2014; Hesse, 2006).

Substance misuse can also have severe legal consequences. Possession of substances such as non-prescription opioids and heroin is illegal in most western jurisdictions. Similarly, many jurisdictions have laws against public intoxication and drunk driving. This means that many people with substance use issues and addictions end up breaking the law, which can result in contact with law enforcement and the criminal justice system, as well as incarceration. These phenomena may contribute to the over-representation of men in the prison population, with men making up over 90% of the incarcerated population in countries such as the USA, the UK, Canada and Australia (Berman & Dar, 2013; Walmsley, 2006).

Substance misuse can also result in tragedies involving others, as it is associated with violence, aggression and accidents. For example, one report indicates that four people a day in Canada are killed in accidents where a car driver is under the influence of drugs and alcohol – which can sometimes involve innocent passengers and bystanders (Vasylchuk, 2019). Intoxication and binge drinking can also lead to violence and aggression, which again can involve harm to innocent bystanders and law enforcement (Branas et al., 2016). In other words, the impact of addictions, SUD, and substance misuse affects individuals, families and society as a whole – making it a major public health issue in need of concerted attention.

3.9 Treatments

Treatment for addictions and substance use disorder can take a variety of forms. First, there are a variety of talk therapies such as cognitive behavioural therapy and motivational interviewing which can be effective interventions, generally delivered by psychologists and other healthcare professionals (Smedslund et al., 2011; Greenfield et al., 2007). Second, there are numerous self-help organizations, for example, Alcoholics Anonymous, delivering group therapies including the well-known 12-step programs (Affleck et al., 2018; Ouimette et al., 1997). Third, there are several inpatient and outpatient detoxification and rehabilitation programs, which often involve a course of medications aiming to decrease craving and withdrawal symptoms, including naltrexone and methadone (King et al., 2013; Day & Strang, 2011; Tidey et al., 2009).

Of note, research indicates that the vast majority of men with a substance use disorder do not get any of the above treatments. For example, Compton et al., (2007) found that the 12-month treatment rates were 30.7% for more severe cases, and 6.1% for less severe cases, though rates were not broken down by gender. Similarly, Wang et al., (2005) found that only 26% of people with any substance use disorder received treatment. McHugh et al., (2018) report that only 11.1% of men with a SUD received treatment, similar to the figures for women (10.4%). Similar rates are witnessed in the 2018 National Survey on Drug Use and Health, which found that 19.3 million Americans experienced a SUD in the last 12 months, but only 2.1 million men had received treatment in that time (SAMHSA, 2019).

Other research indicates that men begin using substances earlier in life than women, but tend to enter treatment later. For example, one study found that men with alcohol-use disorder tend to access treatment an average of four years later than women (Lewis & Nixon, 2014). This treatment-seeking delay in men is concerning as early intervention can foster recovery and prevent worsening of the condition (Drake & Whitley, 2014). Moreover, men tend to have a longer duration of substance use disorder, with a higher average age at remission. This means their quality of life is typically impaired for a longer period.

The reasons for the low rates of treatment and longer delay in help-seeking in men are varied, and can involve generic mental health services issues discussed in greater detail in Chap. 6. But some research indicates that these differential rates may be related to gendered stereotypes and stigma (see Chap. 1) that can deter men from seeking help. For example, research indicates that substance misuse is often viewed as a criminal issue rather than a health issue (Wang et al., 2005). Such a perspective may be gendered through the familiar victim-villain dichotomy, inasmuch as men with mental health issues are more likely to be stereotyped as a villainous threat to the social order, whereas women with mental health issues are more likely to be stereotyped as a helpless victim in need of support (Whitley et al., 2015). This may shape both the wider social climate, as well as the formation and delivery of appropriate health services, especially in relation to substance use disorder, where stigma may be especially severe.

Of note, there are a lack of interventions in the substance use field that are specifically tailored to men. Indeed, Silver & Hur (2020) rightly note that "gender specific interventions are typically synonymous with interventions tailored to women". In fact, there are numerous separate female-only treatment programs for women with substance use disorders, purposely designed to address factors that may be more pertinent for women (Whitley et al., 2008; McHugh et al., 2018). Indeed, a review paper indicates that these programs generally have better outcomes for women than mixed-sex programs (Niv & Hser, 2007), and are also associated with higher satisfaction among female participants (Greenfield et al., 2013). However, similar gender-sensitive male-only programs have not been widely created, implemented or evaluated, with US data indicating that only around 25% of substance abuse treatment programs (that receive state funding) offer any type of specialist service targeted at adult men (Center for Substance Abuse Treatment, 2013). Such deficits in service provision for men with mental health issues, as well as promising male-centred programs and innovative interventions, are discussed in much more detail in Chap. 6.

3.10 Conclusion

This chapter has reviewed considerable literature on the topic of gender and substance misuse, revealing an interesting phenomenon. The word *gender* is a neutral term, and scientific papers with the word 'gender differences' in the title imply a balanced and comprehensive discussion of differences between men and women. However, many of the papers reviewed in this chapter use the words 'gender' and 'women' synonymously, with the phrase 'gender differences' used euphemistically to examine factors specific to women. Sometimes this is done explicitly, while at other times this is done implicitly. For example, McHugh et al., (2018) entitle their paper 'sex and gender differences in substance use disorders', but in paragraph 2 declare that 'we will review…literature specific to females', without any analogous statement about literature specific to males. Similarly, Marsh et al., (2018) entitle their paper 'gender differences in trends for heroin use and nonmedical prescription opioid misuse', but declare in their concluding remarks that 'the need to increase women-centered treatment services is especially compelling…it further calls for continued examination of treatment access…especially for women'. This conclusion seems inconsistent with the findings presented in their paper, which reveals much higher rates of heroin and opioid use in men as compared to women, as well as low service utilization rates in men.

At best, this is a blind spot in some approaches to the study of gender and addictions. At worst, it is a wilful bias, where gender issues are deliberately equated with women's issues, and men's issues are purposely ignored. Whichever, the reality is that men experience substance use and addictions issues at a much higher rate than women, and that this gender differential may be due to social determinants in areas such as education, employment and family life. These high rates typically lead to multiple adverse harms that have negative consequences for the men involved, their families as well as society as a whole. However, men underutilize substance abuse health programs, implying a need for invention and innovation to address these issues. These health service issues are discussed in greater detail in Chap. 6.

References

Substance Abuse and Mental Health Services Administration (SAMHSA). (2019, August). *Key substance use and mental health indicators in the United States: Results from the 2018 National Survey on Drug Use and Health*. U.S. Department of Health & Human Services-Substance Abuse and Mental Health Services Administration. Retrieved April 20, 2020, from https://www.samhsa.gov/data/sites/default/files/cbhsqreports/NSDUHNationalFindingsReport2018/NSDUHNationalFindingsReport2018.pdf.

Affleck, W., Carmichael, V., & Whitley, R. (2018). Men's mental health: Social determinants and implications for services. *Canadian Journal of Psychiatry, 63*(9), 581–589. https://doi.org/10.1177/0706743718762388.

American Psychiatric Association (APA). (2013). Substance-related and addictive disorders. In *Diagnostic and statistical manual of mental disorders* (5th ed.). American Psychiatric Association.

American Psychiatric Association (APA). (2018, June). *Internet gaming*. American Psychiatric Association. Retrieved April 20, 2020, from https://www.psychiatry.org/patients-families/internet-gaming.

Andrews, G., Henderson, S., & Hall, W. (2001). Prevalence, comorbidity, disability and service utilisation: Overview of the Australian National Mental Health Survey. *The British Journal of Psychiatry, 178*(2), 145–153.

Bass, P. F. (2015). Gaming addiction: When going online goes off-kilter. *Contemporary Pediatrics, 32*(11), 16–19.

Beaupré, B., Dryburgh, H., & Wendt, M. (2014, April 23). *Making fathers "count"*. Statistics Canada. Retrieved April 20, 2020, from https://www150.statcan.gc.ca/n1/pub/11-008-x/2010002/article/11165-eng.htm.

Benjet, C., Borges, G., Medina-Mora, M. E., Zambrano, J., & Aguilar-Gaxiola, S. (2009). Youth mental health in a populous city of the developing world: Results from the Mexican adolescent Mental Health survey. *The Journal of Child Psychology and Psychiatry, 50*(4), 386–395. https://doi.org/10.1111/j.1469-7610.2008.01962.x.

Berman, G., & Dar, A. (2013, June 28). *Prison population and statistics*. Antonio Casella. Retrieved April 20, 2020, from http://www.antoniocasella.eu/nume/Berman_2013.pdf.

Blanco, C., Hasin, D. S., Petry, N., Stinson, F. S., & Grant, B. F. (2006). Sex differences in subclinical and DSM-IV pathological gambling: Results from the National Epidemiologic Survey on alcohol and related conditions. *Psychological Medicine, 36*, 943–953. https://doi.org/10.1017/S0033291706007410.

Brady, K. T., & Randall, C. L. (1999). Gender differences in substance use disorders. *The Psychiatric Clinics of North America, 22*(2), 241–252. https://doi.org/10.1016/s0193-953x(05)70074-5.

Branas, C. C., Han, S., & Wiebe, D. J. (2016). Alcohol use and firearm violence. *Epidemiological Reviews, 38*(1), 32–45. https://doi.org/10.1093/epirev/mxv010.

British Columbia Coroners Service (2020, December 21). *Fentanyl-detected illicit drug overdose deaths-January 1, 2012 to April 30, 2017*. Office of the Chief Coroner, Ministry of Public Safety and Solicitor General. Retrieved April 20, 2020, from https://www2.gov.bc.ca/assets/gov/birth-adoption-death-marriage-and-divorce/deaths/coroners-service/statistical/fentanyl-detected-overdose.pdf.

Byrne, A., & Carr, D. (2005). Caught in the cultural lag: The stigma of singlehood. *Psychological Inquiry, 16*(2/3), 84–91. https://doi.org/10.1207/s15327965pli162&3_02.

Canadian Centre on Substance Use and Addiction (2019). *Canada's low-risk alcohol drinking guidelines*. Canadian Centre on Substance Use and Addiction. Retrieved April 20, 2020, from https://www.ccsa.ca/sites/default/files/2019-09/2012-Canada-Low-Risk-Alcohol-Drinking-Guidelines-Brochure-en.pdf.

Case, A., & Deaton, A. (2020). *Deaths of despair and the future of capitalism*. Princeton University Press.

Catalano, R., Dooley, D., Wilson, G., & Hough, R. (1993). Job loss and alcohol abuse: A test using data from the epidemiologic catchment area project. *Journal of Health and Social Behavior, 34*(3), 215–225. https://doi.org/10.2307/2137203.

Center for Substance Abuse Treatment (US). Addressing the Specific Behavioral Health Needs of Men. Rockville (MD): Substance Abuse and Mental Health Services Administration (US). (2013). (Treatment Improvement Protocol (TIP) Series, No. 56.) 1, Creating the Context. Available from: https://www.ncbi.nlm.nih.gov/books/NBK144300/

Centers for Disease Control and Prevention (CDC). (2020). *Fentanyl*. Centers for Disease Control and Prevention. Retrieved April 20, 2020, from https://www.cdc.gov/drugoverdose/opioids/fentanyl.html.

Chen, K. H., Oliffe, J. L., & Kelly, M. T. (2018). Internet gaming disorder: An emergent health issue for men. *American Journal of Men's Health, 12*(4), 1151–1159. https://doi.org/10.1177/1557988318766950.

Cigna (2020). *Loneliness and the workplace*. Cigna. Retrieved April 20, 2020, from https://www.cigna.com/static/www-cigna-com/docs/about-us/newsroom/studies-and-reports/combatting-loneliness/cigna-2020-loneliness-factsheet.pdf.

Compton, W. M., Thomas, Y. F., Stinson, F. S., & Grant, B. F. (2007). Prevalence, correlates, disability, and comorbidity of DSM-IV drug Abuse and dependence in the United States. *JAMA Psychiatry, 64*(5), 566–576. https://doi.org/10.1001/archpsyc.64.5.566.

Crum, R. M., Juon, H.-S., Green, K. M., Robertson, J., Fothergill, K., & Ensminger, M. (2006). Educational achievement and early school behavior as predictors of alcohol-use disorders: 35-year follow-up of the Woodlawn study. *Journal of Studies on Alcohol and Drugs, 67*(1), 75–85. https://doi.org/10.15288/jsa.2006.67.75.

Day, E., & Strang, J. (2011). Outpatient versus inpatient opioid detoxification: A randomized controlled trial. *Journal of Substance Abuse Treatment, 40*(1), 56–66. https://doi.org/10.1016/j.jsat.2010.08.007.

DePaulo, B. (2007). *Singled out: How singles are stereotyped, stigmatized, and ignored, and still live happily ever after*. St Martin's Press.

Dong, G., Wang, Z., Wang, Y., Du, X., & Potenza, M. N. (2019). Gender-related functional connectivity and craving during gaming and immediate abstinence during a mandatory break: Implications for development and progression of internet gaming disorder. *Progress in Neuropsychopharmacology & Biological Psychiatry, 88*, 1–10. https://doi.org/10.1016/j.pnpbp.2018.04.009.

Dooley, D., Catalano, R., & Hough, R. (1992). Unemployment and alcohol disorder in 1910 and 1990: Drift versus social causation. *Journal of Occupational and Organizational Psychology, 65*(40), 277–290. https://doi.org/10.1111/j.2044-8325.1992.tb00505.x.

Drake, R. E., & Whitley, R. (2014). Recovery and severe mental illness: Description and analysis. *Canadian Journal of Psychiatry, 59*(5), 236–242. https://doi.org/10.1177/070674371405900502.

References

Edwards, A. C., Larsson Lönn, S., Sundquist, J., Kendler, K. S., & Sundquist, K. (2018). Associations between divorce and onset of drug Abuse in a Swedish National Sample. *American Journal of Epidemiology, 187*(5), 1010–1018. https://doi.org/10.1093/aje/kwx321.

Erickson, J., El-Gabalawy, R., Palitsky, D., Patten, S., Mackenzie, C. S., Stein, M. B., & Sareen, J. (2016). Educational attainment as a protective factor for psychiatric disorders: Findings from a nationally representative longitudinal study. *Depression and Anxiety, 33*(11), 1013–1022. https://doi.org/10.1002/da.22515.

Esch, P., Bocquet, V., Pull, C., Couffignal, S., Lehnert, T., Graas, M., Fond-Harmant, L., & Ansseau, M. (2014). The downward spiral of mental disorders and educational attainment: A systematic review on early school leaving. *BMC Psychiatry, 14*(1), 237. https://doi.org/10.1186/s12888-014-0237-4.

Fam, J. Y. (2018). Prevalence of internet gaming disorder in adolescents: A meta-analysis across three decades. *Scandinavian Journal of Psychology, 59*(5), 524–531. https://doi.org/10.1111/sjop.12459.

Fothergill, K. E., Ensminger, M. E., Green, K. M., Crum, R. M., Robertson, J., & Juon, H.-S. (2008). The impact of early school behavior and educational achievement on adult drug use disorders: A prospective study. *Drug and Alcohol Dependence, 92*(1-3), 191–199. https://doi.org/10.1016/j.drugalcdep.2007.08.001.

Gonzalez, J. M., Salas-Wright, C. P., Connell, N. M., Jetelina, K. K., Clipper, S. J., & Businelle, M. S. (2016). The long-term effects of school dropout and GED attainment on substance use disorders. *Drug and Alcohol Dependence, 158*, 60–66. j.drugalcdep.2015.11.002.

González-Ortega, I., Echeburúa, E., Corral, P., Polo-López, R., & Alberich, S. (2013). Predictors of pathological gambling severity taking gender differences into account. *European Addiction Research, 19*, 146–154. https://doi.org/10.1159/000342311.

Goodman, A. (1990). Addiction: Definition and implications. *British Journal of Addiction, 85*(11), 1403–1408. https://doi.org/10.1111/j.1360-0443.1990.tb01620.x.

Government of Canada (2019, January 4). Canadian Tobacco, Alcohol and Drugs Survey (CTADS): Summary of results for 2017. Government of Canada. Retrieved April 20, 2020, from https://www.canada.ca/en/health-canada/services/canadian-tobacco-alcohol-drugs-survey/2017-summary.html.

Greenfield, S. F., Brooks, A. J., Gordon, S. M., Green, C. A., Kropp, F., McHugh, R. K., Lincoln, M., Hien, D., & Miele, G. M. (2007). Substance abuse treatment entry, retention, and outcome in women: A review of the literature. *Drug and Alcohol Dependence, 86*(1), 1–21. https://doi.org/10.1016/j.drugalcdep.2006.05.012.

Greenfield, S. F., Back, S. E., Lawson, K., & Brady, K. T. (2010). Substance abuse in women. *Psychiatry Clinics of North America, 33*(2), 339–355. https://doi.org/10.1016/j.psc.2010.01.004.

Greenfield, S. F., Cummings, A. M., Kuper, L. E., Wigderson, S. B., & Koro-Ljungberg, M. (2013). A qualitative analysis of women's experiences in single-gender versus mixed-gender substance abuse group therapy. *Substance Use & Misuse, 48*(9), 750–760. https://doi.org/10.3109/10826084.2013.787100.

Hall, W., Teesson, M., Lynskey, M., & Degenhardt, L. (2002). The 12-month prevalence of substance use and ICD-10 substance use disorders in Australian adults: Findings from the National Survey of Mental Health and Well-Being. *Addiction, 94*(10), 1541–1550. https://doi.org/10.1046/j.1360-0443.1999.9410154110.x.

Hammarström, A. (1994). Health consequences of youth unemployment—Review from a gender perspective. *Social Science & Medicine, 38*(5), 699–709. https://doi.org/10.1016/0277-9536(94)90460-X.

Hasin, D. S., Stinson, F. S., Ogburn, E., & Grant, B. F (2007). Prevalence, correlates, disability, and comorbidity of DSM-IV alcohol abuse and dependence in the United States: Results from the National Epidemiologic Survey on alcohol and related conditions. *Archives of General Psychiatry, 64*(7), 830-842. https://doi.org/10.1001/archpsyc.64.7.830.

Henkel, D. (2011). Unemployment and substance use: A review of the literature (1990-2010). *Current Drug Abuse Reviews, 4*(1), 4–27. https://doi.org/10.2174/1874473711104010004.

Hesse, M. (2006). What does addiction mean to me. *Mens Sana Monographs, 4*(1), 104–126. https://doi.org/10.4103/0973-1229.27609.

Jones, C. M., Logan, J., Gladden, R. M., & Bohm, M. K. (2015). Vital signs: Demographic and substance use trends among heroin users-United States, 2002-2013. *MMWR Morbidity & Mortality Weekly Report, 64*(26), 719–725.

Kelly, S. M., Schwartz, R. P., O'Grady, K. E., Mitchell, S. G., Reisinger, H. S., Peterson, J. A., Agar, M. H., & Brown, B. S. (2009). Gender differences among in- and out-of-treatment opioid-addicted individuals. *American Journal of Drug and Alcohol Abuse, 35*(1), 38–42. https://doi.org/10.1080/00952990802342915.

Kendler, K. S., Lönn, S. L., Salvatore, J., Sundquist, J., & Sundquist, K. (2017). Divorce and the onset of alcohol use disorder: A Swedish population-based longitudinal cohort and co-relative study. *American Journal of Psychiatry, 174*(5), 451–458. https://doi.org/10.1176/appi.ajp.2016.16050589.

Kessler, R. C., McGonagle, K. A., Zhao, S., Nelson, C. B., Hughes, M., Eshelman, S., Wittchen, H. U., & Kendler, K. S. (1994). Lifetime and 12-month prevalence of DSM-III-I psychiatric disorders in the United States. Results from the National Comorbidity Study. *Archives of General Psychiatry, 51*(1), 8–19. https://doi.org/10.1001/archpsyc.1994.03950010008002.

Kestilä, L., Martelin, T., Rahkonen, O., Joutsenniemi, K., Pirkola, S., Poikolainen, K., & Koskinen, S. (2008). Childhood and current determinants of heavy drinking in early adulthood. *Alcohol and Alcoholism, 43*(4), 460–469. https://doi.org/10.1093/alcalc/agn018.

Khan, S. S., Secades-Villa, R., Okuda, M., Wang, S., Pérez-Fuentes, G., Kerridge, B., & Blanco, C. (2013). Gender differences in cannabis use disorders: Results from the National Epidemiologic Survey of alcohol and related conditions. Drug & Alcohol Dependency, 130(0), 101-108. https://doi.org/10.1016/j.drugalcdep.2012.10.015.

King, A. C., Cao, D., Zhang, L., & O'Malley, S. S. (2013). Naltrexone reduction of long-term smoking cessation weight gain in women but not men: A randomized controlled trial. *Biological Psychiatry, 73*, 924–930. https://doi.org/10.1016/j.biopsych.2012.09.025.

King, D. L., Delfabbro, P. H., Wu, A. M. S., Doh, Y. Y., Kuss, D. J., Pallesen, S., Mentzoni, R., Carragher, N., & Sakuma, H. (2017). Treatment of internet gaming disorder: An international systematic review and CONSORT evaluation. *Clinical Psychology Review, 54*, 123–133. https://doi.org/10.1016/j.cpr.2017.04.002.

Kleinfeld, J. (2009). The state of American boyhood. *Gender Issues, 26*(2), 113–129. https://doi.org/10.1007/s12147-009-9074-z.

Legleye, S., Beck, F., Peretti-Watel, P., & Chau, N. (2008). Le rôle du statut scolaire et professionnel dans les usages de drogues des hommes et des femmes de 18 à 25 ans. *Revue d'Épidémiologie et de Santé Publique, 56*(5), 345–355. https://doi.org/10.1016/j.respe.2008.06.262.

Lewis, B., & Nixon, S. J. (2014). Characterizing gender differences in treatment seekers. *Alcoholism: Clinical and Experimental Research, 38*(1), 275–284. https://doi.org/10.1111/acer.12228.

Lin, J. C., Karno, M. P., Grella, C. E., Warda, U., Liao, D. H., Hu, P., & Moore, A. A. (2011). Alcohol, tobacco, and non-medical drug use disorders in U.S. adults aged 65 and older: Data from the 2001-2002 National Epidemiologic Survey of alcohol and related conditions. *American Journal of Geriatric Psychiatry, 19*(3), 292–299. https://doi.org/10.1097/JGP.0b013e3181e898b4.

Marcelo, K. B., Lopez, M. H., & Kirby, E. H. (2007). *Civic engagement among young men and women*. Center for Information & Research on Civic Learning and Engagement (CIRCLE). Retrieved April 20, 2020, from https://files.eric.ed.gov/fulltext/ED495763.pdf.

Marsh, J. C., Park, K., Lin, Y. A., & Bersamira, C. (2018). Gender differences in trends for heroin use and nonmedical prescription opioid use, 2007-2014. *Journal of Substance Abuse Treatment, 87*, 79–85. https://doi.org/10.1016/j.jsat.2018.01.001.

Marshall, K. (2012). Youth neither enrolled nor employed. *Perspectives on Labour and Income, 13*(5), 1–15.

Maynard, B. R., Salas-Wright, C. P., & Vaughn, M. G. (2015). High school dropouts in emerging adulthood: Substance use, mental health problems, and crime. *Community Mental Health Journal, 51*, 289–299. https://doi.org/10.1007/s10597-014-9760-5.

McHugh, R. K., Votaw, V. R., Sugarman, D. E., & Greenfield, S. F. (2018). Sex and gender differences in substance use disorders. *Clinical Psychology Review, 66*, 12–23. https://doi.org/10.1016/j.cpr.2017.10.012.

Merkouris, S. S., Thomas, A. C., Shandley, K. A., Rodda, S. N., Oldenhof, E., & Dowling, N. A. (2016). An update on gender differences in the characteristics associated with problem gambling: A systematic review. *Current Addiction Reports, 3*, 254–267. https://doi.org/10.1007/s40429-016-0106-y.

Myers, J. R., Kisner, S. M., & Fosbroke, D. E. (1998). Lifetime risk of fatal occupational injuries within industries, by occupation, gender, and race. *Human and Ecological Risk Assessment: An International Journal, 4*(6), 1291–1307. https://doi.org/10.1080/10807039891284677.

Niv, N., & Hser, Y. I. (2007). Women-only and mixed-gender drug abuse treatment programs: Service needs, utilization and outcomes. *Drug and Alcohol Dependence, 87*(2-3), 194–201. https://doi.org/10.1016/j.drugalcdep.2006.08.017.

Nolen-Hoeksema, S. (2004). Gender differences in risk factors and consequences for alcohol use and problems. *Clinical Psychology Review, 24*, 981–1010. https://doi.org/10.1016/j.cpr.2004.08.003.

Ouimette, P. C., Finney, J. W., & Moos, R. H. (1997). Twelve-step and cognitive-behavioral treatment for substance abuse: A comparison of treatment effectiveness. *Journal of Consulting and Clinical Psychology, 65*(2), 230–240. https://doi.org/10.1037/0022-006X.65.2.230.

Pearson, C., Janz, T., & Ali, J. (2013, September). *Health at a glance-Mental and substance use disorders in Canada*. Statistics Canada. Retrieved April 20, 2020, from https://www150.statcan.gc.ca/n1/pub/82-624-x/2013001/article/11855-eng.pdf.

Petry, N. M., & O'Brien, C. P. (2013). Internet gaming disorder and the DSM-5. *Addiction, 108*, 1186–1187. https://doi.org/10.1111/add.12162.

Petry, N. M., Rehbein, F., Gentile, D. A., Lemmens, J. S., Rumpf, H.-J., Mößle, T., Bischof, G., Tao, R., Fung, D. S. S., Borges, G., Auriacombe, M., González Ibáñez, A., Tam, P., & O'Brien, C. P. (2014). An international consensus for assessing internet gaming disorder using the new DSM-5 approach. *Addiction, 109*(9), 1399–1406. https://doi.org/10.1111/add.12457.

Plunk, A. D., Syed-Mohammed, H., Cavazos-Rehg, P., Bierut, L. J., & Grucza, R. A. (2014). Alcoholism. *Clinical and Experimental Research, 38*(2), 471–478. https://doi.org/10.1111/acer.12250.

Polak, K., Haug, N. A., Drachenberg, H. E., & Svikis, D. S. (2015). Gender considerations in addiction: Implications for treatment. *Current Treatment Options in Psychiatry, 2*(3), 326–338. https://doi.org/10.1007/s40501-015-0054-5.

Pouget, E. R., Fong, C., & Rosenblum, A. (2018). Racial/ethnic differences in prevalence trends for heroin use and non-medical use of prescription opioids among entrants to opioid treatment programs, 2005-2016. *Substance Use & Misuse, 53*(2), 290–300. https://doi.org/10.1080/10826084.2017.1334070.

Rodda, S. N., Hing, N., & Lubman, D. I. (2014). Improved outcomes following contact with a gambling helpline: The impact of gender on barriers and facilitators. *International Gambling Studies, 14*(2), 318–329. https://doi.org/10.1080/14459795.2014.921721.

Romelsjö, A., Stenbacka, M., Lundberg, M., & Upmark, M. (2004). A population study of the association between hospitalization for alcoholism among employees in different socio-economic classes and the risk of mobility out of, or within, the workforce. *European Journal of Public Health, 14*(1), 53–57. https://doi.org/10.1093/eurpub/14.1.53.

Schepis, T. S., Teter, C. J., & McCabe, S. E. (2018). Prescription drug use, misuse and related substance use disorder symptoms vary by educational status and attainment in U.S. adolescents and young adults. *Drug and Alcohol Dependence, 189*, 172–177. https://doi.org/10.1016/j.drugalcdep.2018.05.017.

Silver, E. R., & Hur, C. (2020). Gender differences in prescription opioid use and misuse: Implications for men's health and the opioid epidemic. *Preventive Medicine, 131*, 105946. https://doi.org/10.1016/j.ypmed.2019.105946.

Smedslund, G., Berg, R. C., Hammerstrøm, K. T., Steiro, A., Leiknes, K. A., Dahl, H. M., & Karlsen, K. (2011). Motivational interviewing for substance abuse. *Campbell Systematic Reviews, 7*(1), 1–126. https://doi.org/10.4073/csr.2011.6.

Smith, C. (2019, March 4). *Addiction in Canada*. Addiction Center. Retrieved April 20, 2020, from https://www.addictioncenter.com/addiction/addiction-in-canada/.

Stinson, F. S., Ruan, W. J., Pickering, R., & Grant, B. F. (2006). Cannabis use disorders in the USA: Prevalence, correlates and co-morbidity. *Psychological Medicine, 36*(10), 1447–1460. https://doi.org/10.1017/S0033291706008361.

Subramaniam, M., Wang, P., Soh, P., Vaingankar, J. A., Chong, S. A., Browning, C. J., & Thomas, S. A. (2015). Prevalence and determinants of gambling disorder among older adults: A systematic review. *Addictive Behaviours, 41*, 199–209. https://doi.org/10.1016/j.addbeh.2014.10.007.

Sussman, S., & Sussman, A. N. (2011). Considering the definition of addiction. *International Journal of Environmental Research and Public Health, 8*(10), 4025–4038. https://doi.org/10.3390/ijerph8104025.

Tanner, Z., Matsukara, M., Ivkov, V., & Buxton, J. (2014, September). *British Columbia Drug Overdose and Alert Partnership (DOAP) report*. BC Center for Disease Control. Retrieved April 20, 2020, from http://www.bccdc.ca/resourcegallery/Documents/Statistics%20and%20Research/ Publications/Epid/Other/FinalDOAPReport2014.pdf.

Tetrault, J. M., Desai, R. A., Becker, W. C., Fiellin, D. A., Concato, J., & Sullivan, L. E. (2008). Gender and non-medical use of prescription opioids: Results from a national US survey. *Addiction, 103*, 258–268. https://doi.org/10.1111/j.1360-0443.2007.02056.x.

Tidey, J. W., Monti, P. M., Rohsenow, D. J., Gwaltney, C. J., Miranda, R., Jr., McGeary, J. E., MacKillop, J., Swift, R. M., Abrams, R. M., Shiffman, S., & Paty, J. A. (2009). Moderators of naltrexone's effects on drinking, urge, and alcohol effects in non-treatment-seeking heavy drinkers in the natural environment. *Alcoholism, Clinical and Experimental Research, 32*(1), 58–66. https://doi.org/10.1111/j.1530-0277.2007.00545.x.

US Bureau of Labor Statistics. (2020a, December 16). Table 1. Fatal occupational injuries by selected demographic characteristics, 2015-19. Retrieved March 12, 2021, from https://www.bls.gov/news.release/cfoi.t01.htm.

US Bureau of Labor Statistics. (2020b, November 4). Table EH1. Number of nonfatal occupational injuries and illnesses involving days away from work by selected worker and case characteristics and medical treatment facility visits, all U.S., private industry, 2019. Retrieved March 12, 2021, from https://www.bls.gov/iif/oshwc/osh/case/cd_eh1_2019.htm.

Vasylchuk, P. (2019). Impaired driving. *RCMP Gazette, 80*(1) https://www.rcmp-grc.gc.ca/en/gazette/impaired-driving.

Vaughn, M. G., Salas-Wright, C. P., & Maynard, B. R. (2014). Dropping out of school and chronic disease in the United States. *Journal of Public Health, 22*, 265–270. https://doi.org/10.1007/s10389-014-0615-x.

Walmsley, R. (2006). *World female imprisonment list* (4th edition). World Prison Brief. Retrieved April 20, 2020, from https://www.prisonstudies.org/sites/default/files/resources/ downloads/world_female_prison_4th_edn_v4_web.pdf.

Wang, P. S., Lane, M., Olfson, M., Pincus, H. A., Wells, K. B., & Kessler, R. C. (2005). Twelve-month use of mental health services in the United States: Results from the National Comorbidity Survey replication. *Archives of General Psychiatry, 62*(2), 629–640. https://doi.org/10.1001/archpsyc.62.6.629.

Whitley, R., Harris, M., & Anglin, J. (2008). Refuge or rehabilitation? Assessing the development of a Women's empowerment center for people with severe mental illness. *Community Mental Health Journal, 44*, 253–260. https://doi.org/10.1007/s10597-008-9125-z.

References

Whitley, R., Adeponle, A., & Miller, A. R. (2015). Comparing gendered and generic representations of mental illness in Canadian newspapers: An exploration of the chivalry hypothesis. *Social Psychiatry and Psychiatric Epidemiology, 50*, 325–333. https://doi.org/10.1007/s00127-014-0902-4.

Wilson, N., Kariisa, M., Seth, P., Smith, H., IV, & Davis, N. L. (2020). Drug and opioid-involved overdose deaths-United States, 2017-2018. *MMWR Morbidity and Mortality Weekly Report, 69*(11), 290–297. https://doi.org/10.15585/mmwr.mm6911a4.

World Health Organization (WHO). (2018). Gaming disorder. In: *International classification of diseases for mortality and morbidity statistics* (11th Rev., ICD-11). World Health Organization.

YouGov (2019). *Friendship*. YouGov. Retrieved April 20, 2020, from https://d25d2506sfb94s.cloudfront.net/cumulus_uploads/document/m97e4vdjnu/Results%20for%20YouGov%20RealTime%20%28Friendship%29%20164%205.7.2019.xlsx%20%20%5BGroup%5D.pdf.

Zimbardo, P. G., & Coulombe, N. (2016). *Man, interrupted: Why young men are struggling what we can do about it*. Red Wheel.

Chapter 4
Attention-Deficit/Hyperactivity Disorder in Young Males: The Medicalization of Boyhood?

Attention-Deficit/Hyperactivity Disorder (ADHD) is a well-researched, much-discussed and somewhat controversial mental disorder. The American Psychiatric Association's *Diagnostic and Statistical Manual of Mental Disorders (2013) Fifth Edition (DSM-5)* contains a whole chapter devoted to ADHD, listing it in the 'neurodevelopmental disorders' section, thus implying that ADHD has a neurological basis that interferes with the developing brain. In contrast to disorders such as major depression, the conceptualization and diagnosis of ADHD is complex. DSM-5 lists three ADHD sub-types (labelled – somewhat confusingly – as 'presentations'), 18 discrete symptoms, and four further conditions that must be met for a diagnosis to be made. On the one hand, this complexity could be considered a conservative framing, laying out several necessary symptoms and conditions for a diagnosis to be made. On the other hand, this complexity could indicate a definitional haze and lack of specificity, making ADHD a malleable and expansive catch-all diagnosis that casts an overly large net. Both these arguments will be considered later in this chapter, which will begin by describing the DSM-5 conceptualization of ADHD in detail, followed by a presentation of epidemiological characteristics and risk factors, with a focus on sex differences. This is followed by a discussion of medication and treatment issues in ADHD. The final part of the chapter will consider some of the critiques of the ADHD concept and its associated treatments by presenting and discussing arguments related to medicalization, social control, overdiagnosis and the allegedly insidious role of 'Big Pharma' vis-à-vis ADHD.

4.1 What Is ADHD?

Attention-Deficit/Hyperactivity Disorder is an umbrella term referring to a persistent and consistent pattern of inattention and/or hyperactivity-impulsivity that negatively interferes with daily functioning and psychosocial development. ADHD is typically considered a disorder of childhood and adolescence, which is where the vast majority of research and action is targeted. As such, this chapter will focus on ADHD in youth under 18. That said, it is worth noting that ADHD can be diagnosed in adults, and this is an area of increasing interest in psychiatry.

Importantly, DSM-5 divides ADHD into two discrete sub-types (labelled as 'presentations'), namely: (i) predominantly inattentive; and (ii) predominantly hyperactive-impulsive. In other words, the oft-omitted forward slash in the phrase *Attention-Deficit/Hyperactivity Disorder* is an important punctuation point representing the 'and/or' rendering of the concept, indicating that the disorder can manifest itself in two distinct ways. This bidimensional rendering of ADHD is evident in the official DSM-5 symptom list, which is divided into two discrete sub-divisions: (i) inattention and (ii) hyperactivity-impulsivity. The symptom list for the inattention subdivision can be seen in Table 4.1, while the symptom list for the hyperactivity-impulsivity subdivision can be seen in Table 4.2. As elucidated later, a third sub-type of ADHD is described in DSM-5, known as 'combined presentation', which refers to a mixture of inattentive symptoms *and* hyperactivity symptoms.

As stated, the process of diagnosis is complex. A clinician must assess symptoms from these two lists, as well as examine the presence and absence of four other conditions. Also, the symptom threshold is slightly higher for children ages 16 and younger, compared to those 17 and older. For an ADHD diagnosis to be made in

Table 4.1 DSM-5 ADHD inattentive sub-type symptoms (APA, 2013)

(a) Makes careless mistakes and lacks attention to detail in schoolwork or other tasks
(b) Has difficulty maintaining attention on tasks or play activities
(c) Often does not appear to listen when spoken to directly
(d) Loses focus and gets sidetracked on tasks such as schoolwork and other activities
(e) Has trouble organizing tasks and activities, e.g. poor time management
(f) Avoids tasks that need mental effort such as schoolwork or homework
(g) Frequently loses task-related materials, e.g. pencils, books, keys, glasses
(h) Gets easily distracted by external stimuli
(i) Forgetfulness in daily activities, e.g. paying bills, keeping appointments

Table 4.2 DSM-5 ADHD hyperactivity-impulsivity sub-type symptoms (APA, 2013)

(a) Frequent fidgeting, for example taps hands/feet or squirms in seat
(b) Often leaves a seat when staying seated is expected, e.g. in the classroom
(c) Restlessness, for example, running or climbing in inappropriate situations
(d) Difficulty in participating in leisure activities quietly
(e) Is frequently 'on the go' behaving as if 'driven by a motor', e.g. trouble being still
(f) Excessive talking
(g) Often blurts out answers before a question has been completed
(h) Difficulties waiting their turn, e.g. in a queue
(i) Often interrupts or intrudes on others in conversation, games or activities

children ages 16 or younger, six or more of the symptoms from one of the two above tables must be present for at least the last 6 months. If six or more symptoms are present from Table 4.1, but less than six are present from Table 4.2, then an inattentive sub-type can be diagnosed. Conversely, if six or more symptoms from Table 4.2 are present, but less than six are present from Table 4.1, then a hyperactivity-impulsivity sub-type can be diagnosed. The 'combined presentation' sub-type can be made when an individual has six or more symptoms from both lists (i.e. 12 or more symptoms). For adults 17 years of age and older, the same process applies; however, only five or more symptoms are required for a sub-type diagnosis, and 10 for diagnosis of combined presentation. The higher symptom threshold for children represents a conservative approach attempting to reduce false positives that conflate boisterous and spirited childhood behaviour with psychopathology, while also reducing the need for psychotropic medication that can affect the developing brain – both phenomena discussed in more detail later in this chapter. Four additional criteria must be met for all three sub-types. These are:

(i) Several symptoms must be present before age 12 years.
(ii) Several symptoms must be present in two or more settings (e.g. home and school).
(iii) Symptoms must negatively impact social, academic or occupational functioning.
(iv) Symptoms are not better explained by another mental disorder.

If the symptom threshold has been reached and the four additional criteria have been met, then a formal diagnosis of ADHD (with the appropriate sub-type) can be made. Of note, the core symptom criteria for ADHD in DSM-5 are very similar to the symptom criteria in DSM-IV. This is important, given that DSM-5 was published in 2013 and DSM-IV was valid from 1994 to 2013. This gives validity to any epidemiological analysis that attempts to examine change over time. That said, three important changes were made to the DSM-5 description of ADHD, namely: (i) the age of onset criteria was raised from 7 to 12 years of age; (ii) the number of symptoms required to diagnose people age 17 and older was reduced; and (iii) a wider range of clinical examples were given to help diagnose older adolescents or adults. All three changes widened the diagnostic net, meaning more people were eligible for an ADHD diagnosis. This expansion of the diagnostic net is discussed in more detail later in the chapter.

4.2 The Epidemiology of ADHD

There is an extensive and nuanced international research literature on ADHD, spanning the 1990s to the present. This research literature converges on three key findings: (i) boys have a much higher prevalence of ADHD than girls, at a rate of around 3:1; (ii) rates of ADHD are rising; (iii) rates of ADHD are higher in the USA compared to Europe and elsewhere. Some of the core studies underpinning these findings are discussed in detail next.

There have been numerous attempts to estimate the global prevalence of ADHD. One systematic review synthesized data from 102 studies from across the world, finding a global prevalence of 5.3% in youth ages 18 or younger (Polanczyk et al., 2007). Many of the studies in this review did not stratify by gender, but a sub-analysis of studies that included gender found a worldwide pooled prevalence of 10% in boys 18 years or younger and just under 5% in girls of the same age.

A similar attempt to measure global prevalence involved a meta-analysis of 96 studies from across the globe (Willcutt, 2012). This revealed a global pooled prevalence of 6% in youth. This meta-analysis did not report differential prevalence levels by gender in percentage terms. Instead, the study reported the M:F ratio for ADHD overall, as well as for the three different sub-types of ADHD. This revealed a M:F ratio of 3.2:1 for ADHD overall in people aged 18 and under. Males had higher rates than females of all three sub-types. The ratio was highest for the hyperactive-impulsivity sub-type, with a M:F ratio of 3.5:1, and lowest for the inattentive sub-type at 1.8:1. The combined sub-type M:F ratio was 2.7:1.

Similar findings were observed in another meta-analysis that had the express intention of examining gender differences in ADHD (Gershon, 2002). This study synthesized data from 38 articles from across the world (mostly published in the 1980s and 1990s) finding that males with ADHD had significantly higher levels of hyperactivity, impulsivity and inattention as compared to females with ADHD. Furthermore, this meta-analysis revealed that males with ADHD have significantly more impairments and more primary symptoms than females with ADHD.

In short, these three comprehensive reviews indicate that males have significantly higher rates of ADHD than females, both overall as well as for the three ADHD sub-types, particularly the hyperactive-impulsive sub-type. These reviews also suggest that males tend to experience the disorder more intensely than females. This is consistent with earlier research indicating that ADHD afflicts males more severely than females (Cantwell, 1996; Gaub & Carlson, 1997).

These international analyses pool together a range of studies of variable quality, some of which lack methodological and epidemiological rigour. For example, some of the included studies contain small sample sizes, while others use nebulous methods of case ascertainment and epidemiological analysis. Moreover, many of the included studies do not stratify by gender. As such, more focused national studies can sometimes give more valid and reliable statistics on prevalence, gender differentials and time trends. Fortunately, there are numerous national studies from a range of western jurisdictions shedding light on ADHD epidemiology. Many rigorous studies originate from Europe; however, researchers in the USA have consistently produced high-quality surveys on ADHD over the last 20 years. These are discussed in detail in the next section.

4.3 US Studies on ADHD

Various agencies of the US Government such as the Centers for Disease Control and Prevention (CDC) conduct regular health-oriented surveys of the US population. These typically involve thousands of randomly selected households, who are asked a series of questions about the health status of household members, as well as other demographic characteristics. These surveys allow for stratification by factors including sex, race and income; and sample numbers are typically sufficient for extrapolation to the wider US population. These surveys include the National Survey of Children's Health (NSCH) and the National Health Interview Survey (NHIS): both include a question for parents, asking if their children (ages under 18) have ever been diagnosed with ADHD by a doctor or other health professional. Different waves also include supplemental questions to allow for in-depth analysis of a certain health condition.

In 2001, the NHIS included the 25-item parent-report Strengths and Difficulties Questionnaire (SDQ): a reliable and validated instrument that measures child and adolescent behaviours including ADHD symptoms (Goodman, 2001). This was administered to over 10,000 randomly selected children ages 4–17 years, giving a firm foundation for a reliable community estimate of ADHD prevalence. Researchers examined this SDQ data, finding a 6-month prevalence of 4.2% in boys, compared to 1.8% in girls (Cuffe et al., 2005). Interestingly, the authors also noted that 6.8% of boys and 2.5% of girls had a parent-reported lifetime ADHD diagnosis, *despite an SDQ score indicating no ADHD*. Some level of mismatch is to be expected when comparing results based on an epidemiological screening instrument with results based on a clinical encounter. That said, this discrepancy raises two other possibilities: (i) a high rate of recovery among those with a lifetime diagnosis; or (ii) a high rate of clinical false positives due to overdiagnosis by clinicians. The issue of false positives is discussed throughout this chapter.

A later purpose-built US study used systematic methods to ascertain lifetime and current prevalence of ADHD overall in over 9000 randomly selected households (Ramtekkar et al., 2010). These methods involved telephone interviews with parents asking about lifetime ADHD symptoms, as well as completion of the Strengths and Weaknesses of ADHD-Symptoms and Normal Behaviour instrument (SWAN) – a validated 18-item questionnaire eliciting information about child behaviour that assesses current symptoms. This study found a current prevalence of ADHD of 12.6% in males, and 5.5% in females aged 7–29; a ratio of 2.28:1. Additionally, the findings indicate that males are more likely to be diagnosed with all sub-types of ADHD, with the highest ratio of 2.89:1 in the combined sub-type. Interestingly, this study also found that boys had a significantly higher number of symptoms across all ages studied compared to girls, with symptom load particularly concentrated in the 7–12-year-old age group. Indeed, this age group had the highest prevalence of ADHD overall, with 15.7% in boys and 7.5% in girls. Of note, the overall prevalence rates reported in this study are over double those of Cuffe et al.'s (2005) earlier study.

A similar prevalence was found in a smaller US study of just under 2000 youth ages 17 or younger in Puerto Rico (Bauermeister et al., 2007). This study elicited parental reports of DSM symptoms through the validated Computerized Diagnostic Interview Schedule for Children (Bravo et al., 2001), which helps ascertain the presence or absence of ADHD. This study found that 10.3% of boys and 4.7% of girls had ADHD, a ratio of 2.3:1. Consistent with the Ramtekkar et al. (2010) study, this study found that boys had higher rates of all three ADHD sub-types.

The previously described studies were conducted more than a decade ago, with much speculation that rates have increased since then. Fortunately, there have been several studies in the last few years which can contribute towards an analysis of time trends. However, these studies have tended to focus on rates of formal diagnosis by health professionals, rather than rates obtained through epidemiological screening. Still, these studies indicate a significant increase in ADHD.

As stated, the CDC has collected periodic data on the prevalence of ADHD since 1997 by collating information from the NHIS – a regular survey of around 35,000 randomly selected households, with the last round of analysed data collected in 2015–2017 (Centers for Disease Control and Prevention, 2019). Results reveal a linear increase in ADHD diagnosis since 1997. For example, the 2015–2017 data indicated that 14.8% of boys and 6.7% of girls had ever been diagnosed with ADHD, while the 1997–1999 figures stood at 9.6% for boys and 3.2% for girls. This represents a 50% increase in diagnosis for boys, and a doubling for girls in the last two decades, with the latest figures suggesting that around one in six boys in the USA had been diagnosed with ADHD at some point in their lives.

The National Survey of Children's Health (NSCH) is another regular survey collecting information from over 40,000 randomly selected US households. Data from the 2016 NSCH wave indicated that 12.9% of boys and 5.6% of girls had received a diagnosis of ADHD. These figures are slightly lower than the 2015–2017 NHIS data, but still higher than the aforementioned earlier community-based surveys (Cuffe et al., 2005; Bauermeister et al., 2007; Ramtekkar et al., 2010). Moreover, a longitudinal analysis of several previous waves of NSCH data indicated a significant increase in diagnosis from 2003 to 2011, with a parent-reported history of ADHD increasing by 42% from 2003 to 2011 (Visser et al., 2014).

In sum, several US studies from different time points using diverse methodologies converge to indicate a significant rise in ADHD diagnosis in the last two decades, with prevalence rates particularly high among school-aged boys. This male preponderance is also seen in European studies, though these studies indicate an overall lower prevalence than the US (Thomas et al., 2015). For example, a population-based survey of over 17,000 randomly selected households in Germany found that 7.9% of boys (under 17 years) and 1.8% of girls (under 17 years) had received an ADHD diagnosis from a health professional (Knopf et al., 2012). Another population-based survey of over 7000 households in France found that 4.7% of boys ages 6–12 years and 2.2% of girls ages 6–12 years screened positive for ADHD following a clinical telephone interview (Lecendreux et al., 2011), with similar figures seen in another French community survey (Caci et al., 2014). In other words, ADHD is being diagnosed with increasing frequency across the western world, but especially in the USA, with school-aged boys being the most affected.

4.4 Risk Factors

There is a rich literature on risk factors for ADHD in male children and adolescents. This literature consistently identifies several factors that increase risk for ADHD including: (i) middle-childhood age; (ii) childhood maltreatment and abuse; (iii) low family income; (iv) low parental education; and (v) living with a single parent (typically a single mother). These factors are discussed in turn in the following subsections.

4.4.1 Middle-Childhood Years

Evidence suggests that boys in the middle-childhood years (approximately 7 years old to 13 years old) have higher rates of ADHD than boys and adolescents of other ages. For example, Ramtekkar et al. (2010) found a prevalence rate of 15.7% in 7–12-year-old boys, higher than the 13.8% observed in 13–17-year-old boys, and 8.6% observed in 18–29-year-old males, also noting that the quantitative number of symptoms tended to decrease with age. Similarly, Cuffe et al. (2005) found a prevalence of 6.3% in boys ages 9–13 years, higher than the 3.1% figure observed in boys ages 4–8 years and the 2.9% figure observed in boys ages 14–17 years. Interestingly, an Australian study found a 18.7% prevalence of ADHD in boys ages 6–13 years, over double the 8.4% prevalence for girls of the same age (Graetz et al., 2005).

4.4.2 Childhood Maltreatment and Neglect

Common to many mental disorders, childhood abuse, neglect and maltreatment have been identified as risk factors for ADHD by a variety of studies (Acosta et al., 2008). For example, a case-control study of over 100 matched pairs found that men with ADHD reported significantly higher scores of childhood neglect and abuse in comparison to male controls (Rucklidge et al., 2006). In this study, 50% of male cases reported moderate to severe emotional abuse, compared to 12.5% in male controls. Similarly, 12.5% of male cases reported moderate to severe sexual abuse compared to 2.5% of male controls.

These findings are consistent with an analysis of data from over 14,000 randomly selected youth participating in the U.S. National Longitudinal Study of Adolescent Mental Health (Ouyang et al., 2008). In Wave III, participants completed an 18-item screening instrument to retrospectively report on the presence and frequency of ADHD symptoms when they were 5–12 years old. Participants also completed a questionnaire on the frequency of maltreatment during these years. The subsequent analysis revealed that ADHD was significantly associated with supervision neglect (OR:1.52; 95% CI: 1.28–1.81), physical neglect (OR:1.97; 95% CI: 1.56–2.50), physical abuse (OR:1.39; 95% CI: 1.16–1.66) and contact sexual abuse (OR:2.31; 95% CI 1.64–3.24). Similar odds ratios have been observed in more recent studies (Stern et al., 2018).

4.4.3 Low Family Income

For some time, ADHD was considered to afflict all social classes equally, and was sometimes even considered a problem of the middle classes. However, the research literature indicates higher rates of ADHD in children from lower-income families. For example, a recent meta-analysis found odds ratios that children from low-income families were 1.85–2.21 more likely to have ADHD than children from high-income families (Russell et al., 2016). These findings of elevated rates among low-income families are consistent with other recent large-scale studies from Sweden (Larsson et al., 2014), the UK (Russell et al., 2014) and the USA (Rowland et al., 2018). In this latter study, Rowland et al. (2018) found an odds ratio of 4.0 (95% CI: 2.6–6.0) when comparing ADHD between low-income families (<$20,000) and high-income families (>$50,000). In sum, the literature indicates that children from low-income families have over twice the risk of developing ADHD compared to high-income families.

4.4.4 Low Parental Education

Relatedly, parental education has been identified as a significant risk factor for ADHD in several studies. For example, Rowland et al. (2018) found that children of parents who had not graduated high school had an odds ratio of 6.0 (95% CI: 3.3–10.7) for ADHD when compared to children of parents with at least some college education. These findings overlap with a UK study which found that children of mothers with a degree or higher were around three times less likely to have ADHD than children of mothers with no educational qualifications (OR:0.32; 95% CI 0.18–0.55) (Russell et al., 2014). Similar results were observed in a Swedish study, which found that levels of maternal education were negatively correlated with offspring ADHD, with an adjusted odds ratio of 2.20 (95% CI: 2.04–2.38) when comparing the least educated mothers to the most educated mothers in the sample (Hjern et al., 2010).

4.4.5 Single-Mother Families

Interestingly, some studies have examined maternal education in tandem with parental marital status, indicating that boys raised by a single parent have an increased risk of ADHD, especially when the said single parent lacks education. Of note, Singh (2004) correctly identifies that the category 'parent' is typically a euphemism for 'mother' in ADHD research, but this is often unspecified in epidemiological research, which typically uses the amorphous category 'single parent' when measuring parental effects in children. However, statistics indicate that over 80% of single-parent households are single mothers (Department of Justice Canada, 2000), meaning that the variable 'single parent household' is generally describing a 'single mother household': an important point discussed in greater detail in Sect. 4.8.3 and Chap. 9, but reviewed briefly next.

For example, a case-control study of 300 children with ADHD and 5000 controls found that low maternal education significantly increased the risk for ADHD in both girls and boys, but most strongly in boys (St. Sauver et al., 2004). This study revealed that a boy raised by a mother with 12 years education or less was more than three times more likely to have ADHD compared to a girl raised by a mother with 12 years education or less. Importantly, this study found that a boy raised by a 'single parent' is four times more likely to be diagnosed with ADHD compared to a girl raised by a single parent.

These findings are consistent with other research. For example, the aforementioned Hjern et al. study (2010) found that children of 'single parents' had an odds ratio of 1.54 (95% CI: 1.47–1.62) for ADHD when compared to children of married parents, with 'single parent' households accounting for 14% of cases. Similar results have been seen in the UK, with a cohort study indicating that children from 'single parent' families are over twice as likely (OR: 2.07; 95% CI: 1.42–3.03) to have ADHD compared to children from two-parent families (Russell et al., 2014). This study also found that maternal smoking during pregnancy doubled the risk of ADHD in children, which is consistent with other research (Rodriguez & Bohlin, 2005; Langley et al., 2005; He et al., 2017). Similarly, evidence suggests that maternal alcohol use during pregnancy can double the risk of offspring ADHD (Mick et al., 2002; Knopik et al., 2006; Eilertsen et al., 2017), while other studies indicate that maternal obesity can significantly increase the risk of ADHD in offspring (Andersen et al., 2018; Chen et al., 2014; Rodriguez et al., 2008).

In short, low maternal education and risky maternal health behaviours are associated with an increased risk of ADHD, with evidence suggesting that male children of low-income single mothers particularly experience elevated rates of ADHD. This implies that father absence may be an important risk factor for ADHD in boys, especially in cases where the mother lacks education. However, Singh (2004) notes that fathers have been systematically excluded from ADHD research, despite related research indicating that father absence leads to a range of negative psychosocial sequalae in children, as described in more detail in Chap. 9 (McLanahan et al., 2013). Given its importance, the role of parenthood in ADHD is revisited later in this chapter.

4.5 Educational Impact

Much research has examined the psychosocial impact of ADHD in the short and long term. By definition, the symptoms of ADHD as listed in Tables 4.1 and 4.2 interfere with schooling, and this is manifest in studies comparing educational outcomes in children with ADHD and children without ADHD. These studies consistently report that children and adolescents with ADHD are more likely to have a negative educational experience including significantly higher rates of suspension, detention, expulsion, grade repetition and school dropout, even while receiving medication (Fleming et al., 2017; Loe & Feldman, 2007; Rucklidge, 2010). For example, one US study of over 1000 school-aged children found that those diagnosed with ADHD were significantly more likely to be: (i) expelled or suspended (OR: 7.1; 95% CI 2.3–10.7); (ii) forced to repeat a grade (OR 3.4; 95% CI 2.1–5.3) and (iii) receive special education (OR 4.1; 95% CI 2.6–6.4) in comparison to non-ADHD pupils (LeFever et al., 2002). Another study of over 500 children in the Netherlands found that over 40% of children with ADHD had repeated a grade and/or had learning problems (Derks et al., 2007). Importantly, some research indicates that rates of these adverse outcomes tend to be higher in boys than in girls.

For example, the aforementioned Bauermeister et al. (2007) study compared outcomes between girls and boys with ADHD, finding that 22.7% of boys with ADHD had been suspended from school, compared to 0% of girls with ADHD. Similarly, 28% of boys with ADHD had failed a grade, compared to 7% of girls with ADHD. Similarly, the aforementioned LeFever et al. (2002) study found that boys with ADHD were significantly more likely to be expelled or suspended than girls with ADHD, with an odds ratio of 4.8 (95% CI: 2.6–8.6). This study also found that boys were more likely to receive special educational services (OR 2.5; 95% CI 1.6–3.8). An Australian study of 300 boys and girls with ADHD revealed that 65% of boys were having problems with schoolwork and grades, compared to 47% of girls (Graetz et al., 2005).

These elevated rates of adverse educational outcomes in boys have been attributed to various factors. First, some research indicates that boys with ADHD tend to have significantly higher rates of hyperactivity, inattention, impulsivity, aggression and externalizing problems compared to girls with ADHD (Gershon, 2002; Abikoff et al., 2002). These problems can disrupt the smooth running of the classroom, leading to disciplinary action from teachers and school administrators. In other words, the more severe typical symptom profile of a boy with ADHD can contribute to more classroom disruption, which in turn can lead to more severe disciplinary measures, resulting in worse outcomes (Cantwell, 1996; Gaub & Carlson, 1997).

Nevertheless, another potential explanation is that teachers and school administrators experience higher rates of annoyance and less tolerance towards boys with ADHD, compared to girls with ADHD. For example, the aforementioned Graetz et al. (2005) study found that 64% of boys with ADHD were rated as annoying or upsetting their teachers compared to 38% of girls with ADHD, despite a similar mean number of symptoms and comparable symptom profiles as elicited by the Diagnostic Interview Schedule for Children: a validated gold standard instrument (Bravo et al., 2001). This could be related to gender stereotypes and the gendered *halo effect* discussed in Chap. 1, where boys with ADHD are perceived as more threatening and disruptive, while girls are perceived as more agreeable and compliant regardless of actual behaviour (see Sect. 4.8.4).

This hypothesis is supported by considerable research indicating that teachers report lower levels of problem behaviours in girls with ADHD and higher levels in boys with ADHD, even when the boys and girls studied have similar symptom profiles and similar rates of disruptive behavioural disorders (Hartung et al., 2002; Biederman et al., 2005; Derks et al., 2007). These studies also indicate a divergence between teacher and parent reports, with parents reporting fewer problem behaviours in sons with ADHD – at a level similar to daughters with ADHD. These important phenomena are discussed later in this chapter, and in much more detail in Chap. 7, which also intensely explores the link between low educational attainment and adult mental health issues.

4.6 Impact into Adulthood

Several studies indicate that ADHD can be a chronic disorder persisting into later life for between 25% and 50% of childhood cases (Hashmi et al., 2017; Dalsgaard, 2013; Kessler et al., 2005). For example, one prospective cohort study of over 5000 individuals indicated that childhood ADHD lasts into adulthood for 29% of cases (Barbaresi et al., 2013). Another Australian cohort study of over 3000 people found higher rates of chronicity in men, with symptoms persisting into adulthood for 63% of males compared to 48% of females (Ebejer et al., 2012).

These and other studies indicate that people with ADHD have an increased risk of various adult difficulties including criminality, incarceration, unemployment, social disadvantage, substance abuse, divorce and low educational attainment (Groenman et al., 2017; Agnew-Blais et al., 2016; Fletcher, 2014; Dalsgaard, 2013; Biederman et al., 2006). Again, these studies indicate that men with ADHD experience some of these difficulties at higher rates than women with ADHD. For example, Biederman et al. (2004) conducted a case-control study, finding significantly higher rates of alcohol and drug abuse in males with ADHD compared to females with ADHD. These findings have been observed in other studies, with one Norwegian study of 600 men and women with ADHD indicating that men (37%) have over double the rate of alcohol abuse compared to women (18%) with ADHD (Rasmussen & Levander, 2009). This study also found considerably higher rates of criminality and drug abuse in men with ADHD compared to women with ADHD. Similarly, 84% of men in this study had an unstable work history, compared to 62% of women.

4.7 Medication Issues

There are a range of US Food and Drug Administration (FDA)-approved medications available for the treatment of ADHD. The two most commonly used medications are psychostimulants: (i) amphetamine compounds, commonly known under the brand name Adderall; and (ii) methylphenidate compounds, commonly known under the brand names of Ritalin or Concerta. Both these forms of psychostimulant medication can be helpful in reducing the symptoms of ADHD, particularly by improving concentration and attention. Indeed, the CDC (2020a) notes that "between 70–80 percent of children with ADHD have fewer ADHD symptoms when they take these fast-acting medications".

These two psychostimulants are commonly used as a first-line treatment for ADHD, though usage varies according to jurisdiction. For example, guild organizations such as the American Academy of Pediatrics (2019) and the American Academy of Child and Adolescent Psychiatry (2007) recommend both these forms of psychostimulants for children ages 6–18 years. However, the UK National Institute for Health Care Excellence (NICE) recommends methylphenidate as a first-line treatment for children and young people ages 5 or older (National Institute for Health Care Excellence, 2018), but amphetamines are not listed as a recommended treatment in the UK NICE guidelines. Indeed, around 90% of prescribed medication for childhood ADHD in Europe is for methylphenidate, while both methylphenidate and amphetamine compounds are commonly used in the USA (Knopf et al., 2012; Zito et al., 2008). This preference for methylphenidates in Europe is based on weighty evidence indicating that methylphenidate is more efficacious in children and adolescents compared to amphetamines, while amphetamines can cause more side effects and adverse events in children compared to methylphenidate (Cortese et al., 2018).

4.7.1 Side Effects and Misuse

In fact, evidence suggests that both amphetamine and methylphenidate can have a range of side effects. This can include decreased appetite, weight loss, mood disturbances and sleep problems (Berman et al., 2009; Cascade et al., 2010). By definition, these stimulant medications can also raise blood pressure and speed up heart rate, thus increasing risk of cardio-vascular issues (Hennissen et al., 2017; Sinha et al., 2016; Martinez-Raga et al., 2013; Westover & Halm, 2012). Some studies have also linked these stimulant medications to behavioural issues including increased hostility, aggression, paranoia and mood swings (Berman et al., 2009). There is also a risk of withdrawal symptoms such as anxiety, nausea and sweating. Moreover, the long-term side effects are largely unknown, with a paucity of studies measuring impact beyond 12 weeks (Cortese et al., 2018). This has led to speculation (sometimes based on animal-research) that the long-term usage of psychostimulants can lead to negative physical, mental and functional sequalae including loss of drive, apathy, and a decline in inner motivation; which has been linked to morphological damage to brain areas including the ventral striatum, particularly the nucleus accumbens (Breggin, 2001; Berman et al., 2009; Whitaker, 2010; Hoekzema et al., 2014; Sax, 2016).

Of note, amphetamine-based psychostimulants can also be used for non-medicinal purposes, and are often sold on the black market. Indeed, there is a brisk trade among university and college students, who use psychostimulants during study periods and exams to improve concentration, with one US study indicating that 39% of university students had misused psychostimulants in this manner (Peralta & Steele, 2010). Moreover, they can be abused for recreational purposes to elevate mood and induce a high (Maturo, 2013). This behaviour is concerning as the FDA notes that psychostimulants can be addictive, and can also have toxic effects, meaning that such non-medicinal use can increase risk of addiction and even overdose. Indeed, such concerns have led some jurisdictions to regulate the diagnosis and treatment of ADHD. In Denmark, for example, only specialists such as child psychiatrists and paediatricians are licensed to initiate treatment, with non-specialists such as general practitioners mainly having a referral role (Dalsgaard, 2013). Similar protections are in place in other European nations including France and Italy (Maturo, 2013; Conrad & Bergey, 2014).

4.7.2 Absolute Gender Differences in Medication Usage

A recent US study examined prevalence of ADHD, as well as associated medication usage, through analysis of data from the 2016 NSCH, a cross-sectional survey that included parent-report data on over 45,000 children (Danielson et al., 2018). This study found that 9.4% of 2–17-year-old children in the USA had received an ADHD diagnosis, totalling 6.1 million people, with double the rate in boys compared to girls. Of note, 62% of children with an ADHD diagnosis were taking medication, totalling over three million young people, which is over 5% of all US children ages 2–17 years. Almost all cases of medication were in school-aged children or adolescents, and rates of usage were higher in boys than girls.

These recent findings are consistent with many other studies showing that boys are significantly more likely to be prescribed medication than girls, in both absolute terms and relative terms. For example, a large-scale three-nation study of over 500,000 pharmacy claims in youth ages 19 or younger compared psychostimulant use for ADHD between boys and girls in the USA, Germany and the Netherlands (Zito et al., 2008). This study found that 6.5% of boys in the USA were prescribed psychostimulants compared to 1.9% of girls. Much lower rates (but similar gender ratios) were observed in the Netherlands, where 2% of Dutch boys and 0.4% of Dutch girls were prescribed psychostimulants, with even lower rates seen in Germany: 1.2% in boys and 0.2% in girls. This translates to a M:F ratio of 3.4:1 in the USA, 4.8:1 in the Netherlands and 5.3:1 in Germany.

These findings overlap with studies focused on a single jurisdiction. For example, one US study examined pharmacy claims for youth under 19 years of age between 2000 and 2005, finding that 6.1% of US boys and 2.6% of US girls were prescribed ADHD medication in 2005, meaning that boys were over twice as likely to receive such medication (Castle et al., 2007). This study also found that boys ages 10–19 years had the highest rate of medication use (8% in 2005), as well as a 10% per year increase in medication usage from 2000 to 2005 in the 0–19-year-old age group. This increase in medication usage has been witnessed in later studies. For example, Zuvekas and Vitiello (2012) found a 3.4% annual growth rate in psychostimulant use for ADHD from 1996 to 2008 in the USA, with usage over 2.5 times greater (OR:2.62; 95% CI: 2.05–3.35) in boys as compared to girls. A more recent analysis of longitudinal NSCH data revealed a 7% annual increase in ADHD medication usage from 2007 to 2011 (Visser et al., 2014). Interestingly, this study found the highest medicated prevalence amongst 11-year-old boys; at 13.3% of all US boys.

4.7.3 Relative Gender Differences in Medication Usage

The previously described studies detail absolute usage of psychostimulant medication, indicating that boys are around two to three times more likely than girls to receive ADHD medication. However, boys are also around two to three times more likely to be diagnosed with ADHD, meaning that patterns of prescription might simply be reflecting differential prevalence. To account for this possibility, several studies have examined gender differences in prescription in youth already diagnosed with ADHD. For example, the aforementioned Bauermeister et al. (2007) study compared gender differences in medication usage among those with an ADHD diagnosis, finding that 9.6% of boys with ADHD had been prescribed medication, compared to 1.8% of girls with ADHD, even though the study revealed similar rates of disruptive behaviour and symptom profiles between boys and girls.

European studies have also found that boys with ADHD are more likely to be prescribed medication than girls with ADHD. For example, a German study examined the prevalence of ADHD medication use in a national sample of over 17,000 youth ages 17 years or younger (Knopf et al., 2012). This study found an overall prevalence of psychostimulant usage of 0.9% – a much lower figure than that seen in US studies. Still, this study revealed important gender differences, with 1.5% (95% CI: 1.2–1.8) of German boys prescribed psychostimulants, compared to 0.3% (95% CI: 0.2–0.5) of German girls – a M:F odds ratio of 5.2:1. This analysis revealed that German boys with ADHD were also more likely to receive medication than German girls with ADHD, with a M:F odds ratio of 1.5:1. Of note, 44% of boys using the medication had used it for 1 year or more, suggesting medium- to long-term usage. This study also found that the rate of adverse reactions in boys (13.2%) was double that of girls (7.4%).

Similar results were found from a seminal Dutch study, which used an innovative methodology to shed light on gender differences in treatment (Derks et al., 2007). In this study, ADHD symptoms, medication usage and school impairment were compared between a sample of 45 boys and 36 girls with ADHD. Moreover, both teachers and parents were asked to independently report on ADHD symptoms and related behaviours in these youth. This study found that 47% of boys with ADHD received medication compared to 6% of girls; a M:F ratio of over 7:1. Findings also revealed similar levels of school impairment in terms of repeating a grade and experiencing learning difficulties. However, the study found that mothers tended to report similar levels of aggression and attention issues in boys and girls with ADHD, while teachers consistently rated boys as having over twice the amount of attention issues and aggression than girls. As previously stated, this variation could be attributed to stereotypes and cognitive biases regarding boys and girls, with girls perceived as better behaved (the so-called halo effect), and boys perceived as more boisterous and unruly, regardless of actual circumstances (see Chap. 1).

Taken together, the research literature indicates that boys per se are significantly more likely to receive ADHD medication than girls per se. Boys with ADHD are also significantly more likely to receive medication than girls with ADHD, with the highest rates in the middle-childhood years. Of note, rates of medication usage are rising, meaning there are more and more medicated school-aged kids (especially boys) throughout western societies. Is this a good or a bad thing?

4.8 The Medicalization Hypothesis

To recap, the voluminous literature on ADHD indicates that: (i) boys have a higher prevalence of ADHD than girls; (ii) boys in general are more likely to receive ADHD medication than girls in general; and (iii) boys with ADHD are more likely to receive medication than girls with ADHD. On the one hand, some scholars have argued that these figures indicate a worryingly high rate of underdiagnosis in girls, with biases in the system negatively impacting girls, leading to a high rate of false negatives in females (e.g. Danielson et al., 2018). In other words, the fact that girls are receiving less diagnosis and medication is considered a problem by some, with concomitant admonitions to increase diagnosis and medication among girls. On the other hand, some scholars have suggested that these figures represent an overdiagnosis in boys, with biases in the system leading to a high rate of false positives, with some even suggesting that ADHD is not a valid construct, and instead simply the relabelling of boisterous and spirited behaviour, especially in boys. This critique centres on the sociological concept of *medicalization*, which is described and analysed below, particularly in relation to ADHD in boys. In a classic work, Conrad states that:

> medicalization describes a process by which nonmedical problems become defined and treated as medical problems, usually in terms of illnesses and disorders. This involves adopting medical language and a medical framework to redefine a problem, while proposing medical (frequently pharmaceutical) interventions to solve the redefined problem (Conrad, 1992)

The medicalization literature points to several examples of conditions that have allegedly been medicalized to buttress their arguments. One strand involves an analysis of medical history, revealing numerous 'deviant' behaviours such as masturbation and homosexuality, which were once considered medical issues and were subject to medical intervention down the ages, but are no longer treated as medical conditions (Engelhardt, 1974). Another strand points to numerous issues and problems that have allegedly been medicalized in recent years including cosmetic issues such as baldness and wrinkles, normative developmental issues such as pregnancy and childbirth, and 'deviant' behavioural issues such as gambling and Internet-gaming usage.

Indeed, numerous scholars have argued that an increasing number of psychiatric disorders are not real illnesses, but simply deviations from social, moral or statistical norms. Put another way, it is argued that some psychiatric illnesses involve the medicalization of everyday life problems. In this argument, critics point to the expanding nature of the DSM, which was first published in 1952, and is currently on its fifth revision. Importantly, each revision includes more and more diagnoses with broader diagnostic criteria. In fact, the current DSM-5 is just under 1000 pages, considerably larger than previous versions (Carlat, 2010; Frances, 2014). This means that a wider diagnostic net is cast with each revision, meaning that more and more people are labelled as mentally ill. Of note, psychiatrists meet and discuss new diagnostic criteria as well as potential new diagnoses before each revision, which involves drawing a somewhat arbitrary threshold between normative and pathological behaviours. Some have argued that psychiatrists are drawing this threshold too low, and are overly keen to label normative behaviours as pathological (Conrad, 2007; Horwitz & Wakefield, 2007). For example, it has been argued that the DSM-5 diagnosis of 'social phobia' involves the medicalization of everyday shyness and introversion (Scott, 2006), while others argue that mild or moderate 'depression' involves the medicalization of everyday sadness and unhappiness (Dowrick & Frances, 2013).

Of primary relevance to this chapter, there has been much debate about medicalization in relation to ADHD. Indeed, some have argued that the ADHD construct involves the 'medicalization of misbehaviour' (Searight & McLaren, 1998), the 'medicalization of underperformance' (Conrad & Potter, 2000) or quite simply 'the medicalization of childhood' (Timimi, 2002). Such concerns are propelled by a variety of factors including:

(i) Evidence that boisterous and spirited behaviour is part of the normal spectrum of behaviour in children and adolescents (especially in boys), but that this has been erroneously pathologized and relabelled as a mental illness.
(ii) Worries that the ADHD construct and diagnostic criteria are ambiguous and overly expansive; meaning considerable overdiagnosis and a large number of false positives caught in an ever-broadening psychiatric net.
(iii) Observations that various interest groups stand to directly benefit from the relabelling and reconceptualizing of 'problem behaviours' as ADHD including

the psychiatric industry, 'Big Pharma', overwhelmed mothers and frustrated teachers all of whom are discussed in detail later in this chapter.

Of note, Conrad (1992) states 'gender is an important factor in understanding medicalization' and may be particularly important in understanding ADHD. Indeed, other scholars have directly argued that the ADHD diagnosis unfairly targets overly energetic boys – who are considered a deviant threat to the harmony and order within modern families and educational institutions (e.g. Sommers, 2015; Sax, 2016). In this argument, it is stated that schools have become particularly unfriendly to boys (see Chap. 7) with statistics indicating a decline in recess time, physical education and gym class, as well as greater intolerance for rough-and-tumble play and similar boy-friendly activities. In the words of Sax (2016), this means that 'boys doing things that boys have always done now gets boys into trouble', and can contribute to an ADHD diagnosis and consequent medication. This would be concerning, given that much research indicates that boys in general are naturally energetic, and that such energy may be evolutionarily adaptive, as it can increase individual fitness by contributing to success in vital energy-intensive activities such as hunting, farming and fishing (Hartmann, 1993).

Indeed, it is common knowledge that humans are sexually dimorphic from conception, meaning that males and females have a differential distribution of sex steroids (e.g. testosterone), lean mass and muscular strength (Wells, 2007; Peper et al., 2009; Jacklin et al., 1984). All this contributes to the well-researched finding that males tend to have more total energy expenditure than females during childhood and adolescence (Ball et al., 2001; Goran et al., 1998). Does this mean we are wrongly singling out overly energetic boys and relabelling them as mentally ill? And is the problem more situated in the schools, which may have become unfriendly to boys, rather than in the mind (or brains) of children diagnosed with ADHD? And who profits from the increasing rate of both ADHD diagnosis and medication usage?

Answering these questions demands a detailed sociological analysis of possible motives for such alleged medicalization. Indeed, it should be noted that medicalization is typically a process of collective action, involving the inter-connected and inter-twining activities of various interest groups, some of whom stand to directly benefit from the relabelling and reconceptualizing of problem behaviours as a mental illness. The sociological literature indicates that five enthusiastic parties may be colluding together to contribute towards a process of medicalization vis-à-vis ADHD, namely: (i) an expansionist psychiatric industry; (ii) profit-driven 'Big Pharma'; (iii) overwhelmed mothers; (iv) frustrated teachers and educationalists; and (v) some affected youth. These five factors are discussed in turn below, in the context of wider social changes regarding educational practice and the family, concluding with a discussion of social control of so-called deviant behaviour, which typically underpins any process of medicalization.

4.8.1 The Psychiatric Industry

In his seminal book entitled *Medical Nemesis*, Ivan Illich (1976) noted that medicine is an industry, and like all industries it is constantly looking to expand into new markets. Similarly, Illich argues that professionals within the medical industry are constantly looking for new roles in order to ensure regular clientele and continuity of employment. On the one hand, this could be considered a humane attempt to serve an already suffering population. On the other hand, it could be considered an expansionist effort to deepen the reservoir of potential clients. What evidence can be marshalled in support of the latter argument?

It has been noted that psychiatrists and psychiatric guild associations such as the American Psychiatric Association (APA) are some of the most enthusiastic proponents of the ADHD construct (Breggin, 2001). In fact, each new revision of the APA's DSM adds new diagnosis and more expansive diagnostic criteria for existing disorders such as ADHD (see Sect. 4.1). In other words, DSM casts a diagnostic net, and this net is capturing more and more people, with research indicating a 50% increase in the prevalence of mental illness after the transition from DSM-III to DSM-III-R, with a similar increase in prevalence of mental illness in the transition from DSM-III to DSM-IV (Newcorn et al., 1989). This means millions of people are transformed overnight from mentally healthy individuals to potential patients in need of treatment, thus increasing overall demand for psychiatric services.

With regard to ADHD, it has been argued that the relabelling of academic underperformance or boisterous misbehaviour as a mental illness brings a never-ending stream of potential patients (or customers) to mental health services, ensuring growth, expansion and employment within the psychiatric industry (Conrad, 1992). Some have argued that this process is facilitated by the official ADHD symptom lists, which some say are ambiguous, malleable and imprecise. For example, it has been noted that the ADHD symptom list involves much subjective interpretation by the diagnosing clinician, as commonly appearing words such as 'often', or specific symptoms such as 'does not seem to listen' are not precisely operationalized (Searight & McLaren, 1998). Just how frequent is 'often'? How can 'does not seem to listen' be validly assessed? Such arguments are sometimes taken even further, noting that this ambiguity may serve a functional purpose, as it ensures that more people are ensnared in the diagnostic net, leading to more business and a growing clientele for the psychiatric profession.

Relatedly, it has been noted (correctly) that the boundaries and symptom lists for ADHD have expanded to include more and more people. This can be witnessed in the addition of adult ADHD to recent versions of DSM. Of note, until the mid-1990s it was widely believed that ADHD symptoms remitted during the transition to adulthood. In other words, ADHD was historically considered a disorder of middle childhood and adolescence. Indeed, the first three versions of the DSM restricted diagnosis of ADHD to children and adolescents, and DSM-II labelled the disorder 'hyperkinetic reaction of childhood'. In 1994, DSM-IV broke with this restriction to allow ADHD to be diagnosed in adults, transforming the disorder from a childhood-specific disorder to one that can affect anyone at any time. DSM-5 led to a further consolidation of this position, with the previously child-centric symptom criteria rewritten to include examples appropriate to adults (e.g. forgetting to pay bills, fails to finish duties in the workplace, etc.).

Similarly, the age of onset criteria was increased to 12 years in DSM-5 (from 7 years in DSM-IV), meaning more people become eligible for a diagnosis. On the one hand, this could be considered a humane research-driven initiative enabling the identification and treatment of adults suffering from a debilitating mental illness. On the other hand, this could be considered a widening of the psychiatric net that is wrongly labelling a psychosocial issue as a psychiatric issue in need of medical treatment and psychiatric medication.

Whichever view is taken, an indubitable fact is that ADHD is big business for the psychiatric profession. Figures from 2013 indicate that US healthcare expenditure for ADHD totalled $23 billion (Dieleman et al., 2016), while figures from the US National Ambulatory Medical Care Survey indicate that there were 13.6 million visits to healthcare providers in 2016 for ADHD-related issues. Of note, boys had around double the rate of visits compared to girls.

4.8.2 Big Pharma

It has been argued that medicalization of a psychosocial issue typically brings concomitant 'pharmaceuticalization', meaning that medication is quickly produced, marketed and used for any medicalized issue (Breggin, 1994). Indeed, British psychiatrist Sami Timimi (Timimi & Taylor, 2004) states that 'ADHD has generated huge profits for the pharmaceutical industry against a background of poor-quality research, publication bias and payments to some of the top academics in this field' (p. 8). In other words, it has been argued that the pharmaceutical industry (sometimes known as 'Big Pharma') has a vested interest in the medicalization of non-medical problems, as this leads to much bigger markets and much larger profits.

While market data on profits are difficult to come by, one market research report noted that the global ADHD medication market was estimated at almost $4 billion in 2010, also predicting an 8% growth in subsequent years (Conrad & Bergey, 2014). This overlaps with a large corpus of research indicating a massive increase in the use of psychostimulants. For example, the 1990s saw an eightfold increase in the use of psychostimulants in the USA (Conrad & Potter, 2000; Zametkin & Ernst, 1999). More recent data examining change from 1993 to 2003 found a threefold increase in ADHD medication use across the world, and a ninefold increase in global spending (Scheffler et al., 2007).

Some recent research indicates a large rise in medication usage in demographic groups that have typically been left untreated with medication. For example, several studies indicate a large rise in ADHD medication usage in children ages 2–5 years: a relatively new yet expanding market for the pharmaceutical companies. One study of insurance claims data shows an increase in children ages 2–5 years receiving clinical care (Visser et al., 2016). Danielson et al. (2017) document a 57% increase (from 1% to 1.57%) in diagnosed ADHD from 2007–2008 to 2011–2012 in 2–5-year-olds. Similarly, Danielson et al. (2018) found that approximately 61,000 children ages 2–5 years were taking ADHD medication in a study of NCSH data. This is somewhat concerning as safety and efficacy in such young children has not been sufficiently researched, and diagnostic validity in this age group is questionable. In fact, some have argued that regular use of psychostimulants in young children may have negative long-term effects on the developing brain, again raising questions about suitability and safety (Sax, 2016; Breggin, 1999; Diller, 1999).

In short, the ADHD construct is expanding from a problem of school-age children to a problem of adults as well as a problem of infants. This expansion in both directions has led to a subtle yet important reconceptualization of ADHD as a lifespan condition that can affect anyone from cradle to grave. Conrad and Potter (2000) note that 'by redefining ADHD as a lifetime disorder, the potential exists for keeping children and adults on medication indefinitely' (p. 568). In other words, the diagnostic expansion of ADHD in both directions (i.e. to older and younger people) opens up new markets for the pharmaceutical companies, and helps ensure healthy profits.

Pharmaceutical expansion has also occurred geographically. For example, evidence suggests that ADHD medication usage is increasing its penetration into jurisdictions that have previously been small markets such as France, Brazil and Germany, partly due to intense marketing efforts by pharmaceutical companies (Conrad & Bergey, 2014; Hinshaw et al., 2011). In fact, research indicates a tenfold increase in psychostimulant prescriptions in Germany between 1998 and 2008 (Conrad & Bergey, 2014). Again, such trends could be considered a humane response to a debilitating disorder. Alternatively, such trends could be considered a cynical ploy by profit-hungry 'Big Pharma' to expand their markets.

4.8.3 Mothers and Medicalization

As stated, an essential element of the medicalization thesis is that the concept of ADHD is simply the relabelling of problem behaviour in school-age children, especially boisterous boys. Indeed, one qualitative study found that some British teachers had a strong antipathy towards medicalizing behavioural problems in children, with teachers making remarks such as 'ADHD is just a label to excuse bad behaviour' (Malacrida, 2004). Traditionally, such 'bad behaviour' was blamed on faulty parenting, typically faulty mothering. Indeed, across human societies, mothers have taken much of the blame (or the credit) for their children's behaviours and educational performance. Such blame for their children's bad behaviour can incur psychosocial costs among mothers, including self-stigma and public stigma in the local community.

Given this situation, it has been argued that mothers have been instrumental in the development, consolidation and perpetuation of the ADHD concept – precisely

4.8 The Medicalization Hypothesis

because this conceptualization can help absolve them of blame for a child's problem behaviours and underperformance at school. In this argument, the ADHD concept provides an exculpatory framework, levelling the blame for problem behaviours on a 'chemical imbalance' or 'brain dysfunction', rather than on incompetent or ineffective mothering.

Indeed, this is one of the principal findings of a seminal qualitative study of American mothers of young boys who had been given an ADHD diagnosis (Singh, 2004). A key finding from this study was that mothers eagerly and enthusiastically bought into the 'brain disease' narrative of problem behaviours, as exemplified by one mother emblematically noting 'it's not his problem, it's his brain's problem' – a sentiment appearing commonly throughout this qualitative dataset.

In addition to providing a conveniently exculpatory framework, this study found that mothers of boys with ADHD self-reported a number of their own psychological issues, which manifested themselves in various dysfunctional behaviours related to anger management and self-control. For example, one mother in this study noted that 'the smallest thing would make me upset and…make me start screaming uncontrollably. I'd shut the door to my room and go bang on something', while another mother noted that 'It made me nuts! I wanted to shake him and hug him and cry all at the same time. I was so frustrated, so upset and angry'. Such perspectives were commonly expressed throughout the dataset with another mother stating that 'I was really starting to dread spending time with him because it was so difficult. It was so hard…'. All this data led Singh to state that 'some mothers began to feel that they hated their sons', suggesting that a contributing problem in some cases may be psychological issues with the mother, rather than psychological issues with the child. This led Singh to ask the rhetorical question 'who benefits more from Ritalin treatment, the child or the mother?' That question has not yet been sufficiently answered by subsequent research, but the core findings from this paper imply that some mothers eagerly buy into the narrative that ADHD is a brain disease in need of psychotropic medication for a variety of functional self-interested reasons.

Of note, Singh (2004) also states that mothers make up the vast majority of parental support, advocacy and educational groups devoted to ADHD, with fathers largely absent from such groups (Singh, 2003). These groups have been instrumental in promoting the acceptance and legitimization of ADHD as an illness category. Importantly, these advocacy and patient groups have received considerable funding from pharmaceutical companies such as Novartis and Ritalin, who have also produced 'educational' materials to spread awareness of ADHD in both traditional and emerging markets (Maturo, 2013). For example, an educational leaflet from Novartis South Africa (n.d.) states that:

> It is important for parents to understand that ADHD is a condition of the brain that makes it difficult for their child to control his or her behaviour. It is not them being a 'bad child' or because of something the parent has done.

The medicalization thesis argues that both pharmaceutical companies and parental advocacy organizations are complicit in pushing the narrative that problem behaviours in children are due to brain chemistry rather than incompetent parenting.

Both have much to gain from societal acceptance of this narrative. In the case of pharmaceutical companies, problems in brain chemistry imply a chemical solution – which means considerably more markets (and profits) for psychotropic medication. In the case of parents (and particularly mothers), problems in brain chemistry shift the blame from problems in parenting, leading to sympathy and empathy rather than opprobrium and reproach. In other words, medicalization is a win-win situation for both mothers as well as pharmaceutical companies.

The literature reviewed earlier indicates that some mothers have difficulty coping with their sons' boisterous behaviour and masculine energy. Given this situation, it could be that some mothers administer psychostimulant medication to their male children to take the edge off this masculine energy. This may be especially so amongst single mother households where the traditional check on a son's boisterous energy (the father) is absent (see Chap. 9). As such, issues of traditional discipline (or lack thereof) and social control may be implicated in maternal behaviour regarding ADHD medication – issues discussed in further detail in Sect. 4.9.

4.8.4 Schools and Education

ADHD has typically been framed as an issue of school-aged children, and several studies indicate that children's problems began or escalated when they entered the school system (Malacrida, 2004). This is further evidenced by the diagnostic criteria of ADHD, which make frequent reference to deficiencies in school performance. This has led some researchers to posit that the educational system plays a key role in the medicalization process, especially as applied to boisterous boys. This has been related to various factors, including macro-level societal changes regarding the disciplining of youth, as well as meso-level changes in common practices in school (Sax, 2016; Zimbardo & Coulombe, 2016).

For example, western societies have become increasingly averse to traditional forms of discipline within families, schools and the judicial system. This is evidenced by widespread prohibitions on corporal punishment within schools and the judicial system, and sometimes even within families in some Scandinavian countries. In the school setting, many educational systems also have a decreased acceptance of other forms of traditional discipline such as suspension and expulsion (see Chap. 7). This means teachers are faced with fewer options when faced with energetic and boisterous pupils, most of whom are boys. Similarly, fathers are typically the disciplinarian of boys within families; however, many young boys across the world are being raised by single mothers, meaning that they may lack traditional male discipline and moral guidance within the home (see Chap. 9).

These two social trends can intertwine, as boys may be coming to school from a home where discipline is lacking, meaning that boisterous behaviour may be the norm for these children. Then at school, teachers may lack the traditional tools to discipline these children, leaving teachers exacerbated and overwhelmed. This may be especially intense in modern American schools, which may be making developmentally inappropriate demands on boys through an early focus on academics, while constraining energy-intensive activities such as physical education, recess and rough-and-tumble play (Sax, 2016; Sommers, 2015). All this means that a diagnosis of ADHD in unruly children may be particularly convenient for teachers, and that concomitant use of psychostimulants (which typically have a calming effect) allows teachers to better control the classroom. In other words, the rise in ADHD diagnosis and medication usage facilitates class order, which may be particularly important given that many scholars have argued that schools have become unfriendly to boys through harsh regulations, inappropriate curricula, and lack of outlets for male energy; all leading to frustrated, irritable or inattentive boys.

This theory is supported by some evidence. For example, Malacrida (2004) found that Canadian teachers played a key role in identifying and labelling pupils with ADHD, despite their lack of qualifications to diagnose mental illness and formulate treatment plans. Indeed, teachers in this study frequently suggested to mothers that ADHD was a likely explanation for disruptive behaviour in the classroom, with teachers further suggesting medication as a viable and effective treatment. Put another way, this study found that teachers actively promoted use of the ADHD construct and associated medication. Such concern may have come from a desire to placate disruptive children and make their classes easier to manage. These findings overlap with results from another study, which found that teachers and school personnel were the first to suggest a diagnosis of ADHD in over 50% of potential cases, followed by parents in 30% of potential cases, and primary care physicians in 11% of potential cases (Sax & Kautz, 2003). In other words, teachers were most enthusiastic about labelling a child as having ADHD.

Relatedly, some research indicates that teachers (who are overwhelmingly female: see Chap. 7) tend to stereotype boys and girls in their classrooms, which can play a role in any hypothesized medicalization of (mis)behaviours. As stated in Chap. 1, some evidence suggests a *halo effect* for girls at school, with teachers minimizing or overlooking disruptive behaviours in girls, while overly attending to disruptive behaviours in boys. In practice, this means that girls are frequently perceived to be more benign and harmless, while boys are perceived to be more disruptive and unruly, regardless of actual behaviours on the ground.

For example, Bauermeister et al. (2007) found that boys with ADHD were more likely than girls with ADHD to be suspended from school, perhaps indicating the aforementioned *halo effect* for girls with ADHD. Similarly, several studies find that teachers routinely report that boys with ADHD are more disruptive and impaired than girls with ADHD, but mothers routinely report that boys and girls have similar levels of impairment and disruptive behaviours (Gaub & Carlson, 1997; Gershon, 2002). Indeed, Hartung et al. (2002) averaged teacher and mother reports of disruptive behaviours and impairment in a sample of US elementary school children diagnosed with ADHD, comparing averages between boys and girls. When averaged, mothers reported no significant difference between boys and girls, while teachers reported that boys had almost twice the level of disruptive behaviours compared to girls. This begs the question: who is right and who is wrong in their assessment – the teachers or the mothers? It could be that teachers perceive girls to be less disruptive due to the *halo effect*, while perceiving boys to be more disruptive due to the negative stereotypes of males discussed in Chap. 1.

To end this section of the chapter, it is worth tying together a few strands from the previous sections. It has been mentioned that both the pharmaceutical and psychiatric industries benefit from the ADHD construct in multifarious ways. In this chapter, it has been argued that teachers also benefit from the construct. However, there are another group of people who benefit from the ADHD construct, and this includes special educators, educational psychologists and associated support staff. In fact, the ADHD construct has spawned a whole sub-industry comprising of individuals whose jobs depend on the framing of boisterous behaviour and underperformance as a medical illness. Everybody working in this sub-industry benefits from this framing, as do teachers at the primary and secondary level. In other words, teachers, educationalists and allied professionals may all have contributed to any medicalization associated with ADHD.

4.8.5 People with an ADHD Diagnosis

Several scholars have argued that the medicalization of a trait or behaviour can bring a series of benefits to the group being medicalized. For example, Conrad and Potter (2000) note that 'a diagnosis of ADHD puts an individual into the larger category of having a 'disability', which can serve as a gateway to potential claims to certain benefits and accommodations' (p. 574). Under legislation such as the Americans with Disabilities Act, a diagnosis of mental illness gives the right to reasonable accommodations in the workplace and other settings. Adults with ADHD may also receive disability benefits, which can be a source of financial security.

In the educational context, possession of an ADHD diagnosis can lead to the receipt of special services as well as special accommodations for tests and exams, which may be particularly important in secondary and tertiary education. Reflecting on the weighty ADHD literature, Maturo (2013) notes that 'in competitive US universities, strategic use of ADHD diagnosis can be witnessed: students use psychostimulants in order to improve their academic performance, …there are students who strategically get themselves diagnosed, by exaggerating their symptoms' (pp. 175–183). In other words, psychostimulant medication can help improve academic performance, and give students a competitive advantage over other students.

Another potential benefit relates to what has been called 'medical excusing' (Halleck, 1971) or 'the dislocation of responsibility' (Conrad, 1992). This refers to the typical shift in culpability that comes from framing a behaviour or trait as an illness rather than a characterological issue. This controversial argument implies that people with ADHD and associated advocacy organizations (often funded by pharmaceutical companies) collude together in promoting the medicalization of the set of behaviours associated with ADHD, as this gives the individuals diagnosed a series of functional and social advantages. Such advantages would be absent if this set of behaviours were framed as a characterological flaw or a lack of self-discipline.

Of note, this argument regarding self-interest has mainly been applied to tertiary students or adults with ADHD. School-aged children rarely self-present when faced with ADHD symptoms, and are not typically involved in ADHD advocacy organizations. On the contrary, they may resist the labelling (and associated stigma) that comes with an ADHD diagnosis, and may be less than willing to participate in the whole ADHD infrastructure (Ringer, 2020).

4.9 Social Control

A theme running through many of the previously described factors underpinning the process of medicalization is *social control*. Sociologists have long argued that for a society to function, there must be shared moral frameworks, with concomitant social control and disciplinary mechanisms for 'deviants' who transgress moral boundaries (Foucault, 1975; Durkheim, 1984). Historically, religion provided a moral framework, delineating acceptable and unacceptable behaviours through concepts such as 'sin', 'evil' and 'immorality'. In religious countries such as Ireland, there were strict laws and social conventions about behaviours that contravened Roman Catholic precepts such as abortion, homosexuality, divorce, contraception and extramarital sex. This has led many scholars to conclude that religion is an instrument of *social control,* especially of so-called deviant behaviours. Another instrument of social control has traditionally been the nuclear family. More specifically, the father typically acted as head of household, setting out behavioural boundaries for his children and meting out the appropriate discipline when such boundaries were violated (Mansfield, 2006).

Importantly, a large corpus of research indicates the decline of religion and the decline of nuclear families in western societies. For example, rates of attendance at places of worship have dropped precipitously, as have rates of belief in God per se (Pew Research Center, 2015, 2019). Similarly, divorce rates have increased dramatically, reaching around 40% in countries such as Canada, the UK and the USA (Ghosh, 2019; Statistics Canada, 2020; CDC, 2020b). Importantly, mothers typically win custody of children after a divorce (see Chap. 9), with Canadian figures indicating that the mother wins primary custody in over 80% of contested cases (Department of Justice Canada, 2000). This means that more and more children are growing up without the influence of religion or a father, meaning they lack two of the traditional instruments of social control.

Some sociologists have argued that the decline of religion and the nuclear family has left a moral vacuum, which has been filled by medicine. In this argument, medicine (specifically psychiatry) has become an instrument of social control by demarcating acceptable (or normative) and unacceptable (or pathological) behaviours. This has shaped wider social perspectives, meaning that psychiatry can effortlessly engage in the surveillance and intervention of 'deviants' who engage in unacceptable/pathological behaviour, with public support for this endeavour (Zola, 1972; Conrad, 1992). Indeed, Timimi and Taylor (2004) alleges that their fellow psychiatrists are often 'acting as agents of social control and stifling diversity in children, we are victimising millions of children...by putting them on highly addictive drugs that have no proven long-term benefit' (p. 8). This is consistent with the views of Thomas Szasz (2006), another psychiatrist who has critiqued the expansionist nature of psychiatry, with Szasz wryly stating that 'psychiatry is a branch of the law, not a branch of medicine'.

In this argument, psychiatrists become a source of moral authority, and take over the disciplinary functions that were once the purview of priests, fathers and other local pillars of the moral order. Instead of social control through religiously inspired moral frameworks and disciplinary action, psychiatry could be said to exert social control vis-à-vis ADHD by three different steps. First, it draws a line between normative and pathological behaviour, categorizing boisterous and spirited children as mentally ill. Second, it engages in medical surveillance to identify those on the wrong side of the line, aided and abetted by teachers and mothers frustrated by children's behaviour. Third, action is taken through dispensing psychostimulant medication, which controls and reigns in the problem behaviours, particularly among boys, who make up the bulk of ADHD patients. The argument that ADHD involves the *medicalization of boyhood* is controversial; however, it must be seriously considered given the accumulating evidence.

4.10 Conclusion

ADHD can be perceived in two distinct ways. On the one hand, it can be perceived as a legitimate brain disease causing severe psychosocial impairment, particularly in school-aged boys, which can be treated by effective psychostimulant medication. This framing is typically favoured by powerful stakeholders, including the psychiatric industry and the pharmaceutical industry, who incidentally profit from such an explanation in a variety of ways. It can also be a preferred explanation of mothers, as this argument absolves them of blame and responsibility, and by teachers whose lives may be made easier by having medicated children in the classroom.

On the other hand, ADHD can be perceived as a fictional man-made category, involving the medicalization of a set of normative behaviours that have been relabelled as pathological. This has been called the 'medicalization of misbehaviour' (Searight & McLaren, 1998), the 'medicalization of underperformance' (Conrad & Potter, 2000), or 'the medicalization of childhood' (Timimi, 2002). The present chapter has entertained the possibility that this may represent 'the medicalization of boyhood'. Such medicalization can lead to the targeting of boisterous and spirited boys in particular, leading to treatment with powerful mind-altering psychostimulant medication, which can help to control and reign in any disruptive behaviour. As stated, such processes could be related to wider social trends, including the rise of single-mother households, a decline in religion, and changes in the nature and delivery of education.

Many arguments around ADHD in boys are controversial, and discussions about this matter will undoubtedly continue in the progress of time. But one thing is for sure. More and more boys are being given an ADHD diagnosis, and more and more boys are receiving psychostimulant medication. Whether this is a positive or negative phenomenon is still a matter of debate.

References

Abikoff, H. B., Jensen, P. S., Arnold, L. E., Hoza, B., Hechtman, L., Pollack, S., Martin, D., Alvir, J., March, J. S., Hinshaw, S., Vitiello, B., Newcorn, J., Greiner, A., Cantwell, D. P., Conners, C. K., Elliott, G., Greenhill, L. L., Kraemer, H., Pelham, W. E., Jr., … Wigal, T. (2002). Observed classroom behavior of children with ADHD: Relationship to gender and comorbidity. *Journal of Abnormal Child Psychology, 30*(4), 349–359. https://doi.org/10.1023/A:1015713807297

Acosta, M. T., Castellanos, F. X., Bolton, K. L., Balog, J. Z., Eagen, P., Nee, L., Jones, J., Palacio, L., Sarampote, C., Russell, H. F., Berg, K., Arcos-Burgos, M., & Muenke, M. (2008). Latent class subtyping of attention-deficit/hyperactivity disorder and comorbid conditions. *Journal of the American Academy of Child & Adolescent Psychiatry, 47*(7), 797–807. https://doi.org/10.1097/CHI.0b013e318173f70b

Agnew-Blais, J. C., Polanczyk, G. V., Danese, A., Wertz, J., Moffitt, T. E., & Arseneault, L. (2016). Evaluation of the persistence, remission, and emergence of attention-deficit/hyperactivity disorder in young adulthood. *JAMA Psychiatry, 73*(7), 713–720. https://doi.org/10.1001/jamapsychiatry.2016.0465

American Academy of Child and Adolescent Psychiatry. (2007). Practice parameter for the assessment and treatment of children and adolescents with attention-deficit/hyperactivity disorder. *Journal of the American Academy of Child & Adolescent Psychiatry, 46*(7), 894–921. https://doi.org/10.1097/chi.0b013e318054e724

American Academy of Pediatrics' Subcommittee on Attention-Deficit/Hyperactivity Disorder, Steering Committee on Quality Improvement and Management. (2019). ADHD: Clinical practice guideline for the diagnosis, evaluation, and treatment of attention-deficit/hyperactivity disorder in children and adolescents. *Pediatrics, 144*(4), e20192528. https://doi.org/10.1542/peds.2019-2528

American Psychiatric Association (APA). (2013). Substance-related and addictive disorders. In *Diagnostic and statistical manual of mental disorders* (5th ed.). American Psychiatric Association.

Andersen, C. H., Thomsen, P. H., Nohr, E. A., & Lemcke, S. (2018). Maternal body mass index before pregnancy as a risk factor for ADHD and autism in children. *European Child & Adolescent Psychiatry, 27*(2), 139–148. https://doi.org/10.1007/s00787-017-1027-6

Ball, E. J., O'Connor, J., Abbott, R., Steinbeck, K. S., Davies, P. S., Wishart, C., Gaskin, K. J., & Baur, L. A. (2001). Total energy expenditure, body fatness, and physical activity in children aged 6–9 y. *The American Journal of Clinical Nutrition, 74*(4), 524–528. https://doi.org/10.1093/ajcn/74.4.524

Barbaresi, W. J., Colligan, R. C., Weaver, A. L., Voigt, R. G., Killian, J. M., & Katusic, S. K. (2013). Mortality, ADHD, and psychosocial adversity in adults with childhood ADHD: A prospective study. *Pediatrics, 131*(4), 637–644. https://doi.org/10.1542/peds.2012-2354

Bauermeister, J. J., Shrout, P. E., Chávez, L., Rubio-Stipec, M., Ramírez, R., Padilla, L., Anderson, A., García, P., & Canino, G. (2007). ADHD and gender: Are risks and sequela of ADHD the same for boys and girls? *Journal of Child Psychology and Psychiatry, 48*(8), 831–839. https://doi.org/10.1111/j.1469-7610.2007.01750.x

Berman, S., Kuczenski, R., McCracken, J., & London, E. D. (2009). Potential adverse effects of amphetamine treatment on brain and behavior: A review. *Molecular Psychiatry, 14*, 123–142. https://doi.org/10.1038/mp.2008.90

Biederman, J., Faraone, S. V., Monuteaux, M. C., Bober, M., & Cadogen, E. (2004). Gender effects on attention-deficit/hyperactivity disorder in adults, revisited. *Biological Psychiatry, 55*(7), 692–700. https://doi.org/10.1016/j.biopsych.2003.12.003

Biederman, J., Kwon, A., Aleardi, M., Chouinard, V.-A., Marino, T., Cole, H., Mick, E., & Faraone, S. V. (2005). Absence of gender effects on attention deficit hyperactivity disorder: Findings in nonreferred subjects. *The American Journal of Psychiatry, 162*(6), 1083–1089. https://doi.org/10.1176/appi.ajp.162.6.1083

Biederman, J., Monuteaux, M. C., Mick, E., Spencer, T., Wilens, T. E., Silva, J. M., Synder, L. E., & Faraone, S. V. (2006). Young adult outcome of attention deficit hyperactivity disorder: A controlled 10-year follow-up study. *Psychological Medicine, 36*(2), 167–179. https://doi.org/10.1017/S0033291705006410

Bravo, M., Ribera, J., Rubio-Stipec, M., Canino, G., Shrout, P., Ramírez, R., Fábregas, L., Chavez, L., Alegría, M., Bauermeister, J. J., & Martínez Taboas, A. (2001). Test-retest reliability of the Spanish version of the Diagnostic Interview Schedule for Children (DISC-IV). *Journal of Abnormal Child Psychology, 29*(5), 433–444. https://doi.org/10.1023/A:1010499520090

Breggin, P. R. (1994). *Toxic psychiatry: Why therapy, empathy and love must replace the drugs, electroshock, and biochemical theories of the "new psychiatry"*. Macmillan.

Breggin, P. R. (1999). Psychostimulants in the treatment of children diagnosed with ADHD: Risks and mechanism of action. *International Journal of Risk & Safety in Medicine, 12*(1), 3–35.

Breggin, P. R. (2001). *Talking back to Ritalin: What doctors aren't telling you about stimulants and ADHD*. Da Capo Press.

Caci, H., Doepfner, M., Asherson, P., Donfrancesco, R., Faraone, S. V., Hervas, A., & Fitzgerald, M. (2014). Daily life impairments associated with self-reported childhood/adolescent attention-deficit/hyperactivity disorder and experiences of diagnosis and treatment: Results from the European Lifetime Impairment Survey. *European Psychiatry, 29*(5), 316–323. https://doi.org/10.1016/j.eurpsy.2013.10.007

Cantwell, D. P. (1996). Attention deficit disorder: A review of the past 10 years. *Journal of the American Academy of Child & Adolescent Psychiatry, 35*(8), 978–987. https://doi.org/10.1097/00004583-199608000-00008

Carlat, D. J. (2010). *Unhinged: The trouble with psychiatry-A doctor's revelations about a profession in crisis*. Free Press.

Cascade, E., Kalali, A. H., & Wigal, S. B. (2010). Real-world data on: Attention deficit hyperactivity disorder medication side effects. *Psychiatry (Edgmont (Pa Township)), 7*(4), 13–15.

Castle, L., Aubert, R. E., Verbrugge, R. R., Khalid, M., & Epstein, R. S. (2007). Trends in medication treatment for ADHD. *Journal of Attention Disorders, 10*(4), 335–342. https://doi.org/10.1177/1087054707299597

Centers for Disease Control and Prevention (CDC). (2019). *Health conditions among children under age 18, by selected characteristics: United States, average annual, selected years 1997–1999 through 2015–2017*. Centers for Disease Control and Prevention (CDC). Retrieved November 23, 2020, from https://www.cdc.gov/nchs/data/hus/2018/012.pdf

Centers for Disease Control and Prevention (CDC). (2020a, September 21). *Treatment of ADHD*. Centers for Disease Control and Prevention (CDC). Retrieved November 23, 2020, from https://www.cdc.gov/ncbddd/adhd/treatment.html

Centers for Disease Control and Prevention (CDC). (2020b). *Marriage and divorce*. Centers for Disease Control and Prevention (CDC). Retrieved November 23 2020, from https://www.cdc.gov/nchs/products/nvsr.htm

Chen, Q., Sjölander, A., Långström, N., Rodriguez, A., Serlachius, E., D'Onofrio, B. M., Lichtenstein, P., & Larsson, H. (2014). Maternal pre-pregnancy body mass index and offspring attention deficit hyperactivity disorder: A population-based cohort study using a sibling-comparison design. *International Journal of Epidemiology, 43*(1), 83–90. https://doi.org/10.1093/ije/dyt152

Conrad, P. (1992). Medicalization and social control. *Annual Review of Sociology, 18*, 209–232. https://doi.org/10.1146/annurev.so.18.080192.001233

Conrad, P. (2007). *The medicalization of society: On the transformation of human conditions into treatable disorders*. Johns Hopkins University Press.

Conrad, P., & Bergey, M. R. (2014). The impending globalization of ADHD: Notes on the expansion and growth of a medicalized disorder. *Social Science & Medicine (1982), 122*, 31–43. https://doi.org/10.1016/j.socscimed.2014.10.019

Conrad, P., & Potter, D. (2000). From hyperactive children to ADHD adults: Observations on the expansion of medical categories. *Social Problems, 47*(4), 559–582. https://doi.org/10.2307/3097135

Cortese, S., Adamo, N., Del Giovane, C., Mohr-Jensen, C., Hayes, A. J., Carucci, S., Atkinson, L. Z., Tessari, L., Banaschewski, T., Coghill, D., Hollis, C., Simonoff, E., Zuddas, A., Barbui, C., Purgato, M., Steinhausen, H.-C., Shokraneh, F., Xia, J., & Cipriani, A. (2018). Comparative efficacy and tolerability of medications for attention-deficit hyperactivity disorder in children, adolescents, and adults: A systematic review and network meta-analysis. *The Lancet Psychiatry, 5*(9), 727–738. https://doi.org/10.1016/S2215-0366(18)30269-4

Cuffe, S. P., Moore, C. G., & McKeown, R. E. (2005). Prevalence and correlates of ADHD symptoms in the national health interview survey. *Journal of Attention Disorders, 9*(2), 392–401. https://doi.org/10.1177/1087054705280413

Dalsgaard, S. (2013). Attention-deficit/hyperactivity disorder (ADHD). *European Child & Adolescent Psychiatry, 22*, 43–48. https://doi.org/10.1007/s00787-012-0360-z

Danielson, M. L., Visser, S. N., Gleason, M. M., Peacock, G., Claussen, A. H., & Blumberg, S. J. (2017). A national profile of attention-deficit hyperactivity disorder diagnosis and treatment among US children aged 2 to 5 years. *Journal of Developmental and Behavioral Pediatrics, 38*(7), 455–464. https://doi.org/10.1097/DBP.0000000000000477

Danielson, M. L., Bitsko, R. H., Ghandour, R. M., Holbrook, J. R., Kogan, M. D., & Blumberg, S. J. (2018). Prevalence of parent-reported ADHD diagnosis and associated treatment among U.S. children and adolescents, 2016. *Journal of Clinical Child and Adolescent Psychology, 47*(2), 199–212. https://doi.org/10.1080/15374416.2017.1417860

Department of Justice Canada. (2000). *Selected statistics on Canadian families and family law* (2nd edn.). Department of Justice Canada. Retrieved November 12, 2020, from https://www.justice.gc.ca/eng/rp-pr/fl-lf/famil/stat2000/index.html#a01

Derks, E., Hudziak, J., & Boomsma, D. (2007). Why more boys than girls with ADHD receive treatment: A study of Dutch twins. *Twin Research and Human Genetics, 10*(5), 765–770. https://doi.org/10.1375/twin.10.5.765

Dieleman, J. L., Baral, R., Birger, M., Bui, A. L., Bulchis, A., Chapin, A., Hamavid, H., Horst, C., Johnson, E. K., Joseph, J., Lavado, R., Lomsadze, L., Reynolds, A., Squires, E., Campbell, M., DeCenso, B., Dicker, D., Flaxman, A. D., Gabert, R., ... Murray, C. J. L. (2016). US spending on personal health care and public health, 1996-2013. *JAMA, 316*(24), 2627–2646. https://doi.org/10.1001/jama.2016.16885

Diller, L. H. (1999). Assessment of Adderall in ADHD. *Journal of the American Academy of Child and Adolescent Psychiatry, 38*(1), 2. https://doi.org/10.1097/00004583-199901000-00002

Dowrick, C., & Frances, A. (2013). Medicalising unhappiness: New classification of depression risks more patients being put on drug treatment from which they will not benefit. *BMJ, 347*, f7140. https://doi.org/10.1136/bmj.f7140

Durkheim, E. (1984). *The division of labor in society*. Macmillan.

Ebejer, J. L., Medland, S. E., van der Werf, J., Gondro, C., Henders, A. K., Lynskey, M., Martin, N. G., & Duffy, D. L. (2012). Attention deficit hyperactivity disorder in Australian adults: Prevalence, persistence, conduct problems and disadvantage. *PLoS One, 7*(10), e47404. https://doi.org/10.1371/journal.pone.0047404

Eilertsen, E. M., Gjerde, L. C., Reichborn-Kjennerud, T., Ørstavik, R. E., Knudsen, G. P., Stoltenberg, C., Czajkowski, N., Røysamb, E., Kendler, K. S., & Ystrom, E. (2017). Maternal alcohol use during pregnancy and offspring attention-deficit hyperactivity disorder (ADHD): A prospective sibling control study. *International Journal of Epidemiology, 46*(5), 1633–1640. https://doi.org/10.1093/ije/dyx067

Engelhardt, H. T. (1974). The disease of masturbation: Values and the concept of disease. *Bulletin of the History of Medicine, 48*(2), 234–248.

Fleming, M., Fitton, C. A., Steiner, M. F., McLay, J. S., Clark, D., King, A., Mackay, D. F., & Pell, J. P. (2017). Educational and health outcomes of children treated for attention-deficit/ hyperactivity disorder. *JAMA Pediatrics, 171*(7), e170691–e170691. https://doi.org/10.1001/jamapediatrics.2017.0691

Fletcher, J. M. (2014). The effects of childhood ADHD on adult labor market outcomes. *Health Economics, 23*(2), 159–181. https://doi.org/10.1002/hec.2907

Foucault, M. (1975). *Discipline and punish: The birth of the prison*. Pantheon Books.

Frances, A. (2014). *Saving normal: An insider's revolt against out-of-control psychiatric diagnosis, DSM-5, big pharma, and the medicalization of ordinary life*. William Morrow Paperbacks.

Gaub, M., & Carlson, C. L. (1997). Gender differences in ADHD: A meta-analysis and critical review. *Journal of the American Academy of Child & Adolescent Psychiatry, 36*(8), 1036–1045. https://doi.org/10.1097/00004583-199708000-00011

Gershon, J. (2002). A meta-analytic review of gender differences in ADHD. *Journal of Attention Disorders, 5*(3), 143–154. https://doi.org/10.1177/108705470200500302

Ghosh, K. (2019, November 29). *Divorces in England and Wales: 2018*. Office for National Statistics. Retrieved November 12, 2020, from https://www.ons.gov.uk/peoplepopulationandcommunity/birthsdeathsandmarriages/divorce/bulletins/divorcesinenglandandwales/2018

Goodman, R. (2001). Psychometric properties of the strengths and difficulties questionnaire. *Journal of the American Academy of Child & Adolescent Psychiatry, 40*(11), 1337–1345. https://doi.org/10.1097/00004583-200111000-00015

Goran, M., Gower, B., Treuth, M., & Nagy, T. R. (1998). Prediction of intra-abdominal and subcutaneous abdominal adipose tissue in healthy pre-pubertal children. *International Journal of Obesity, 22*, 549–558. https://doi.org/10.1038/sj.ijo.0800624

Graetz, B. W., Sawyer, M. G., & Baghurst, P. (2005). Gender differences among children with DSM-IV ADHD in Australia. *Journal of the American Academy of Child & Adolescent Psychiatry, 44*(2), 159–168. https://doi.org/10.1097/00004583-200502000-00008

Groenman, A. P., Janssen, T. W., & Oosterlaan, J. (2017). Childhood psychiatric disorders as risk factor for subsequent substance abuse: A meta-analysis. *Journal of the American Academy of Child & Adolescent Psychiatry, 56*(7), 556–569. https://doi.org/10.1016/j.jaac.2017.05.004

Halleck, S. L. (1971). *The politics of therapy*. Science House.

Hartmann, T. (1993). *Attention deficit disorder: A different perception*. Underwood Books.

Hartung, C. M., Willcutt, E. G., Lahey, B. B., Pelham, W. E., Loney, J., Stein, M. A., & Keenan, K. (2002). Sex differences in young children who meet criteria for attention deficit hyperactivity disorder. *Journal of Clinical Child and Adolescent Psychology, 31*(4), 453–464. https://doi.org/10.1207/S15374424JCCP3104_5

Hashmi, A. M., Imran, N., Ali, A. A., & Shah, A. A. (2017). Attention-deficit/hyperactivity disorder in adults: Changes in diagnostic criteria in DSM-5. *Psychiatric Annals, 47*(6), 291–295. https://doi.org/10.3928/00485713-20170509-02

He, Y., Chen, J., Zhu, L.-H., Hua, L.-L., & Ke, F.-F. (2017). Maternal smoking during pregnancy and ADHD: Results from a systematic review and meta-analysis of prospective cohort studies. *Journal of Attention Disorders, 24*(12), 1637–1647. https://doi.org/10.1177/1087054717696766

Hennissen, L., Bakker, M. J., Banaschewski, T., Carucci, S., Coghill, D., Danckaerts, M., Dittmann, R. W., Hollis, C., Kovshoff, H., McCarthy, S., Nagy, P., Sonuga-Barke, E., Wong, I. C. K., Zuddas, A., Rosenthal, E., & Buitelaar, J. K. (2017). Cardiovascular effects of stimulant and non-stimulant medication for children and adolescents with ADHD: A systematic review and meta-analysis of trials of methylphenidate, amphetamines and atomoxetine. *CNS Drugs, 31*(3), 199–215. https://doi.org/10.1007/s40263-017-0410-7

References

Hinshaw, S. P., Scheffler, R. M., Fulton, B. D., Aase, H., Banaschewski, T., Cheng, W., Mattos, P., Holte, A., Levy, F., Sadeh, A., Sergeant, J. A., Taylor, E., & Weiss, M. D. (2011). International variation in treatment procedures for ADHD: Social context and recent trends. *Psychiatric Services, 62*(5), 459–464. https://doi.org/10.1176/ps.62.5.pss6205_0459

Hjern, A., Weitoft, G., & Lindblad, F. (2010). Social adversity predicts ADHD-medication in school children – A national cohort study. *Acta Paediatrica, 99*(6), 920–924. https://doi.org/10.1111/j.1651-2227.2009.01638.x

Hoekzema, E., Carmona, S., Ramos-Quiroga, J. A., Canals, C., Moreno, A., Fernández, V. R., ... Vilarroya, O. (2014). Stimulant drugs trigger transient volumetric changes in the human ventral striatum. *Brain Structure and Function, 219*(1), 23–34. https://doi.org/10.1007/s00429-012-0481-7

Horwitz, A. V., & Wakefield, J. C. (2007). *The loss of sadness: How psychiatry transformed normal sorrow into depressive disorder.* Oxford University Press.

Illich, I. (1976). *Medical nemesis.* Pantheon Books.

Jacklin, C. N., Maccoby, E. E., Doering, C. H., & King, D. R. (1984). Neonatal sex-steroid hormones and muscular strength of boys and girls in the first three years. *Developmental Psychobiology, 17*(3), 301–310. https://doi.org/10.1002/dev.420170309

Kessler, R. C., Adler, L. A., Barkley, R., Biederman, J., Conners, C. K., Faraone, S. V., Greenhill, L. L., Jaeger, S., Secnik, K., Spencer, T., Üstün, T. B., & Zaslavsky, A. M. (2005). Patterns and predictors of attention-deficit/hyperactivity disorder persistence into adulthood: Results from the national comorbidity survey replication. *Biological Psychiatry, 57*(11), 1442–1451. https://doi.org/10.1016/j.biopsych.2005.04.001

Knopf, H., Hölling, H., Huss, M., & Schlack, R. (2012). Prevalence, determinants and spectrum of attention-deficit hyperactivity disorder (ADHD) medication of children and adolescents in Germany: Results of the German health interview and examination survey (KiGGS). *BMJ Open, 2*(6), e000477. https://doi.org/10.1136/bmjopen-2011-000477

Knopik, V. S., Heath, A. C., Jacob, T., Slutske, W. S., Bucholz, K. K., Madden, P. A., Waldron, M., & Martin, N. G. (2006). Maternal alcohol use disorder and offspring ADHD: Disentangling genetic and environmental effects using a children-of-twins design. *Psychological Medicine, 36*(10), 1461–1471. https://doi.org/10.1017/S0033291706007884

Langley, K., Rice, F., van den Bree, M. B., & Thapar, A. (2005). Maternal smoking during pregnancy as an environmental risk factor for attention deficit hyperactivity disorder behaviour. A review. *Minerva Pediatrica, 57*(6), 359–371.

Larsson, H., Sariaslan, A., Långström, N., D'Onofrio, B., & Lichtenstein, P. (2014). Family income in early childhood and subsequent attention deficit/hyperactivity disorder: A quasi-experimental study. *Journal of Child Psychology and Psychiatry, 55*(5), 428–435. https://doi.org/10.1111/jcpp.12140

Lecendreux, M., Konofal, E., & Faraone, S. V. (2011). Prevalence of attention deficit hyperactivity disorder and associated features among children in France. *Journal of Attention Disorders, 15*(6), 516–524. https://doi.org/10.1177/1087054710372491

LeFever, G. B., Villers, M. S., Morrow, A. L., & Vaughn, E. S., III. (2002). Parental perceptions of adverse educational outcomes among children diagnosed and treated for ADHD: A call for improved school/provider collaboration. *Psychology in the Schools, 39*(1), 63–71. https://doi.org/10.1002/pits.10000

Loe, I. M., & Feldman, H. M. (2007). Academic and educational outcomes of children with ADHD. *Journal of Pediatric Psychology, 32*(6), 643–654. https://doi.org/10.1093/jpepsy/jsl054

Malacrida, C. (2004). Medicalization, ambivalence and social control: Mothers' descriptions of educators and ADD/ADHD. *Health, 8*(1), 61–80. https://doi.org/10.1177/1363459304038795

Mansfield, H. C. (2006). *Manliness.* Yale University Press.

Martinez-Raga, J., Knecht, C., Szerman, N., & Martinez, M. I. (2013). Risk of serious cardiovascular problems with medications for attention-deficit hyperactivity disorder. *CNS Drugs, 27*(1), 15–30. https://doi.org/10.1007/s40263-012-0019-9

Maturo, A. (2013). The medicalization of education: ADHD, human enhancement and academic performance. *Italian Journal of Sociology of Education, 5*(3), 175–188. https://doi.org/10.14658/pupj-ijse-2013-3-10

McLanahan, S., Tach, L., & Schneider, D. (2013). The causal effects of father absence. *Annual Review of Sociology, 39*(1), 399–427. https://doi.org/10.1146/annurev-soc-071312-145704

Mick, E., Biederman, J., Faraone, S. V., Sayer, J., & Kleinman, S. (2002). Case-control study of attention-deficit hyperactivity disorder and maternal smoking, alcohol use, and drug use during pregnancy. *Journal of the American Academy of Child & Adolescent Psychiatry, 41*(4), 378–385. https://doi.org/10.1097/00004583-200204000-00009

National Institute for Health Care Excellence (NICE). (2018, March 18). *Attention deficit hyperactivity disorder: Diagnosis and management*. National Institute for Health Care Excellence (NICE). Retrieved November 23, 2020, from https://www.nice.org.uk/guidance/ng87/chapter/Recommendations

Newcorn, J. H., Halperin, J. M., Healey, J. M., O'Brien, J. D., Pascualvaca, D. M., Wolf, L. E., Morganstein, A., Sharma, V., & Young, J. G. (1989). Are ADDH and ADHD the same or different? *Journal of the American Academy of Child & Adolescent Psychiatry, 28*(5), 734–738. https://doi.org/10.1097/00004583-198909000-00015

Novartis South Africa. (n.d.). *ADHD. What does that mean to you?* Novartis South Africa. Retrieved November 12, 2020, from https://www.novartis.co.za/sites/www.novartis.co.za/files/10090-ADHD%20Ritalin%20Health%2024%20Landing%20Page_V6%20FA.pdf

Ouyang, L., Fang, X., Mercy, J., Perou, R., & Grosse, S. D. (2008). Attention-deficit/hyperactivity disorder symptoms and child maltreatment: A population-based study. *The Journal of Pediatrics, 153*(6), 851–856. https://doi.org/10.1016/j.jpeds.2008.06.002

Peper, J. S., Brouwer, R. M., Schnack, H. G., van Baal, G. C., van Leeuwen, M., van den Berg, S. M., Delemarre-Van de Waal, H. A., Boomsma, D. I., Kahn, R. S., & Hulshoff Pol, H. E. (2009). Sex steroids and brain structure in pubertal boys and girls. *Psychoneuroendocrinology, 34*(3), 332–342. https://doi.org/10.1016/j.psyneuen.2008.09.012

Peralta, R. L., & Steele, J. L. (2010). Nonmedical prescription drug use among US college students at a Midwest university: A partial test of social learning theory. *Substance Use & Misuse, 45*(6), 865–887. https://doi.org/10.3109/10826080903443610

Pew Research Center. (2015, November 3). *U.S. public becoming less religious*. Pew Research Center. Retrieved November 24, 2020, from https://www.pewforum.org/2015/11/03/u-s-public-becoming-less-religious/

Pew Research Center. (2019, October 17). *In U.S., decline of Christianity continues at rapid pace*. Pew Research Center. Retrieved November 24, 2020, from https://www.pewforum.org/2019/10/17/in-u-s-decline-of-christianity-continues-at-rapid-pace/

Polanczyk, G., De Lima, M. S., Horta, B. L., Biederman, J., & Rohde, L. A. (2007). The worldwide prevalence of ADHD: A systematic review and metaregression analysis. *American Journal of Psychiatry, 164*(6), 942–948. https://doi.org/10.1176/ajp.2007.164.6.942

Ramtekkar, U. P., Reiersen, A. M., Todorov, A. A., & Todd, R. D. (2010). Sex and age differences in attention-deficit/hyperactivity disorder symptoms and diagnoses: Implications for DSM-V and ICD-11. *Journal of the American Academy of Child & Adolescent Psychiatry, 49*(3), 217–228. https://doi.org/10.1016/j.jaac.2009.11.011

Rasmussen, K., & Levander, S. (2009). Untreated ADHD in adults: Are there sex differences in symptoms, comorbidity, and impairment? *Journal of Attention Disorders, 12*(4), 353–360. https://doi.org/10.1177/1087054708314621

Ringer, N. (2020). Living with ADHD: A meta-synthesis review of qualitative research on children's experiences and understanding of their ADHD. *International Journal of Disability, Development and Education, 67*(2), 208–224. https://doi.org/10.1080/1034912X.2019.1596226

Rodriguez, A., & Bohlin, G. (2005). Are maternal smoking and stress during pregnancy related to ADHD symptoms in children? *Journal of Child Psychology and Psychiatry, 46*(3), 246–254. https://doi.org/10.1111/j.1469-7610.2004.00359.x

Rodriguez, A., Miettunen, J., Henriksen, T. B., Olsen, J., Obel, C., Taanila, A., Ebeling, H., Linnet, K. M., Moilanen, I., & Järvelin, M.-R. (2008). Maternal adiposity prior to pregnancy is associated with ADHD symptoms in offspring: Evidence from three prospective pregnancy cohorts. *International Journal of Obesity (2005), 32*(3), 550–557. https://doi.org/10.1038/sj.ijo.0803741

Rowland, A. S., Skipper, B. J., Rabiner, D. L., Qeadan, F., Campbell, R. A., Naftel, A. J., & Umbach, D. M. (2018). Attention-deficit/hyperactivity disorder (ADHD): Interaction between socioeconomic status and parental history of ADHD determines prevalence. *Journal of Child Psychology and Psychiatry, 59*(3), 213–222. https://doi.org/10.1111/jcpp.12775

Rucklidge, J. J. (2010). Gender differences in attention-deficit/hyperactivity disorder. *The Psychiatric Clinics of North America, 33*(2), 357–373. https://doi.org/10.1016/j.psc.2010.01.006

Rucklidge, J. J., Brown, D. L., Crawford, S., & Kaplan, B. J. (2006). Retrospective reports of childhood trauma in adults with ADHD. *Journal of Attention Disorders, 9*(4), 631–641. https://doi.org/10.1177/1087054705283892

Russell, G., Ford, T., Rosenberg, R., & Kelly, S. (2014). The association of attention deficit hyperactivity disorder with socioeconomic disadvantage: Alternative explanations and evidence. *Journal of Child Psychology and Psychiatry, and Allied Disciplines, 55*(5), 436–445. https://doi.org/10.1111/jcpp.12170

Russell, A. E., Ford, T., Williams, R., & Russell, G. (2016). The association between socioeconomic disadvantage and attention deficit/hyperactivity disorder (ADHD): A systematic review. *Child Psychiatry & Human Development, 47*(3), 440–458. https://doi.org/10.1007/s10578-015-0578-3

Sax, L. (2016). *Boys adrift*. Basic Books.

Sax, L., & Kautz, K. J. (2003). Who first suggests the diagnosis of attention-deficit/hyperactivity disorder? *The Annals of Family Medicine, 1*(3), 171–174. https://doi.org/10.1370/afm.3

Scheffler, R. M., Hinshaw, S. P., Modrek, S., & Levine, P. (2007). The global market for ADHD medications. *Health Affairs (Project Hope), 26*(2), 450–457. https://doi.org/10.1377/hlthaff.26.2.450

Scott, S. (2006). The medicalisation of shyness: From social misfits to social fitness. *Sociology of Health & Illness, 28*(2), 133–153. https://doi.org/10.1111/j.1467-9566.2006.00485.x

Searight, H. R., & McLaren, A. L. (1998). Attention-deficit hyperactivity disorder: The medicalization of misbehavior. *Journal of Clinical Psychology in Medical Settings, 5*(4), 467–495. https://doi.org/10.1023/A:1026263012665

Singh, I. (2003). Boys will be boys: Fathers' perspectives on ADHD symptoms, diagnosis, and drug treatment. *Harvard Review of Psychiatry, 11*(6), 308–316. https://doi.org/10.1080/714044393

Singh, I. (2004). Doing their jobs: Mothering with Ritalin in a culture of mother-blame. *Social Science & Medicine, 59*(6), 1193–1205. https://doi.org/10.1016/j.socscimed.2004.01.011

Sinha, A., Lewis, O., Kumar, R., Yeruva, S. L., & Curry, B. H. (2016). Adult ADHD medications and their cardiovascular implications. *Case Reports in Cardiology, 2016*(8), 1–6. https://doi.org/10.1155/2016/2343691

Sommers, C. H. (2015). *The war against boys: How misguided feminism is harming our young men*. Simon and Schuster.

St. Sauver, J. L., Barbaresi, W. J., Katusic, S. K., Colligan, R. C., Weaver, A. L., & Jacobsen, S. J. (2004). Early life risk factors for attention-deficit/hyperactivity disorder: A population-based cohort study. *Mayo Clinic Proceedings, 79*(9), 1124–1131. https://doi.org/10.4065/79.9.1124

Statistics Canada. (2020). Divorce rates, by year of marriage. *Statistics Canada*. Retrieved November 23, 2020, from https://www150.statcan.gc.ca/t1/tbl1/en/tv.action?pid=3910002801

Stern, A., Agnew-Blais, J., Danese, A., Fisher, H. L., Jaffee, S. R., Matthews, T., Polanczyk, G. V., & Arsenault, L. (2018). Associations between abuse/neglect and ADHD from childhood to young adulthood: A prospective nationally-representative twin study. *Child Abuse & Neglect, 81*, 274–285. https://doi.org/10.1016/j.chiabu.2018.04.025

Szasz, T. S. (2006). *Psychiatry: A branch of the law*. The Freeman. https://fee.org/articles/psychiatry-a-branch-of-the-law/

Thomas, R., Sanders, S., Doust, J., Beller, E., & Glasziou, P. (2015). Prevalence of attention-deficit/hyperactivity disorder: A systematic review and meta-analysis. *Pediatrics, 135*(4), e994–e1001. https://doi.org/10.1542/peds.2014-3482

Timimi, S. (2002). *Pathological child psychiatry and the medicalization of childhood*. Brunner-Routledge.

Timimi, S., & Taylor, E. (2004). ADHD is best understood as a cultural construct. *British Journal of Psychiatry, 184*(1), 8–9. https://doi.org/10.1192/bjp.184.1.8

Visser, S. N., Danielson, M. L., Bitsko, R. H., Holbrook, J. R., Kogan, M. D., Ghandour, R. M., Perou, R., & Blumberg, S. J. (2014). Trends in the parent-report of health care provider-diagnosed and medicated attention-deficit/hyperactivity disorder: United States, 2003-2011. *Journal of the American Academy of Child & Adolescent Psychiatry, 53*(1), 34–46. https://doi.org/10.1016/j.jaac.2013.09.001

Visser, S. N., Danielson, M. L., Wolraich, M. L., Fox, M. H., Grosse, S. D., Valle, L. A., Holbrook, J. R., Claussen, A. H., & Peacock, G. (2016). Vital signs: National and state-specific patterns of attention deficit/hyperactivity disorder treatment among insured children aged 2-5 years – United States, 2008-2014. *Morbidity and Mortality Weekly Report, 65*, 443–450. https://doi.org/10.15585/mmwr.mm6517e1

Wells, J. C. (2007). Sexual dimorphism of body composition. *Best Practice & Research. Clinical Endocrinology & Metabolism, 21*(3), 415–430. https://doi.org/10.1016/j.beem.2007.04.007

Westover, A. N., & Halm, E. A. (2012). Do prescription stimulants increase the risk of adverse cardiovascular events?: A systematic review. *BMC Cardiovascular Disorders, 12*(1), 41. https://doi.org/10.1186/1471-2261-12-41

Whitaker, R. (2010). *Anatomy of an epidemic: Magic bullets, psychiatric drugs, and the astonishing rise of mental illness in America*. Crown Publishers/Random House.

Willcutt, E. G. (2012). The prevalence of DSM-IV attention-deficit/hyperactivity disorder: A meta-analytic review. *Neurotherapeutics, 9*(3), 490–499. https://doi.org/10.1007/s13311-012-0135-8

Zametkin, A. J., & Ernst, M. (1999). Problems in the management of attention-deficit-hyperactivity disorder. *New England Journal of Medicine, 340*(1), 40–46. https://doi.org/10.1056/NEJM199901073400107

Zimbardo, P. G., & Coulombe, N. (2016). *Man, interrupted: Why young men are struggling what we can do about it*. Red Wheel.

Zito, J. M., Safer, D. J., de Jong-van den Berg, L. T. W., Janhsen, K., Fegert, J. M., Gardner, J. F., Glaeske, G., & Valluri, S. C. (2008). A three-country comparison of psychotropic medication prevalence in youth. *Child and Adolescent Psychiatry and Mental Health, 2*(1), 26. https://doi.org/10.1186/1753-2000-2-26

Zola, I. K. (1972). Medicine as an institution of social control. *The Sociological Review, 20*(4), 487–504. https://doi.org/10.1111/j.1467-954X.1972.tb00220.x

Zuvekas, S. H., & Vitiello, B. (2012). Stimulant medication use in children: A 12-year perspective. *The American Journal of Psychiatry, 169*(2), 160–166. https://doi.org/10.1176/appi.ajp.2011.11030387

Chapter 5
Risk Factors and Rates of Depression in Men: Do Males Have Greater Resilience, or Is Male Depression Underrecognized and Underdiagnosed?

Everyone experiences a range of emotions and moods in response to the changing circumstances of life. This can typically include occasional and short-lived periods of sadness and low mood. Such sadness and low mood are part of the human condition, and these experiences do not necessarily represent psychopathology, especially if they dissipate within a short space of time.

However, this sadness and low mood can sometimes become particularly intense and persistent, enveloping the whole life experience to severely affect daily functioning in an all-encompassing manner. This atypical experience is commonly known as *clinical depression* or more technically *Major Depressive Disorder* (MDD). The American Psychiatric Association devotes a whole chapter of the *Diagnostic and Statistical Manual of Mental Disorders Fifth Edition (DSM-5)* to MDD, with several pages giving a description of the diagnostic criteria. These criteria include nine specific symptoms said to characterize MDD, listed in Table 5.1:

For a diagnosis to be made, five or more of the above symptoms must have been present most of the day, nearly every day, over the preceding two weeks, and must cause significant distress and impairment. Moreover, one symptom must be depressed mood or loss of interest or pleasure.

Major depression can range from a single episode once in a lifetime, to a reoccurring persistent chronic disorder. Several epidemiological studies note that the average duration of a depressive episode is around 3 to 6 months, depending on factors such as severity and treatment (Richards 2011). Relatedly, the research literature indicates that the majority of people with depression make a full recovery within one year. For example, the large-scale Epidemiological Catchment Area study noted that 50% of first episode cases make a full recovery within one year, while 35% experience recurring episodes, and 15% experience a chronic disorder (Eaton et al. 2008).

Table 5.1 DSM-5 symptom list of MDD (APA, 2013)

	Symptom
a	Depressed mood and persistent sadness
b	Loss of interest or pleasure
c	Significant change in weight or appetite
d	Insomnia or hypersomnia
e	Psychomotor retardation or agitation
f	Fatigue or loss of energy
g	Feelings of worthlessness or guilt
h	Impaired concentration or indecisiveness
i	Suicidal ideation, suicide attempt or thoughts of death

5.1 The Prevalence of Depression

A recent systematic review of prevalence studies from across the world estimated a global point prevalence of depression of 4.7% (Ferrari et al. 2013). This study also found an increasing rate of depression over the preceding decades indicating a worsening situation. These findings are consistent with another large-scale cross-national study which found that over 250 million people across the globe experienced clinical depression in the last 12 months (James et al. 2018).

In the USA, the 2018 National Survey on Drug Use and Health (NSDUH) collected information from around 70,000 Americans on mental health and drug use through systematic and validated procedures. This includes questions based on the above-described MDD diagnostic criteria, allowing for reliable case ascertainment. This methodology provides a strong foundation for reliable national estimates of MDD prevalence. This survey found that 7.2% of adults (ages 18+ years) reached the criteria for MDD in the past year, which translates to around 18 million Americans. Again, this survey found an increasing rate of MDD, with the 7.2% figure higher than all of the preceding 20 years. This figure is also considerably higher than the aforementioned 4.7% global estimate, and is also higher than recent estimates from Canada.

In Canada, data from the large-scale and equally rigorous Canadian Community Health Survey - Mental Health indicates that the 12-month prevalence of MDD is 4.7%, making this the most common mental disorder in Canada (Pearson et al. 2013). This survey also indicates a lifetime prevalence of 11.3%, meaning that around 3.2 million Canadians have experienced MDD at some point in their lives. In contrast to some of the aforementioned US and global studies, this survey found that the rate of depression remained stable between 2002 and 2012.

Clinical depression is also one of the leading causes of disability and ill health worldwide. A recent study noted that MDD is the third leading cause of disability across the globe (James et al. 2018). Importantly, this paper indicates that disability associated with depression has increased over 50% since 1990, consistent with other literature suggesting that the prevalence and impact of MDD is worsening. Of note, clinical depression can have a devastating effect on quality of life, often involving severe functional impairment in domains such as education (see Chapter 7), employment (see Chapter 8) and family life (see Chapter 9). For example, longitudinal research indicates that people with depression are much more likely to be unemployed or drop out of education (Jefferis et al., 2011; Quiroga et al., 2013). Indeed, the 2018 NSDUH assessed the impact and levels of impairment of MDD on four important life domains, namely: (i) work life; (ii) home life; (iii) social relationships; and (iv) wider social life. Analysis revealed that 11.5 million US adults (4.7%) had a severe impairment in one or more of the above life domains due to MDD, and again this percentage was notably higher than the preceding 20 years.

5.2 Gender Differentials in Prevalence and Treatment

Interestingly, evidence suggests that men have a much lower prevalence of depression than women. Indeed, a systematic review of prevalence studies across the world found that the 12- month prevalence of depression was 7.2% for females and 3.9% for males (Ferrari et al., 2013). Other epidemiological surveys routinely indicate that adult women are around two times more likely to be diagnosed with depression compared to adult men.

In the USA, the 2018 NSDUH estimates that 11.5 million adult women have experienced a major depressive episode in the last year, compared to 6.3 million adult men. These numbers translate to 9% of adult women, and 5.3% of adult men, meaning a female-to-male ratio of just under 2:1. A similar ratio is seen when comparing men and women severely impaired by MDD, with 7.5 million adult women (5.9%) experiencing such impairment, as compared to 4 million adult men (3.4%). In Canada, the aforementioned large-scale Canadian Community Health Survey - Mental Health indicates a similar gender differential, with a 12-month prevalence of depression of 5.8% for females, and 3.6% for males, with females having higher rates across all age groups (Pearson et al., 2013).

Interestingly, a large corpus of research indicates that men with MDD are much less likely to receive treatment from a health professional compared to women with MDD. For example, the 2018 NSDUH estimated 6.3 million adult male cases of MDD, but only 3.7 million of these (57%) received treatment from a health professional. This means that over 2.5 million American men with MDD are going untreated. In contrast, the NSDUH estimated 11.5 million adult female cases of MDD, with 7.9 million of these (70%) receiving treatment. In other words, 43% of adult men with MDD are not receiving treatment, compared to 30% of adult women with MDD.

These findings are consistent with another large-scale US study finding that men with MDD were half as likely to utilize services compared to women with MDD (Wang et al., 2005). Moreover, data from the US National Health Interview Survey 2010–2013 indicates that nearly 9% of men had daily feelings of depression or anxiety, but less than half sought any type of treatment (Blumberg et al., 2015). Of note, this survey found that 33% took medication, while 26% had seen a mental health professional in the last month, showing low rates of engagement with official health services – a phenomena discussed in greater detail in Chap. 6.

Similar results are found in other jurisdictions. For example, the Canadian Chronic Disease Surveillance System captures data from official health service registries to assess health service utilization. It found that around 10% of Canadians (3.5 million people) used health services for mood and anxiety disorders during a 12-month period, consisting of 2.2 million females and 1.3 million males (Public Health Agency of Canada 2016). This translates to a 1.7:1 female:male ratio of health service use for mood and anxiety disorders.

Importantly, evidence suggests that people with MDD are significantly more likely to use illicit drugs, binge drink and smoke cigarettes compared to the general population, with particularly elevated rates in men (Davis et al. 2008; Degenhardt and Hall 2001). Indeed, the 2018 NSDUH indicates that over one in three people with major depressive disorders use cannabis, indicating a degree of self-medication for MDD, particularly among men (see Chap. 3).

In sum, converging evidence from a variety of sources and surveys indicates that rates of depression are considerably and significantly higher in women compared to men. Moreover, these surveys show that rates of health service utilization for MDD are considerably lower for men compared to women. These observed gender differences have led to speculation that:

(i) Men may be more resilient to depression than women.
(ii) Gender differentials in prevalence are largely artefactual, with male cases missed due to systematic measurement and diagnostic biases in both research and clinical practice.
(iii) Men experience an atypical but real *male depressive syndrome* (or *masked depression*), which is unrecognized and undetected by existing epidemiological measures and diagnostic criteria.

All three of these factors are discussed in more detail in the following sections.

5.3 Male Resilience

One hypothesis regarding the gender differential in prevalence is that men tend to have a more effective set of responses and reactions when they begin to feel depressed in comparison to women, allowing men to nip depression in the bud and prevent a full-blown MDD episode.

This thesis was championed by Susan Nolen-Hoeksema, who conducted decades of research indicating that men and women tend to employ different coping mechanisms during the initial stages of a low mood (Nolen-Hoeksema, 1987, 2003; Nolen-Hoeksema & Girgus, 1994). In this research, Nolen-Hoeksema notes that men and women frequently experience periods of low mood, as well as feelings of psychosocial distress. However, men are more likely to engage in distracting behavioural activities such as exercise or hobbies. These activities can foster a strong sense of agency and internal locus of control, while distracting from negative rumination and catastrophizing of the situation. According to Nolen-Hoeksema, this strategy can 'dampen' a period of low mood, blunting its impact and allowing it to dissipate in a short passage of time.

In contrast to this active style of dealing with an initial low mood, Nolen-Hoeksema marshals considerable evidence indicating that women tend to adopt a cognitively driven approach and are more likely to passively ruminate over the causes and consequences of low mood and distress. This can intensify and amplify the experience while contributing to a sense of helplessness and a perceived external locus of control. Put another way, women tend to 'think too much' about causes and consequences when they begin to feel depressed, which can deepen and prolong the experience, trapping them into inaction and further distress (Nolen-Hoeksema, 2003).

Importantly, negative rumination has been implicated in a variety of other psychological factors that have been linked to depression and which differ in prevalence between men and women. For example, evidence suggests that males are more likely to be satisfied with their bodies in comparison to females, engaging in less rumination about body image issues (Grogan, 2017; Furnham et al., 2002). Importantly, some research indicates that such body dissatisfaction is a risk factor for depression (Karazsia et al., 2017). By the same token, men are less likely to engage in body monitoring and have less appearance anxiety than women, both of which can lead to negative rumination, and have been identified as risk factors contributing to higher rates of depression in women (Szymanski & Henning, 2007). Similarly, surveys indicate that men tend to have higher levels of self-esteem compared to women, with low self-esteem a proven risk factor for depression that may also contribute to higher rates in women (McMullin & Cairney, 2004).

Much of the above-described findings can be related to a quest for approval and validation from others, which can involve constant self-evaluation and considerable impression management. This can become pathological when taken to an extreme, especially, as external validation may not always be forthcoming. All this can combine to deepen negative rumination about the self and the world, which can further lower self-esteem and may contribute towards the onset of depression (Sargent et al., 2006). In sum, research indicates that preoccupations with body image, appearance and external validation are less common among men than women, and that this can protect against low self-esteem and the onset of depression (Grogan, 2017; Nolen-Hoeksema & Girgus, 1994; McMullin & Cairney, 2004).

These findings are important, especially given that the American Psychological Association's (2018) recently released *Guidelines for Psychological Practice with Boys and Men* tends to pathologize traditional male modalities of coping with mental distress (see Chap. 10). In contrast, the above-described evidence implies that men tend to possess robust and protective psychological orientations and coping mechanisms that can protect against depression while promoting wider psychological resilience. This includes:

(i) Engaging in distracting activities that prevent negative rumination
(ii) Avoiding constant self-evaluations that can damage self-esteem
(iii) Lowered sensitivity and less of a need for approval and validation from others

These common aspects of male psychology have sometimes been considered weaknesses in the mental health literature, and labelled unfavourably as 'escapism' or 'avoidance' (APA 2018). However, an alternative perspective is that these traits and tendencies should be considered strengths that may contribute towards lower rates of depression in men compared to women. Far from being exemplars of a putatively pathological masculinity, men with such traits could be considered as exemplars of a mentally healthy masculinity, and such traits could be encouraged in both men and women to improve their mental health.

5.4 An Artefactual Difference?

The evidence for gender differences in depression is strong, and some have argued that these differences are due to differential coping and resilience mechanisms in men and women. But some scholars are forcefully arguing that the epidemiological surveys are flawed, and that male depression is underdiagnosed and underrecognized due to a variety of factors, meaning that the true rates of male depression are much higher and much closer to the rates observed for women. This view is consistent with the so-called gender paradox in suicide rates. As explored in detail in Chap. 2, depression is one of the strongest predictors of suicide, but men have low rates of depression as compared to women. However, men make up around 75% of completed suicides in jurisdictions such as Canada and the USA. The disconnect between low rates of male depression and high rates of male suicide has been used to support the view that conventional measures of depression may be missing the mark when it comes to identifying male cases. Indeed, numerous factors may be biasing the statistics, with scholarly attention focused on: (i) the socio-cultural framing of depression; (ii) response bias in men experiencing low mood; and (iii) bias in the official diagnostic criteria.

To start, there is a common impression across society that depression is a woman's disease, manifesting itself in diverse venues including media, advertising and medical education. For example, media coverage of depression predominantly features females (Bengs et al., 2008), and advertisements for antidepressants overwhelmingly feature women (Munce et al., 2004). Similarly, the medical literature on depression throughout the twentieth century has typically featured case studies of women and rarely discussed men, meaning that depression as a clinical category developed largely without reference to the male experience (Hirshbein, 2006). This medical literature, frequently used in both medical education and clinical practice, continues to be infused with a female focus up to the present (Smith et al., 2018). All this can perpetuate the impression that depression is a woman's disease, which in turn can permeate into both lay and clinical perspectives – which may shape the practice of clinical staff, as well as men in distress.

Indeed, qualitative research indicates that men often consider depression to be a woman's illness (Whitley, 2013; Johnson et al., 2012). This can lead men to ignore or minimize symptoms and features of psychological distress, decreasing the likelihood of acknowledging and disclosing possible symptoms of depression. On the one hand, this could be considered part of the adaptive distracting coping mechanism identified by Nolen-Hokesema (2003). On the other hand, this may impede service utilization and contribute to the low rates of treatment for men with MDD. Such reluctance to acknowledge and disclose may also be consistent with dominant notions of masculinity, which tend to emphasize male strength, stoicism and control in the face of adversity (Oliffe & Phillips, 2008). In other words, societal stereotypes may interact with dominant notions of masculinity to inhibit recognition, disclosure and service utilization vis-à-vis male depression.

All this means that epidemiological surveys of sex differences in depression may be coloured by a significant response bias in men, with men failing to acknowledge symptoms due to a social desirability bias and other socio-cultural factors prompting men to show 'true grit' masculinity in the face of adversity. This means that these surveys may contain significant numbers of false negatives, where men with actual depression are miscategorized as mentally healthy. This can result in inaccurately low prevalence rates of male depression.

5.5 Bias in Diagnostic Criteria: A Male Depressive Syndrome?

The socio-cultural framing of depression as a women's disease combined with men's reluctance to disclose may contribute towards diagnostic error in the clinic, with doctors commonly failing to detect the presence of depression in men. However, this process may be compounded by an even greater factor, related to the official diagnostic criteria. In short, it has been convincingly argued that depression can manifest itself very differently in men, in a way that substantially deviates from the generic DSM-5 criteria. Because of its atypical nature, this form of male depression can largely go unrecognized in research and practice, thus contributing to the low observed rates of depression in men.

This form of atypical depression is sometimes known as *masked depression* or *male depressive syndrome* with scholars arguing that it is characterized by 'acting out' behaviours such as alcohol and drug misuse, excessive risk-taking, poor impulse control, anger attacks, aggression and irritability (Hart, 2000; Winkler et al., 2005). It has been argued that these acting-out behaviours are *depressive equivalents* masking a pathological sadness, despair and loneliness in the affected men (Addis, 2008). Of note, many such 'acting out' behaviours are significantly more common in men compared to women (Martin et al., 2013). For example, men account for around 75% of people experiencing substance use disorder and severe substance misuse issues (see Chap. 3). Similarly, anger attacks and aggression are around three times more common in men as compared to women, and men also have higher rates of irritability (Winkler et al., 2006). These acting-out behaviours could be considered pathological attempts to distract (or escape) from depressive moods and thoughts. Importantly, such 'acting-out' behaviours are not part of the official DSM-5 diagnostic criteria for depression, and are not contained in commonly used epidemiological instruments attempting to measure population rates of depression.

Relatedly, evidence suggests that women tend to 'act in' when faced with psychosocial adversity and low mood, focusing their energy and attention inwards. This can manifest itself in crying, sadness and negative rumination, accompanied by feelings of worthlessness, helplessness and guilt. Such behaviours are core to the official diagnostic criteria and are typically included in epidemiological instruments that measure depression. Of note, this 'acting-in' response to low mood and psychosocial adversity is less common among men (Nolen-Hoeksema, 2003).

If men experience depression differently than women, then conventional approaches to the diagnosis of depression in men will be flawed. Indeed, untold cases of male depression will be missed by existing methods of diagnosis, as well as by instruments often used in epidemiological surveys. Again, this may interact with the socio-cultural framing of depression as a women's disease, meaning that clinicians may be more attuned to detecting depression in women as compared to men (Smith et al., 2018). In other words, rates of male depression will be significantly underestimated if the phenomena of *masked depression* or *male depressive syndrome* is considered a real diagnostic entity, and individual cases will be missed in physician consults leading to a high rate of false negatives in the community and in the clinic.

In an attempt to shed light on this situation, a team of US researchers set out to assess 'masked depression' using an innovative and groundbreaking methodology (Martin et al., 2013). This involved the creation of new epidemiological instruments comprised of eight items that included hypothesized depressive equivalents as well as conventional markers of depression, namely: (i) stress; (ii) irritability; (iii) anger attacks/aggression; (iv) sleep problems; (v) alcohol/ drug use; (vi) loss of interest; (vii) risk-taking; and (viii) hyperactivity. These were completed by over 5000 US adults, with results compared between men and women. The findings revealed that men in this survey scored significantly higher in terms of risk-taking, aggression/ anger attacks and substance abuse compared to women, consistent with the literature on 'acting-out'. In contrast, women had higher rates of stress, sleep problems, and loss of interest in line with the literature on 'acting-in'. The authors then treated these depressive equivalents as symptoms of depression, tallying their frequency within individuals, scoring those with five or more 'symptoms' as cases of depression. Twenty-six percent of men in the sample had five or more 'symptoms', compared to 22% of women. In other words, the prevalence of depression between men and women is similar if the diagnostic criteria are widened to include 'acting-out' depressive equivalents.

In sum, when depression is conceptualized and measured more broadly, and includes depressive equivalents said to characterize 'masked depression', the rates of depression between men and women even out. If this is accepted as a valid approach, it means that the rates of depression commonly found in conventional epidemiological studies are artefactual, and mask a large amount of suffering and distress experienced by men in the community.

5.6 Risk Factors

The scientific literature documents several prominent and well-established risk factors for DSM-5-defined MDD in men. These tend to overlap with some of the prominent and well-established risk factors for suicide and substance use disorder discussed in previous chapters, including low educational attainment (see Chap. 7), unemployment (see Chap. 8) and separation/divorce (see Chap. 9). That said, the literature indicates that some men at low risk of substance abuse or suicide are particularly vulnerable to depression, for example new fathers. Six core risk factors are discussed next, namely: (i) low educational attainment; (ii) unemployment and financial strain; (iii) disability; (iv) homosexual orientation; (v) divorce; and (vi) ethno-racial status. This is followed by an in-depth case study of *paternal postpartum depression*, which ties together many of the strands weaved throughout this chapter.

5.6.1 *Low Educational Attainment*

Several studies have indicated an inverse dose-response relationship between educational attainment and depression, with more education protective against MDD. Indeed, a large-scale meta-analysis noted that 35 out of 51 studies reviewed found a significant association between low socio-economic status (SES) and depression, with low SES individuals having an overall odds ratio of 1.8 (95% CI, 1.57–2.10) when compared to high SES individuals (Lorant et al., 2003). Importantly, 37 of the 51 studies used level of education as a proxy for socio-economic status. This study also found that the odds of being depressed decreased by 3% for each additional year of education.

Similarly, a longitudinal analysis of data from the US National Epidemiologic Survey on Alcohol and Related Conditions (NESARC) (N=34,653; 87% response rate) found that those with a graduate, professional or bachelor degree had the lowest rates of depression, while those with a high-school diploma or less had the highest rates of these disorders (Erickson et al., 2016). Indeed, educational attainment at wave 1 was negatively associated with incident depression at wave 2, and those with less than high school education had a 65% to 70% higher rate of depression and anxiety compared to those with a graduate or professional degree. Such findings are consistent with a systematic review, which found that high school dropouts had higher rates of depression than high school graduates at the age of expected graduation, as well as more anxiety in young adulthood per se (Esch et al., 2014). The authors attributed these elevated rates to the lack of vocational opportunities for high school dropouts, as well as more precarious living conditions due to lower income and fewer resources.

In sum, low educational attainment increases risk for depression while high educational attainment decreases risk. As explained in much more detail in Chap. 7, considerable research indicates large gender differences in educational attainment, with males typically performing worse at all levels of education. This means that educational attainment is a distal yet modifiable risk factor which could be the target for prevention and promotion activities aiming to improve men's mental health.

5.6.2 Unemployment and Financial Strain

A large corpus of research indicates that unemployment and financial strain are risk factors for depression. For example, van der Noordt et al. (2014) examined 33 prospective studies finding that employed people had lower rates of depression than the unemployed (OR=0.52; 95% CI 0.33–0.83). Similarly, Modini et al. (2016) conducted a meta-review of 11 relevant reviews, again concluding that employment protected against depression, particularly when there are favourable workplace conditions and good-quality supervision.

Importantly, several studies indicate that unemployment and financial strain are stronger risk factors for male depression than for female depression. For example, a cross-sectional study of over 4,000 individuals in Spain compared depression symptoms by gender and employment status (Artazcoz et al., 2004). This study found that unemployed men had an adjusted odds ratio of 2.98 (95% CI 2.30–3.87) for high levels of depressive symptoms compared to employed men, while unemployed women had an adjusted odds ratio of 1.51 (95% CI 1.11–2.06) for high levels of depressive symptoms compared to employed women.

Similarly, another seminal study of over 1,000 opposite-sex dizygotic twin pairs examined sex differences in pathways to depression, finding that past-year stressful life events related to legal, financial and employment issues were strong risk factors for male depression, but not for female depression (Kendler & Gardner, 2014). This is consistent with studies from a variety of western jurisdictions indicating a significantly greater risk of depression among men experiencing job insecurity or financial strain (Meltzer et al., 2010; Ross & Mirowsky, 2006; Inaba et al., 2005; Diala & Muntaner, 2003). Financial strain can take many forms but can include severe debt, mortgage repayment difficulties and bankruptcy, which have all been shown to increase risk of male depression (e.g. Gathergood, 2012; Gili et al., 2013).

Interestingly, one UK study found that downward social mobility over the life course increased risk of depression for men, but not for women (Tiffin et al., 2005), while other studies found that men living in disadvantaged districts are at higher risk of depression, in particular deprived rural areas. For example, one UK cohort study of over 20,000 individuals living in the rural county of Norfolk demonstrated that men living in districts with high unemployment were over 75% more likely to have depression (RR: 1.77; 95% CI: 1.16–2.71) than men living in districts with low unemployment (Remes et al., 2019). Interestingly, this study found no relationship between risk of depression and district deprivation in women, again indicating a gendered effect. This is consistent with US research indicating that men living in rural areas have a higher rate of depression than men living in urban areas (Diala & Muntaner, 2003).

The reasons behind this gender differential in impact of unemployment and financial strain are discussed in detail in Chap. 7. In brief, research indicates that men derive considerable purpose and meaning from their employment and their role as a successful breadwinner, which is often necessary to support themselves and their families. Thus, the disruption of employment success, financial stability and fulfilment of the family breadwinner role can have a significant impact on standard of living and quality of life. Of note, radical changes in the economy, specifically the decline in blue-collar and manufacturing jobs, is leaving large swathes of men unemployed, financially strained and bereft of wider meaning and purpose in life (Case & Deaton, 2020). The implications of these changes vis-à-vis mental health are discussed in more detail in Chap. 7.

5.6.3 Disability

The research literature consistently indicates that disability and long-term medical conditions increase the risk of male depression. For example, Patten (2001) found that a long-term medical condition doubled the risk of developing major depression, while the aforementioned Remes et al. (2019) study found that men with a disability experienced depression at double the rate of men without a disability. By definition, a disability can negatively affect the ability to fulfil functional roles, and disabled men are often unable to fully participate in the workforce, with unemployment rates over double that of people without a disability (Office for National Statistics, 2019). This means that men with a disability are often deprived of the financial rewards and sense of purpose and meaning associated with participation in the workforce discussed in section 5.6.2.

In fact, many disabilities are a consequence of workplace injury, which are much more common amongst men than women. For example, US Bureau of Labor Statistics (2020a) data indicates that men accounted for 92% of workplace fatalities in 2019 (4,896 male fatalities compared to 437 female fatalities). In terms of serious workplace injuries, men accounted for 75% of all injuries requiring an overnight stay in a hospital (32,620 men compared to 10,440 women), with men taking 10 days off work on average after such an injury, compared to 7 days for women (US Bureau of Labor Statistics 2020b). This differential in workplace injuries is reflected in disability beneficiaries, with 220,850 American men receiving disability benefits due to injuries, compared to 116,804 women (US Social Security Administration, 2020).

Moreover, disability and long-term medical conditions can cause chronic pain, which can be incapacitating and contribute to further isolation and despair. Such pain can be mitigated by prescription opioids, but these have severe side effects such as drowsiness, confusion and fatigue which can further impair the ability to participate in activities that mitigate against the onset of depression, such as employment and education. These opioids can also be addictive, with other serious consequences, as outlined in detail in Chap. 3.

5.6.4 Homosexual Orientation

Certain disabilities and long-term medical conditions also incur stigma and can lead to prejudice and social exclusion, for example HIV/AIDS. In fact, numerous studies show that men living with HIV/AIDS have significantly higher rates of depression than the general population (Rabkin, 2008), with one study indicating a 42% rate of depression in men with HIV/AIDS (Horberg et al., 2008). Of note, gay men make up over 70% of men with HIV/AIDS (Hess et al., 2017), and these men may suffer a double stigma associated with their illness status and their homosexuality.

Indeed, a consistent finding in the literature is that gay and bisexual men have a significantly higher risk of depression than heterosexual men (King et al., 2008). For example, data from a large sample of US adults found that gay and bisexual men were 3.5 times more likely to have MDD compared to heterosexual men. Interestingly, this survey found no significant difference between rates of depression for heterosexual women and lesbian women. These elevated rates in gay men have been linked to many factors including internal/external stigma, issues surrounding HIV/AIDS, victimization and bullying (Lee et al., 2017). These findings indicate the importance of treating gay and bisexual men as a specific demographic, rather than lumping people together in an amorphous 'LGBTQIA+' category. Using this amorphous umbrella category can dilute the experience of gay and bisexual men and implicitly fails to recognize their unique stressors.

Interestingly, some research indicates that single gay men have higher rates of depression than gay men who are legally married. This is an important finding, given that gay marriage is not legal in some jurisdictions. For example, one large-scale study examined differential rates of psychological distress by marital status in California, finding that single gay men had much higher rates than married gay men (Wight et al., 2013). This could be related to loneliness and social isolation among single gay men, as well as the protective influence of familial social support and stability among gay men who are married. Indeed, these findings overlap with other research indicating that single men per se (regardless of sexual orientation) have higher rates of depression than married men per se, discussed in the next section.

5.6.5 Divorce

Evidence suggests that single, divorced, and separated people have higher rates of depression than married people. For example, a US cohort study of over 2,000 midlife individuals found that 22% of individuals who had become separated or divorced had experienced past-year MDD, compared to 8.4% of those who had been continuously married. This translates to an adjusted odds ratio of 2.29 (95% CI, 1.41–3.75) of MDD for the separated and divorced, compared to those who were continuously married (Sbarra et al., 2014). However, this study did not stratify outcomes by sex, but this weakness has been overcome by a variety of other studies elsewhere.

For example, the aforementioned Remes et al. (2019) study found MDD in 1.7% of married men, 3.6% of never-married men and 6.3% of divorced, separated, or widowed men. This translates to an adjusted odds ratio of 3.66 (95% CI: 2.53–5.28) of MDD for divorced, separated, or widowed men compared to married men. The odds ratio of MDD for never-married men (compared to married men) was less potent, at 1.46 (95% CI: 0.76–2.83). Analogous rates for females were 2.7% of married women, 2.4% of never married women and 5.6% of divorced, separated and widowed women. This translates to an adjusted odds ratio of 2.56 (95% CI: 2.00–3.27) for divorced, separated, or widowed women as compared to married women. The odds ratio for never-married women (compared to the married) was 0.93 (95% CI: 0.48–1.78). In other words, this study found that divorce, separation and widowhood were more potent risk factors for male depression than female depression.

These findings are consistent with earlier studies. For example, a cross-sectional survey of around 35,000 people from 15 different countries found that depression was significantly associated with divorce, while marriage was a protective factor (Scott et al., 2010). This study found that the adjusted odds ratio for the onset of MDD was 2.8 (95% CI: 1.8–3.0) for divorced men compared to married men. The analogous adjusted odds ratio for the onset of MDD in divorced women was 1.7 (95% CI: 1.5–2.0) as compared to married women. Again, divorce was a significant risk factor for depression for both men and women, but risk was considerably higher among divorced men. Interestingly, this study also found that the adjusted odds ratio for the onset of MDD was 0.8 (95% CI: 0.6–0.9) for married men, compared to never-married men, indicating that marriage is protective for men and that never-married men had a slightly increased risk of major depression.

Similarly, a Canadian longitudinal study of over 15,000 adults participating in the National Population Health Survey found that men whose marriages ended were at higher risk of being diagnosed with depression compared to their female peers (Rotermann, 2007). In this study, the adjusted odds ratio for the onset of MDD in the past two years for divorced and separated men was 3.3 (95% CI 1.7–6.5) compared to men who remained married. For divorced and separated women, the adjusted odds ratio was 2.4 (95% CI 1.6–3.5). Interestingly, sub-analysis indicated that men who were separated from their children after marital dissolution had a higher risk than men who were not separated (OR 1.9: 95% CI: 0.9–4.2), while men whose social support had decreased also had a higher risk than men whose social support had not decreased (OR=2.3: 95% CI 1.3–3.9). In short, this study confirms that divorced and separated men are at particular risk, especially those who are separated from their children and experience decreased social support.

The reasons behind these gender differentials are discussed in detail in Chap. 9. In short, several elements of the research literature indicate that the psychosocial experience of divorce can be particularly painful for men, acting as an acute stressor with chronic consequences. For example, men are significantly more likely to be separated from their children after a divorce, leading to a massive void and sense of loss (Grall, 2016; Department of Justice Canada, 2000). Moreover, divorced or separated men often have financially responsibility for two households: their own and that of their ex-spouse and children. This burden may place intolerable limits on a man's financial and psychosocial resources leading to a maladaptive response (Kposowa, 2003).

5.6.6 *Ethno-Racial Status*

A final risk factor found across the literature relates to race and ethnicity, with much research indicating that white men in western jurisdictions have higher lifetime rates of depression than minority men. One large-scale epidemiological study found that the lifetime rate of depression in white men was 16.2% – over double the 7% rate found for African-American men (Williams et al., 2007). Similarly, a large-scale US study found that 3.8% of white men felt depressed every day, compared to 2.9% of black and Hispanic men (Blumberg et al., 2015). These ethno-racial differences have been attributed to variations in religiosity, social support, ethnic identity, hopefulness and resilience between ethno-racial communities, with some research indicating that all of the above tend to be lower among white men (Bailey et al., 2019).

5.7 Paternal Postpartum Depression

The birth of a child is generally a time of great joy for both mother and father alike. However, the advent of parenthood creates a new set of onerous financial and caregiving responsibilities for both parents. New parenthood can also lead to biological changes including extreme fatigue, sleep deprivation, and hormonal fluctuations. All of the above can become stressors and combine with other pre-existing vulnerabilities to increase risk of postpartum depression.

Traditionally, postpartum depression (like depression in general) has been perceived as a women's disorder mainly afflicting new mothers, and issues surrounding paternal postpartum depression were largely ignored by clinicians and researchers (Cox, 2005). However, a growing body of research indicates that the onset of

5.7 Paternal Postpartum Depression

fatherhood is a risk factor for male depression, and that new fathers have elevated rates of depression compared to other men.

For example, a meta-analysis revealed that around 10% of fathers experience prenatal and/or postpartum depression (Paulson & Bazemore, 2010). Interestingly, this meta-analysis found that US studies revealed an average rate of 14%, whereas the average rate found elsewhere was 8%. This is consistent with previously described research indicating higher rates of depression in the USA compared to other countries. Notably, this meta-analysis found the highest rates of paternal postpartum depression during the 3- to 6-month postnatal period, with over 25% of fathers meeting the diagnostic criteria for MDD during this stage.

These high rates of paternal postpartum depression can be attributed to various factors. As said, both parents can experience sleep deprivation and extreme fatigue, which has been linked to postpartum depression in men and women (Scarff, 2019). Moreover, some research indicates that fathers undergo hormonal changes after the birth of a child, including decreased testosterone and increased estrogen (Kim & Swain, 2007). While these changes can increase father-child bonding, decreased testosterone has been linked to an increased risk of depression in men via effects on mood, appetite and libido (Walther et al., 2019; Zarrouf et al., 2009). In other words, men (like women) can experience dramatic hormonal changes in the postpartum period, which can interact with psychosocial factors to lower mood and increase risk.

Indeed, much research indicates that psychosocial factors play a significant role in the aetiology of paternal postpartum depression. For example, one large US population study found that paternal unemployment was the strongest risk factor for paternal postpartum depression, with an adjusted odds ratio of 6.49 (95% CI 4.12–10.22), while poor paternal physical health had an adjusted odds ratio of 3.31 (95% CI 2.50–4.38) (Rosenthal et al., 2013). These findings overlap with the previously described literature on generic depression in men, indicating that disability and unemployment are prominent risk factors that can increase risk of male depression. Of note, these risk factors may be relatively tolerable for childless men, who might become habituated to their own physical and social suffering. But such issues may become particularly conspicuous for new fathers, whose ability to care and provide for their child may be impaired by disability and unemployment, while raising new existential issues about competence and self-worth.

Furthermore, some research indicates that an unintended or unwanted pregnancy can increase risk of paternal postnatal depression (Leathers & Kelley, 2010; Nishimura & Ohashi, 2010). Such pregnancies (and resultant change of parental status) are not always a time of great joy, as they may bring unwanted financial and caregiving obligations that can be very difficult to meet. Of note, a pregnant mother has a right to choose whether she keeps the baby, with numerous options for women unwilling to take on this major new life responsibility, such as abortion or adoption. In contrast, men lack such a right to choose and may be forced to become fathers against their will. Such unwilling fathers may experience a sense of entrapment and defeat, with no escape from these new and unwanted financial and caregiving obligations. Of note, a variety of studies indicate that experiences of entrapment and defeat are risk factors for depression; suggesting a causal mechanism explaining higher rates of paternal postpartum depression among fathers of children arising from an unintended or unwanted pregnancy (Gilbert & Allan, 1998; Panagioti et al., 2012; Kendler et al., 2003).

Despite the increasing research, there remains considerable ignorance about the phenomenon of paternal postpartum depression in clinical practice, as well as in the public mind (Scarff, 2019). For example, paternal postpartum depression is not recognized as an official sub-category of DSM-5, meaning there are no official diagnostic criteria beyond those for MDD. This can have a knock-on effect in clinical training and practice, where issues of paternal postnatal depression are rarely considered (Cox, 2005). Indeed, a recent general population survey found that 97% of respondents were able to identify vignettes of women with postpartum depression, while only 76% identified vignettes of men with postpartum depression – indicating greater public ignorance about paternal postpartum depression (Swami et al., 2019). Of note, respondents possessed more positive attitudes towards female vignettes than male vignettes, implying that men with paternal postpartum depression might incur less empathy and more stigma than women with postpartum depression. All these findings may be indicative of the *gender empathy gap* and the *male gender blindness* discussed in detail in Chap. 1.

In sum, a growing corpus of evidence suggests that paternal postpartum depression is a reality for a notable proportion of men, and is associated with factors such as poor physical health, unemployment and unwanted pregnancies. However, this form of depression is not well-known to the public, and is under-researched and under-acknowledged in clinical practice. This means that there are few specific treatments and a large number of fathers are likely suffering in silence.

5.8 Conclusion

A large corpus of epidemiological research indicates a differential prevalence of depression by gender, with men experiencing depression at about half the rate of women. On the one hand, some researchers have argued that this is a true difference, with men being more resilient to depression due to adaptive coping mechanisms and protective psychological orientations. On the other hand, others have argued that the differential rates are largely artefactual, due to diagnostic and measurement biases failing to capture men with depression. This has led to lively debate about the true nature and prevalence of male depression, leading to the development of new concepts such as *male depressive syndrome* and *paternal postpartum depression*. This debate will continue with the course of time, hopefully shedding more light on a serious disorder that is affecting growing numbers of men in our societies.

References

Addis, M. E. (2008). Gender and depression in men. *Clinical Psychology: Science and Practice, 15*(3), 153–168. https://doi.org/10.1111/j.1468-2850.2008.00125.x

American Psychiatric Association (APA). (2013). Substance-related and addictive disorders. In *In Diagnostic and statistical manual of mental disorders* (5th ed.). Association.

American Psychological Association (APA). (2018, August). APA guidelines for psychological practice with boys and men. *American Psychological Association*. Retrieved July 23, 2020, from https://www.apa.org/about/policy/boys-men-practice-guidelines.pdf

Artazcoz, L., Benach, J., Borrell, C., & Cortès, I. (2004). Unemployment and mental health: Understanding the interactions among gender, family roles, and social class. *American Journal of Public Health (AJPH), 94*(1), 82–88. https://doi.org/10.2105/AJPH.94.1.82

Bailey, R. K., Mokonogho, J., & Kumar, A. (2019). Racial and ethnic differences in depression: Current perspectives. *Neuropsychiatric Disease and Treatment, 15*, 603–609. https://doi.org/10.2147/NDT.S128584

Bengs, C., Johansson, E., Danielsson, U., Lehti, A., & Hammarström, A. (2008). Gendered portraits of depression in Swedish newspapers. *Qualitative Health Research, 18*(7), 962–973. https://doi.org/10.1177/1049732308319825

Blumberg, S. J., Clarke, T. C., Blackwell, D. L. (2015). *Racial and ethnic disparities in men's use of mental health treatments. NCHS data brief no. 206.* National Center for Health Statistics (NCHS). Retrieved July 23, 2020, from https://www.cdc.gov/nchs/data/databriefs/db206.pdf

Case, A., & Deaton, A. (2020). *Deaths of despair and the future of capitalism.* Princeton University Press.

Cox, J. (2005). Postnatal depression in fathers. *The Lancet, 366*(9490), 982. https://doi.org/10.1016/S0140-6736(05)67372-2

Davis, L., Uezato, A., Newell, J., & Frazier, E. (2008). Major depression and comorbid substance use disorders. *Current Opinion in Psychiatry, 21*(1), 14–18. https://doi.org/10.1097/YCO.0b013e3282f32408

Degenhardt, L., & Hall, W. (2001). The relationship between tobacco use, substance-use disorders and mental health: Results from the National Survey of Mental Health and Well-being. *Nicotine & Tobacco Research, 3*(3), 225–234. https://doi.org/10.1080/14622200110050457

Department of Justice Canada. (2000). *Selected statistics on Canadian families and family law: 2nd.* Department of Justice Canada. Retrieved April 20, 2021 from https://www.justice.gc.ca/eng/rp-pr/fl-lf/famil/stat2000/pdf/stats.pdf

Diala, C. C., & Muntaner, C. (2003). Mood and anxiety disorders among rural, urban, and metropolitan residents in the United States. *Community Mental Health Journal, 39*(3), 239–252. https://doi.org/10.1023/A:1023342307323

Eaton, W. W., Shao, H., Nestadt, G., Lee, B. H., Bienvenu, J., & Zandi, P. (2008). Population-based study of first onset and chronicity in major depressive disorder. *JAMA Psychiatry, 65*(5), 513–520. https://doi.org/10.1001/archpsyc.65.5.513

Erickson, J., El-Gabalawy, R., Palitsky, D., Patten, S., Mackenzie, C. S., Stein, M. B., & Sareen, J. (2016). Educational attainment as a protective factor for psychiatric disorders: Findings from a nationally representative longitudinal study. *Depression and Anxiety, 33*(11), 1013–1022. https://doi.org/10.1002/da.22515

Esch, P., Bocquet, V., Pull, C., Couffignal, S., Lehnert, T., Graas, M., Fond-Harmant, L., & Ansseau, M. (2014). The downward spiral of mental disorders and educational attainment: A systematic review on early school leaving. *BMC Psychiatry, 14*(1), 237. https://doi.org/10.1186/s12888-014-0237-4

Ferrari, A. J., Somerville, A. J., Baxter, A. J., Norman, R., Patten, S. B., Vos, T., & Whiteford, H. A. (2013). Global variation in the prevalence and incidence of major depressive disorder: A systematic review of the epidemiological literature. *Psychological Medicine, 43*(3), 471–481. https://doi.org/10.1017/S0033291712001511

Furnham, A., Badmin, N., & Sneade, I. (2002). Body image dissatisfaction: Gender differences in eating attitudes, self-esteem, and reasons for exercise. *The Journal of Psychology, 136*(6), 581–596. https://doi.org/10.1080/00223980209604820

Gathergood, J. (2012). Debt and depression: Causal links and social norm effects. *The Economic Journal, 122*(563), 1094–1114. https://doi.org/10.1111/j.1468-0297.2012.02519.x

Gilbert, P., & Allan, S. (1998). The role of defeat and entrapment (arrested flight) in depression: An exploration of an evolutionary view. *Psychological Medicine, 28*(3), 585–598. https://doi.org/10.1017/s0033291798006710

Gili, M., Roca, M., Basu, S., McKee, M., & Stuckler, D. (2013). The mental health risks of economic crisis in Spain: Evidence from primary care centres, 2006 and 2010. *European Journal of Public Health, 23*(1), 103–108. https://doi.org/10.1093/eurpub/cks035

Grall, T. (2016, January). *Custodial mothers and fathers and their child support: 2013*. United States Census Bureau. Retrieved April 20, 2021, from https://www.census.gov/content/dam/Census/library/publications/2016/demo/P60-255.pdf

Grogan, S. (2017). *Body image: Understanding body dissatisfaction in men, women and children* (3rd ed.). Routledge.

Hart, A. D. (2000). *Unmasking male depression: Recognize the root cause to many problem behaviors such as anger, resentment, abusiveness, silence and sexual compulsions*. Thomas Nelson.

Hess, K., Johnson, S., Hu, X., Li, J., Wu, B., Yu, C., Zhu, H., Jin, C., Chen, M., Gerstle, J., Morgan, M., Friend, M., Satcher Johnson, A., Siddiqi, A., Hernandez, A., the HIV Incidence and Case Surveillance Branch, & the Data Management Team of the Quantitative Sciences and Data Management Branch. (2017). *HIV surveillance report, volume 29. Diagnoses of HIV infection in the United States and dependent areas, 2017*. Centers for Disease Control and Prevention (CDC). Retrieved July 23, 2020, from https://www.cdc.gov/hiv/pdf/library/reports/surveillance/cdc-hiv-surveillance-report-2017-vol-29.pdf

Hirshbein, L. D. (2006). Science, gender, and the emergence of depression in American psychiatry, 1952–1980. *Journal of the History of Medicine and Allied Sciences, 61*(2), 187–216. https://doi.org/10.1093/jhmas/jrj037

Horberg, M. A., Silverberg, M. J., Hurley, L. B., Towner, W. J., Klein, D. B., Bersoff-Matcha, S., Weinberg, W. G., Antoniskis, D., Mogyoros, M., Dodge, W. T., Dobrinich, R., Quesenberry, C. P., & Kovach, D. A. (2008). Effects of depression and selective serotonin reuptake inhibitor use on adherence to highly active antiretroviral therapy and on clinical outcomes in HIV-infected patients. *Journal of Acquired Immune Deficiency Syndromes, 47*(3), 384–390. https://doi.org/10.1097/QAI.0b013e318160d53e

Inaba, A., Thoits, P. A., Ueno, K., Gove, W. R., Evenson, R. J., & Sloan, M. (2005). Depression in the United States and Japan: Gender, marital status, and SES patterns. *Social Science & Medicine, 61*(11), 2280–2292. https://doi.org/10.1016/j.socscimed.2005.07.014

James, S. L., Abate, D., Abate, K. H., Abay, S. M., Abbafati, C., Abbasi, N., Abbastabar, H., Abd-Allah, F., Abdela, J., Abdelalim, A., Abdollahpour, I., Abdulkader, R. S., Abebe, Z., Abera, S. F., Abil, O. Z., Abraha, H. N., Abu-Raddad, L. J., Abu-Rmeileh, N. M. E., Accrombessi, M. M. K., et al. (2018). Global, regional, and national incidence, prevalence, and years lived with disability for 354 diseases and injuries for 195 countries and territories, 1990–2017: A systematic analysis for the Global Burden of Disease Study 2017. *The Lancet, 392*(10159), 1789–1858. https://doi.org/10.1016/S0140-6736(18)32279-7

Jefferis, B. J., Nazareth, I., Marston, L., Moreno-Kustner, B., Bellón, J. Á., Svab, I., Rotar, D., Geerlings, M. I., Xavier, M., Goncalves-Pereira, M., Vincente, B., Saldivia, S., Aluoja, A., Kalda, R., & King, M. (2011). Associations between unemployment and major depressive disorder: evidence from an international, prospective study (the predict cohort). *Social Science & Medicine, 73*(11), 1627–1634. https://doi.org/10.1016/j.socscimed.2011.09.029

Johnson, J. L., Oliffe, J. L., Kelly, M. T., Galdas, P., & Ogrodniczuk, J. S. (2012). Men's discourses of help-seeking in the context of depression. *Sociology of Health & Illness, 34*(3), 345–361. https://doi.org/10.1111/j.1467-9566.2011.01372.x

References

Karazsia, B. T., Murnen, S. K., & Tylka, T. L. (2017). Is body dissatisfaction changing across time? A cross-temporal meta-analysis. *Psychological Bulletin, 143*(3), 293–320. https://doi.org/10.1037/bul0000081

Kendler, K. S., & Gardner, C. O. (2014). Sex differences in the pathways to major depression: a study of opposite-sex twin pairs. *American Journal of Psychiatry, 171*(4), 426–435. https://doi.org/10.1176/appi.ajp.2013.13101375

Kendler, K. S., Hettema, J. M., Butera, F., Gardner, C. O., & Prescott, C. A. (2003). Life event dimensions of loss, humiliation, entrapment, and danger in the prediction of onsets of major depression and generalized anxiety. *JAMA Psychiatry, 60*(8), 789–796. https://doi.org/10.1001/archpsyc.60.8.789

Kim, P., & Swain, J. E. (2007). Sad dads: Paternal postpartum depression. *Psychiatry (Edgmont), 4*(2), 35–47.

King, M., Semlyen, J., Tai, S. S., Killaspy, H., Osborn, D., Popelyuk, D., & Nazareth, I. (2008). A systematic review of mental disorder, suicide, and deliberate self harm in lesbian, gay and bisexual people. *BMC Psychiatry, 8*, 70. https://doi.org/10.1186/1471-244X-8-70

Kposowa, A. J. (2003). Divorce and suicide risk. *Journal of Epidemiology & Community Health, 57*(12), 993. https://doi.org/10.1136/jech.57.12.993

Leathers, S. J., & Kelley, M. A. (2010). Unintended pregnancy and depressive symptoms among first-time mothers and fathers. *American Journal of Orthopsychiatry, 70*(4), 523–531. https://doi.org/10.1037/h0087671

Lee, C., Oliffe, J. L., Kelly, M. T., & Ferlatte, O. (2017). Depression and suicidality in gay men: Implications for health care providers. *American Journal of Men's Health, 11*(4), 910–919. https://doi.org/10.1177/1557988316685492

Lorant, V., Deliège, D., Eaton, W., Robert, A., Philippot, P., & Ansseau, M. (2003). Socioeconomic inequalities in depression: A meta-analysis. *American Journal of Epidemiology, 157*(2), 98–112. https://doi.org/10.1093/aje/kwf182

Martin, L. A., Neighbors, H. W., & Griffith, D. M. (2013). The experience of symptoms of depression in men vs women: Analysis of the National Comorbidity Survey Replication. *JAMA Psychiatry, 70*(10), 1100–1106. https://doi.org/10.1001/jamapsychiatry.2013.1985

McMullin, J. A., & Cairney, J. (2004). Self-esteem and the intersection of age, class, and gender. *Journal of Aging Studies, 18*(1), 75–90. https://doi.org/10.1016/j.jaging.2003.09.006

Meltzer, H., Bebbington, P., Brugha, T., Jenkins, R., McManus, S., & Stansfeld, S. (2010). Job insecurity, socio-economic circumstances and depression. *Psychological Medicine, 40*(8), 1401. https://doi.org/10.1017/S0033291709991802

Modini, M., Joyce, S., Mykletun, A., Christensen, H., Bryant, R. A., Mitchell, P. B., & Harvey, S. B. (2016). The mental health benefits of employment: Results of a systematic meta-review. *Australasian Psychiatry, 24*(4), 331–336. https://doi.org/10.1177/1039856215618523

Munce, S. E., Robertson, E. K., Sansom, S. N., & Stewart, D. E. (2004). Who is portrayed in psychotropic drug advertisements? *The Journal of Nervous and Mental Disease, 192*(4), 284–288. https://doi.org/10.1097/01.nmd.0000120887.30063.9b

Nishimura, A., & Ohashi, K. (2010). Risk factors of paternal depression in the early postnatal period in Japan. *Nursing & Health Sciences, 12*(2), 170–176. https://doi.org/10.1111/j.1442-2018.2010.00513.x

Nolen-Hoeksema, S. (1987). Sex differences in unipolar depression: Evidence and theory. *Psychological Bulletin, 101*(2), 259–282. https://doi.org/10.1037/0033-2909.101.2.259

Nolen-Hoeksema, S. (2003). *Women who think too much: How to break free of overthinking and reclaim your life.*. Macmillan.

Nolen-Hoeksema, S., & Girgus, J. S. (1994). The emergence of gender differences in depression during adolescence. *Psychological Bulletin, 115*(3), 424–443. https://doi.org/10.1037/0033-2909.115.3.424

Office for National Statistics (2019, December 2). *Disability and employment, UK: 2019*. Office for National Statistics. Retrieved July 23, 2020, from https://www.ons.gov.uk/peoplepopulationandcommunity/healthandsocialcare/disability/bulletins/disabilityandemploymentuk/2019#:~:

text=Labour%20Force%20Survey%20(LFS)%20data,%25%20for%20non%2Ddisabled%20 people.

Oliffe, J. L., & Phillips, M. J. (2008). Men, depression and masculinities: A review and recommendations. *Journal of Men's Health, 5*(3), 194–202. https://doi.org/10.1016/j.jomh.2008.03.016

Panagioti, M., Gooding, P., & Tarrier, N. (2012). Hopelessness, defeat, and entrapment in post-traumatic stress disorder: Their association with suicidal behavior and severity of depression. *The Journal of Nervous and Mental Disease, 200*(8), 676–683. https://doi.org/10.1097/NMD.0b013e3182613f91

Patten, S. B. (2001). Long-term medical conditions and major depression in a Canadian population study at waves 1 and 2. *Journal of Affective Disorders, 63*(1-3), 35–41. https://doi.org/10.1016/S0165-0327(00)00186-5

Paulson, J. F., & Bazemore, S. D. (2010). Prenatal and postpartum depression in fathers and its association with maternal depression: A meta-analysis. *JAMA, 303*(19), 1961–1969. https://doi.org/10.1001/jama.2010.605

Pearson, C., Janz, T., & Ali, J. (2013, September). *Health at a glance: Mental and substance use disorders in Canada*. Statistics Canada. Retrieved July 23, 2020, from https://www150.statcan.gc.ca/n1/en/pub/82-624-x/2013001/article/11855-eng.pdf?st=zKUFXIsh

Public Health Agency of Canada. (2016, June 2). *Report from the Canadian Chronic Disease Surveillance System: Mood and anxiety disorders in Canada, 2016*. Government of Canada. Retrieved July 23, 2020, from https://www.canada.ca/en/public-health/services/publications/diseases-conditions/report-canadian-chronic-disease-surveillance-system-mood-anxiety-disorders-canada-2016.html

Quiroga, C. V., Janosz, M., Bisset, S., & Morin, A. J. S. (2013). Early adolescent depression symptoms and school dropout: Mediating processes involving self-reported academic competence and achievement. *Journal of Educational Psychology, 105*(2), 552–560. https://doi.org/10.1037/a0031524

Rabkin, J. G. (2008). HIV and depression: 2008 review and update. *Current HIV/AIDS Reports, 5*, 163–171. https://doi.org/10.1007/s11904-008-0025-1

Remes, O., Lafortune, L., Wainwright, N., Surtees, P., Khaw, K. T., & Brayne, C. (2019). Association between area deprivation and major depressive disorder in British men and women: A cohort study. *BMJ Open, 9*(11), 1–12. https://doi.org/10.1136/bmjopen-2018-027530

Richards, D. (2011). Prevalence and clinical course of depression: a review. *Clinical Psychology Review, 31*(7), 1117–1125. https://doi.org/10.1016/j.cpr.2011.07.004

Rosenthal, D. G., Learned, N., Liu, Y., & Weitzman, M. (2013). Characteristics of fathers with depressive symptoms. *Maternal and Child Health Journal, 17*, 119–128. https://doi.org/10.1007/s10995-012-0955-5

Ross, C. E., & Mirowsky, J. (2006). Sex differences in the effect of education on depression: Resource multiplication or resource substitution? *Social Science & Medicine, 63*(5), 1400–1413. https://doi.org/10.1016/j.socscimed.2006.03.013

Rotermann, M. (2007). Marital breakdown and subsequent depression. *Health Reports, 18*(2), 33–44.

Sargent, J. T., Crocker, J., & Luhtanen, R. K. (2006). Contingencies of self-worth and depressive symptoms in college students. *Journal of Social and Clinical Psychology, 25*(6), 628–646. https://doi.org/10.1521/jscp.2006.25.6.628

Sbarra, D. A., Emery, R. E., Beam, C. R., & Ocker, B. L. (2014). Marital dissolution and major depression in midlife: A propensity score analysis. *Clinical Psychological Science, 2*(3), 249–257. https://doi.org/10.1177/2167702613498727

Scarff, J. R. (2019). Postpartum depression in men. *Innovations in Clinical Neuroscience, 16*(5-6), 11–14.

Scott, K. M., Wells, J. E., Angermeyer, M., Brugha, T. S., Bromet, E., Demyttenaere, K., de Girolamo, G., Gureje, O., Haro, J. M., Jin, R., Nasser Karam, A., Kovess, V., Lara, C., Levinson, D., Ormel, J., Posada-Villa, J., Sampson, N., Takeshima, T., Zhang, M., & Kessler, R. C. (2010). Gender and the relationship between marital status and first onset of mood,

References

anxiety and substance use disorders. *Psychological Medicine, 40*(9), 1495–1505. https://doi.org/10.1017/S0033291709991942

Smith, D. T., Mouzon, D. M., & Elliott, M. (2018). Reviewing the assumptions about men's mental health: An exploration of the gender binary. *American Journal of Men's Health, 12*(1), 78–89. https://doi.org/10.1177/1557988316630953

Swami, V., Barron, D., Smith, L., & Furnham, A. (2019). Mental health literacy of maternal and paternal postnatal (postpartum) depression in British adults. *Journal of Mental Health, 29*(2), 217–224. https://doi.org/10.1080/09638237.2019.1608932

Szymanski, D. M., & Henning, S. L. (2007). The role of self-objectification in women's depression: A test of objectification theory. *Sex Roles, 56*, 43–53. https://doi.org/10.1007/s11199-006-9147-3

Tiffin, P., Pearce, M., & Parker, L. (2005). Social mobility over the lifecourse and self reported mental health at age 50: Prospective cohort study. *Journal of Epidemiology & Community Health, 59*(1), 870–872. https://doi.org/10.1136/jech.2005.035246

US Bureau of Labor Statistics. (2020a, December 16). Table 1. Fatal occupational injuries by selected demographic characteristics, 2015-19. Retrieved March 12, 2021, from https://www.bls.gov/news.release/cfoi.t01.htm

US Bureau of Labor Statistics. (2020b, November 4). Table EH1. Number of nonfatal occupational injuries and illnesses involving days away from work by selected worker and case characteristics and medical treatment facility visits, all U.S., private industry, 2019. Retrieved March 12, 2021, from https://www.bls.gov/iif/oshwc/osh/case/cd_eh1_2019.htm

US Social Security Administration. (2020, October). *Annual statistical report on the social security disability insurance program, 2019.* Retrieved March 12, 2021, from https://www.ssa.gov/policy/docs/statcomps/di_asr/2019/

van der Noordt, M., Ijzelenberg, H., Droomers, M., & Proper, K. I. (2014). Health effects of employment: A systematic review of prospective studies. *Occupational and Environmental Medicine, 71*(10), 730–736. https://doi.org/10.1136/oemed-2013-101891

Walther, A., Breidenstein, J., & Miller, R. (2019). Association of testosterone treatment with alleviation of depressive symptoms in men: A systematic review and meta-analysis. *JAMA Psychiatry, 76*(1), 31–40. https://doi.org/10.1001/jamapsychiatry.2018.2734

Wang, P. S., Berglund, P., Olfson, M., Pincus, H. A., Wells, K. B., & Kessler, R. C. (2005). Failure and delay in initial treatment contact after first onset of mental disorders in the National Comorbidity Survey Replication. *Archives of General Psychiatry, 62*(6), 603–613. https://doi.org/10.1001/archpsyc.62.6.603

Whitley, R. (2013). Fear and loathing in New England: Examining the health-care perspectives of homeless people in rural areas. *Anthropology & Medicine, 20*(3), 232–243. https://doi.org/10.1080/13648470.2013.853597

Wight, R. G., LeBlanc, A. J., & Badgett, M. V. L. (2013). Same-sex legal marriage and psychological well-being: Findings from the California Health Interview Survey. *American Journal of Public Health, 103*(2), 339–346. https://doi.org/10.2105/AJPH.2012.301113

Williams, D. R., González, H. M., Neighbors, H., Nesse, R., Abelson, J. M., Sweetman, J., & Jackson, J. S. (2007). Prevalence and distribution of major depressive disorder in African Americans, Caribbean Blacks, and Non-Hispanic Whites: Results from the National Survey of American Life. *Archives of General Psychiatry, 64*(3), 305–315. https://doi.org/10.1001/archpsyc.64.3.305

Winkler, D., Pjrek, E., & Kasper, S. (2005). Anger attacks in depression–Evidence for a male depressive syndrome. *Psychotherapy and Psychosomatics, 74*, 303–307. https://doi.org/10.1159/000086321

Winkler, D., Pjrek, E., & Kasper, S. (2006). Gender-specific symptoms of depression and anger attacks. *Journal of Men's Health, 3*(1), 19–24. https://doi.org/10.1016/j.jmhg.2005.05.004

Zarrouf, F. A., Artz, S., Griffith, J., Sirbu, C., & Martin, K. (2009). Testosterone and depression: Systematic review and meta-analysis. *Journal of Psychiatric Practice, 15*(4), 289–305. https://doi.org/10.1097/01.pra.0000358315.88931.fc

Chapter 6
Why Do Men Have Low Rates of Formal Mental Health Service Utilization? An Analysis of Social and Systemic Barriers to Care and Discussion of Promising Male-Friendly Practices

Health care is typically divided into the informal (or popular) sector and the formal (or professional) sector (Brown et al., 2014; World Health Organization, 2003; Kleinman, 1980). The informal healthcare sector consists of advice, remedies, or services provided by lay nonprofessionals including family, friends, religious organizations, ethnocultural healing, alternative medicine, or peer services delivered by grassroots bottom-up community organizations. An example of an informal healthcare service is Alcoholics Anonymous and similar 12-step peer support programs. Another example is spiritual ceremonies common in Aboriginal communities such as sweat lodges and healing circles. Evidence suggests that a substantial number of people with mental health difficulties use aspects of the informal sector of health care including self-help groups, folk remedies, and spiritual healing (Barnes et al., 2004; Unützer et al., 2000; Eisenberg et al., 1998).

In contrast to such lay nonprofessional approaches, formal health care is typically delivered by a range of accredited and licensed professionals with formal training and advanced degrees. These professionals typically work from formal clinics or hospitals and often receive public funding for their work, meaning their activity is officially supported and sanctioned by the state. In the case of mental health, these professionals include psychiatrists, psychologists, social workers, therapists, general practitioners, and a variety of other adjunct professionals.

Formal health care is often divided into primary care, secondary care, and tertiary care. Typically, the first point of contact for people with mental health difficulties is *primary care* clinics staffed by general practitioners or family doctors. These clinics will often manage more moderate cases of mental illness such as anxiety and depression (known as *common mental disorders*), mainly by dispensing the appropriate medication alongside concomitant lifestyle advice. More serious cases of mental disorder such as schizophrenia, bipolar disorder, or major depression (known as *severe mental illnesses*) are typically referred to *secondary care* services staffed by specialist clinicians such as psychiatrists, psychologists, and social workers, who are equipped to give the appropriate diagnosis and treatment. These are typically delivered from dedicated small-scale clinics and are often focused on the delivery of specialist outpatient services including talk therapies, polypharmacy, and psychosocial interventions. *Tertiary care* services are typically delivered from large-scale mental hospitals, or acute care psychiatric wards within general hospitals, and mainly deal with psychiatric crises through emergency inpatient care. They are typically staffed by psychiatrists and psychiatric nurses, focusing on stabilization during acute episodes or psychiatric crises.

Interestingly, evidence suggests that less than half of people with a mental illness use any of the above-described formal mental health services to help with their disorder. In a seminal large-scale US epidemiological study, Wang et al. (2005) found that only 41% of people with a mental disorder received some treatment in the last 12 months. These results overlap with another large-scale US study finding that only 33% of people with a mental disorder received treatment (Kessler et al., 2005). Another landmark large-scale US study found that less than 40% of people with substance use disorder received any treatment for their disorder (Compton et al., 2007). A large-scale Canadian study found that only 45% of people self-reporting depression had contact with the health system for mental health reasons in the past 12 months (Smith et al., 2013). More recently, the US National Survey on Drug Use and Health indicates that 46% of young adults get no treatment for any mental disorder, while 36% percent of adults per se get no treatment for severe mental illnesses (Substance Abuse and Mental Health Services Administration, 2019). These data indicate that people with more severe mental illnesses such as schizophrenia are more likely to receive treatment, in comparison with common mental disorders such as anxiety and depression.

Importantly, there are clear gender differentials in formal mental health service utilization, with considerable research indicating that males underutilize formal mental health services when compared with females, even when controlling for the presence of mental disorder (Addis & Mahalik, 2003). Precise figures describing gender differentials in formal mental health service use for depression (see Chap. 5) and substance use disorder (see Chap. 3) were described in detail in previous chapters, but a quick recap will be given here as a refresher. In sum, research from a variety of jurisdictions indicates that men with a mental illness are much less likely to use formal mental health services than females with a mental illness. For example, a large-scale Canadian study of over 100,000 individuals found odds ratios showing that females were 2.7 times more likely (95% CI: 2.3–3.1) to use mental health services than males (McDonald et al., 2017). These data are consistent with another Canadian study noting that 22% of women with depression had used a mental health service in the past year, compared with 13% of men, meaning that females were more than 60% more likely to use these services (Smith et al., 2013). In the United States, the aforementioned Wang et al. (2005) study found that women with a mental illness were 60% more likely than men to receive treatment for mental illness in the last 12 months, while the Kessler et al. (2005) study also found that women were 70% more likely to receive services (OR 1.7; 95% CI: 1.4–1.9). An Australian study revealed a massive gender disparity in service use, finding that only 13% of young men (aged 16–24) sought help for a mental health issue, compared with 31% of similarly aged young women (Slade et al., 2009). Another

Australian study of all age groups indicated that 55% of women with a substance use disorder (SUD) use mental health services (95% CI: 51.6%–57.9%), compared with 40% of men with a SUD (95% CI: 36.1%–44.3%), meaning that women in this study were 37% more likely than men to receive treatment for a SUD (Harris et al., 2015). A review of the British literature notes that around one woman in four with depression will receive treatment, compared with one man in ten (Wilkins, 2015). Moreover, stratified analysis within several of the aforementioned studies indicates that this gender differential exists across all ages, socioeconomic backgrounds and ethno-racial groups, meaning that underutilization is an issue affecting many men from many different demographics (Addis & Mahalik, 2003).

6.1 Masculinity and Men's Formal Service Use

Formal mental health service underutilization in men is typically attributed to dominant notions of masculinity that are internalized by men, leading them to avoid these mental health services (Oliffe & Phillips, 2008; Möller-Leimkühler, 2003; Courtenay, 2000a, 2000b). Indeed, this is perhaps the most common explanation of mental health service underutilization in men in both the professional literature and the popular mind. According to this argument, dominant notions of masculinity are part of the collective consciousness and circulate throughout society, which colors the beliefs and actions of individual men of all backgrounds (Canetto & Sakinofsky, 1998). These dominant notions are mainly centered on the idea that the "ideal man" is strong, stable, and self-sufficient, displaying "true grit" resilience in the face of adversity. It has been argued that such notions are internalized by many men, leading them to respond to mental distress with an allegedly dysfunctional silence and stoicism. In this argument, men are stubbornly opposed to using mental health services as such usage could be considered a sign of weakness and an implicit acknowledgement that a man has failed to live up to masculine norms of strength and self-sufficiency. For example, a man with depression may be socially conditioned to feel that "real men" shut-up and "man-up" in the face of adversity, rather than disclose and discuss their issues with clinicians, family, or friends.

In this argument, the responsibility for mental health service underutilization is put squarely on men's shoulders, inasmuch as they are depicted as self-destructively stubborn and silent in the face of adversity. This is sometimes intensified by a parallel and related discourse that focuses on men's alleged lack of mental health literacy or absence of emotional awareness. For example, the authors of a small study in Ireland state that barriers to men's help-seeking for mental health include "denial of emotions and low mental health literacy…gender socialization and macho ideals further inhibit propensities to seek help" (Lynch et al., 2018, p. 139). Similarly, Smith et al. (2013) speculate that women had higher rates of health service use for self-reported depression than men because "women may be more health conscious, more aware of symptoms and may be better at translating feelings of distress into problem recognition" (p. 1568).

This discourse often adopts monocausal language, with male underutilization overwhelmingly attributed to men's alleged psychological deficits, deriving from warped gender norms that create a dysfunctional "toxic" masculinity. This narrow deficit-based focus has been criticized by a growing number of scholars working in men's health research in recent years. For example, Englar-Carlson (2019) reports that too much research on men's mental health is "skewed towards negative traits and the negative functioning of men." As explained in more detail in Chap. 1, other scholars have argued that this deficit-based discourse can sometimes adopt an unhelpful finger-pointing victim-blaming approach that ignores the wider social determinants of men's tendency to under-utilize mental health services (Whitley, 2018). Indeed, a growing body of research indicates that male underutilization of formal mental health care is caused by a variety of factors, which are insufficiently considered in narrow discussions focused on notions of masculinity. Two factors are particularly important. First, wider contextual issues related to mental health stigma can colour and shape men's willingness to engage with mental health services. Second, the nature and configuration of many formal mental health services may be unappealing to men, leading them to explore and utilize alternatives in the informal healthcare sector. These factors are explored below, moving the focus beyond these mythically stubborn, silent, and stoical men to examine important aspects of social context.

6.2 Stigma

Mental illness and the associated use of mental health services still incurs considerable stigma (Gaebel et al., 2017). This stigma is commonly divided into two dimensions: internal (or self) stigma and external (or public) stigma (Link & Phelan, 2001). Internal stigma refers to private feelings of shame and worthlessness held by stigmatized individuals, often leading to social withdrawal and low self-esteem. External stigma refers to negative attitudes and prejudicial stereotypes held by the community at large, often leading to rejection and discrimination. A key finding from the research literature is that men with mental health issues may face particularly intense stigma (Chatmon, 2020).

As previously stated, much discourse on men's mental health focuses on the internal psychology of affected men, who are often depicted as self-destructively stubborn and silent in the face of mental illness. This implies that men with mental health issues experience high-levels of internal self-stigma. While this may be true, wider research indicates that internal self-stigma is often determined by external public stigma (Stuart et al., 2014; Whitley & Campbell, 2014). In other words, internal stigma is downstream of external stigma; however, this has not been properly acknowledged or documented in the men's mental health literature. This is important to discuss, given that evidence suggests that external stigma toward men with mental health issues exists across various influential sectors of society such as: (i) the media, (ii) the workplace. (iii) the family, and (iv) healthcare providers. Negative attitudes and prejudicial stereotypes in these environments may be playing an underacknowledged role in deterring men from disclosing their mental health issues and seeking help from services. As such, they are discussed in detail in the following subsections.

6.2.1 Stigma in the Media

Research implies that media portrayals of socioeconomic groups can shape wider public beliefs and attitudes (Wahl, 2012). In fact, considerable research indicates that the media has contributed to negative stereotypes and prejudices toward all people with mental illness, regardless of gender (Corrigan et al., 2004). However, some research indicates that men with mental illness are portrayed very differently to women with mental illness in the media. For example, a study of Swedish newspaper coverage of depression found that the media tended to criticize, belittle, and berate men for their silence and unwillingness to seek help, while offering more empathic portrayals of women with depression (Bengs et al., 2008). Similarly, a Canadian study found that articles about women with mental illness tended to be much more positive and empathic, while articles about men with mental illness tended to contain much more stigmatizing content, and linked men's mental illness to crime and violence (Whitley et al., 2015).

This is an important finding, as these media portrayals can contribute to a wider climate of fear where men with mental health issues are stereotyped as a physical threat with the potential to "snap" at any moment. Indeed, an Australian study found that the public tended to express more stigmatizing and fearful attitudes toward vignettes of men with mental illness in comparison with vignettes of women with mental illness (Reavley & Jorm, 2011). Given this situation, men may legitimately worry that their family, friends, and colleagues will react with fear, suspicion, and rejection if they reveal mental health issues. Indeed, this is a common sentiment among men with mental illness (Whitley, 2016) poignantly summarized in a quote from a study participant:

> People, they have fear....They think, "That man there, he is crazy. He could kill us!" They think, "He is not like us!" They think you are lower than them. If I say to some, "Yes, I am schizophrenic," for sure they are going to have another idea of me. I am scared of saying that to people. I do not want them to judge me.

Such legitimate worries of rejection may deter disclosure to others and formal mental healthcare service utilization among men with mental health issues. These issues of stereotyping and rejection are core to the next sections of this chapter as well.

6.2.2 Stigma in the Workplace

Another sector of society, which may contribute toward men's reluctance to use mental health services, is the workplace. As explained in greater detail in Chap. 8, men are still typically the primary breadwinner for themselves and their families, and their income is necessary to rear children, pay bills, and repay a mortgage (Klesment & Van Bavel, 2015). Maintaining gainful employment and being considered a productive and reliable employee is thus a key priority for working-age men. This priority can affect formal mental health service use for many men in a variety of ways.

To start, many men experience heavy workloads and onerous demands in the workplace, with research indicating that the average man works significantly more hours per week than the average woman. For example, one Canadian study found that men work 40 hours per week on average, while women work 33 hours per week (Statistics Canada, 2007). Men with mental health issues may be justifiably worried that taking time off to access mental health services will affect their income, their reputation, and their career prospects. Indeed, evidence suggests that employers may resent men taking time off for mental health reasons, fueled by stereotypes that equate mental illness with malingering, hypochondria, and laziness (Ashfield & Gouws, 2019).

Such stereotypes can be compounded in certain male-dominated workplaces such as the police and the military, where people with mental health difficulties may be considered physically dangerous, unpredictable, a threat to unit morale, and unfit for service (Dallaire, 2019; Linford, 2013). Indeed, a mental health issue in the military or the police will often be noted on an individual's employment file and monitored by superior officers. This can lead to negative outcomes including redeployment to undesired tasks or being overlooked for promotion, which can lead to general professional stagnation or even medical discharge. Such processes of rejection – fueled by the above-described media-driven stereotypes – may occur in other male-dominated occupations where there is access to hazardous materials and a reliance on harmonious teamwork such as mining, oil/gas, transport, manufacturing, or security (Scheid, 2005; Seaton et al., 2019).

In other words, men in mental distress may have legitimate fears that emotional disclosure and the associated use of formal mental health services can severely damage their employment status and future job opportunities. This can negatively affect their job retention, promotion prospects, and career advancement. Men can be well aware that seeking help may have these dire secondary consequences and may make a calculated cost-benefit analysis, deciding that the social costs of using services outweighs the potential mental health benefits. Again, these processes have been overlooked in the men's mental health literature, which has instead taken a deficit-based approach by focusing on the alleged negative impact of workplace "masculine culture" and the "constraints of masculinity" as deterrents for service use in working men (O'Brien et al., 2005).

6.2.3 Stigma in the Family

Another sector of society, which may affect men's desire to disclose mental health issues and use formal mental health services, is the family. To be sure, some research indicates that the immediate family can be an important source of support and solace for people with mental illness and can be an active agent in the recovery process (Aldersey & Whitley, 2015). That said, evidence suggests that some family members can perceive mental illness as a source of shame that is potentially ruinous to familial reputation. This can lead to attempts to deny or conceal any mental health difficulties, again deterring disclosure or help-seeking in the affected men.

Parents, siblings, and even spouses can be complicit in this silence. For example, Affleck et al. (2018) conducted a research study finding that husbands with mental illness frequently reported negative and unsympathetic comments from their wives. This was especially so if the mental illness interfered with the man's bread-winning abilities. In fact, wives seemed acutely aware that mental health difficulties would lead to stigma in the workplace, which could affect family income and economic security. As such, they exerted pressure on their husbands to "man up" and conceal the illness. Some men in the study reported that they tried but failed to continue life as normal in order to appease their wives, with devastating consequences as evidenced in the following quote:

> I lost the respect of my wife as I continue to fail in my duties. She lost trust in me. I am extremely sad when I hear the sentence "Are you a man?" and "Are you a husband?" from my wife. I want to die. I want to commit suicide.

6.2.4 Stigma in Health Services

A final yet obviously important sector of society that can affect men's mental health service utilization relates to the nature and configuration of formal health services. Worryingly, some research indicates that formal healthcare providers themselves can hold stigmatizing attitudes toward people with mental illness, which may be particularly intense toward males in distress.

For example, a study found that 44% of mental health service users report major discrimination in their interactions with the UK mental healthcare system (Gabbidon et al., 2014). In a study of low-income men with mental distress living in rural New England, participants reported several negative encounters with healthcare professionals, with one stating that "whenever I would go in there [a local hospital], they treated me like a drunk, and I don't drink!" (Whitley, 2013).

Indeed, a growing literature indicates that a massive factor explaining men's under-utilization of formal mental health services is the nature and configuration of such services. Again, this has been underplayed and underemphasized in both the scientific literature and the popular mind, which has instead focused on concepts of "masculinity" as the key factor explaining such underutilization. Given this literature, the rest of this chapter will focus on mental health services in detail, examining underlying issues, and key findings vis-à-vis provision of services for men.

6.3 Formal Mental Health Services: An Unwelcoming Environment?

A growing corpus of research indicates that the environment, language, and ambience of much formal mental health care is "feminized." Indeed, prominent Canadian researchers recently concluded from decades of relevant research that "a lot of guys have the perception that current mental health services are set up mainly to serve women...there are aspects of how services are delivered, and even the language that is used, that fail to resonate with men" (Ogrodniczuk et al., 2016). This argument has been made elsewhere. In 2014, a team of UK researchers wrote a stimulating academic paper entitled "Are mental health services inherently feminised?" (Morison et al., 2014). In this paper, the authors note that the mental health workforce is female-dominated, which can contribute to a "feminised" environment, which may be off-putting to some men. For example, they marshal statistics from the United Kingdom indicating that around 80% of clinicians who provide formal psychological services are women. This lack of male clinicians has been identified as problematic by the British Psychological Society, which has officially categorized men as an underrepresented group among clinical psychologists, making conscious effort to recruit more men into that field (Bullen & Hughes, 2016). Such efforts have met with limited success, as a recent report indicates that men make up around 15% of new clinical psychology trainees in the United Kingdom (Liddon et al., 2018). This situation means that the many men with mental health issues who prefer to consult a male clinician may have difficulties meeting their preference.

Similar issues have been raised regarding the primary care environment, which is often the first point of access for men with mental health issues. For example, Banks (2001) discusses the typical GP clinic in the United Kingdom, stating that men "often find it male unfriendly. There are few male receptionists and practice nurses...waiting rooms display all the propaganda of women's and children's health, but there are few if any examples for men." Such a finding is consistent with the results from a thematic analysis of interviews with key players involved in men's mental health in the United Kingdom, with experts stating that mental health services including GP practices were "feminised or unfamiliar environments and therefore off-putting for many men and boys" (Robertson et al., 2015). A similar conclusion was made by men's mental health researchers in Canada, with Oliffe & Phillips (2008) stating that "men's experiences of healthcare institutions and interactions with professionals may dissuade them from accessing services."

The aforementioned literature describes how the "face" of services and the general ambience of formal mental health care (including GPs) tends to be "feminized," but what happens to men who make it through the door to an official clinical consult? Interestingly, research indicates that men are typically treated differently to women during a clinician–patient interaction. For example, clinicians tend to spend significantly more time (on average) in a consultation with women than with men, and men are significantly less likely to receive detailed explanation or advice about changing behaviors (Barry et al., 2019; Courtenay, 2000a). Indeed, Courtenay (2000a) details a whole corpus of research that consistently indicates that clinicians:

(i) Spend more time with female patients than male patients.
(ii) Provide shorter and fewer explanations to male patients compared with female patients.
(iii) Give more advice to female patients than male patients.

This review of the literature led Courtenay (2000a) to conclude that "no study has ever found that women received less information from physicians than men" (p. 1395), a finding that holds true in the present (Barry et al., 2019).

The reasons why men tend to be treated more curtly than women are manifold. Researchers from the UK Men's Health Forum argue that the whole mental health infrastructure is typically insensitive to men's needs, concluding that "the structure and style of services has tended to become better attuned to the needs of women" (Wilkins, 2015). Furthermore, it has been noted that there is little training in men's mental health for mental health clinicians, and attention to gender issues in clinical training and education typically means attention to women's issues (Whitley, 2018). This means that clinicians are not trained to recognize and address men's issues in the clinic and the preponderance of female clinicians means a lack of lived experience of men's issues. This can signify and perpetuate the male gender blindness discussed in Chap. 1, where men's issues and unique life experiences are overlooked or ignored in clinical care (Seager & Barry, 2019). Indeed, this was a key finding from a focus group study, with Ellis et al. (2013) finding that young men had a range of negative attitudes to mental health professionals, who they perceived to be out of touch, with different life experiences and rarely "down-to-earth." They also doubted their ability to help, believing they could get similar support for free from the informal healthcare sector, including friends, family, or online support.

Worse still, numerous authors have noted that clinicians can sometimes adopt a finger-pointing attitude toward male patients with mental health issues, a manifestation of the aforementioned victim-blaming approach that plagues men's mental health. This can be seen in the recently released (and much criticized) American Psychological Association (2018) guidelines for psychological practice with boys and men, which takes a deficit-based approach to men's mental health by consistently pathologizing elements of traditional masculinity such as "achievement," "adventure," and "success." Such documents can guide clinicians to take a "blaming and shaming" approach, which can be a dissonant experience for a man seeking help. Indeed, one expert notes that "too often, service providers start from a position that men are to blame for their predicament and enter the work with an agenda to fix the problem that is men…men will intuitively uncover this value base and either not engage or promptly disengage" (Robertson et al., 2018).

6.4 The Different Modalities of Healing

Decades of research indicate that there are many different modalities of healing in the face of mental distress. In formal mental health care, the two most commonly employed modalities of healing are prescription medication (which aims to reduce symptoms) and a variety of one-on-one talk-therapies (such as cognitive-behavioral therapy), which allow patients to talk about their experiences and feelings, as well as set goals and plans for the future. In the case of informal mental health care, there are many different modalities of healing including self-help groups, religious/spiritual healing, physical exercise/activity, and various "ecotherapies" such as wilderness/bushcraft activities, horticultural therapy, and animal-assisted therapies.

Importantly, a variety of surveys indicate that men and women tend to have different preferences regarding these various forms of mental healing. In short, women tend to show a preference for formal approaches such as talk-therapies and prescription medications, while men tend to prefer informal approaches such as self-help groups and action-oriented forms of healing (Bilsker et al., 2018). For example, Liddon et al. (2018) conducted a survey finding that women (52%) were significantly more likely than men (27%) to want to use prescription medication, also finding that women prefer psychotherapy, counselling, and talking with friends more than men. These findings are consistent with a variety of other studies indicating that women have significantly more positive attitudes toward seeking formal psychological help compared with men, as well as significantly greater openness to talking about their issues (Mackenzie et al., 2006). In other words, many women prefer to talk, while many men prefer to act.

In fact, considerable research indicates that men in mental distress prefer interventions focused on "doing," particularly those that are: (i) action oriented, (ii) solution-focused, (iii) informal, (iv) group oriented, and (v) involve the acquisition of new skills (Ellis et al., 2013; Robertson et al., 2018; Patrick & Robertson, 2016; Sagar-Ouriaghli et al., 2019; Liddon et al., 2018; Struszczyk et al., 2019). For example, Emslie et al. (2007) conducted a qualitative study of men with depression, finding that participants prefer practical and problem-focused interventions, rather than simply talking about their feelings and emotional disclosure. Similarly, Lynch et al. (2018) note that young men prefer more informal action-oriented interventions to address mental health issues (such as youth clubs), which can provide a "supportive informal environment [that] could tackle service-related and personal barriers." These findings are consistent with several recent review papers, which concluded that men frequently prefer informal goal-directed action-oriented interventions that focus on "doing" as much as "talking" (Brown et al., 2019; Seidler et al., 2019; Wilkins, 2015; Wyllie et al., 2012). This can include interventions that are exercise-based, sports-based, crafts-based, or adventure-based, which are often considered preferable than the face-to-face talking that is dominant in formal mental healthcare settings.

Indeed, Robertson et al. (2018) note that "for most men, an initial focus on activity rather than talking is a safer way to facilitate engagement," and experts Dr John

Barry and Dr Damien Ridge note that "it is helpful if the focus of group work be on doing activities, rather than group talking. This allows men to open up and talk gradually and naturally" (quoted in Robertson et al., 2015). Indeed, a review of male suicide prevention interventions notes that informal action-based or community-based interventions are particularly engaging to men, precisely because they adopt a subtle and discrete approach to mental health that emphasizes the activities per se, rather than talking about feelings and emotion (Struszczyk et al., 2019). This is sometimes known as a "health by stealth" approach, as it foregrounds the activities and potential psychosocial benefits, rather than emphasizing "mental health" per se. In sum, action-oriented interventions can provide multiple benefits including:

(i) Tapping into typical male interests and drives that can engage men to join in.
(ii) Providing a hook that can entice men into a supportive mental health promoting setting, while removing initial pressure to rapidly talk and open up.
(iii) Imparting valuable social connectedness and peer support when such activities occur in a group setting.

Importantly, many of the aforementioned studies indicate the importance of group activity to promote men's mental health. These interventions typically have a double-benefit inasmuch as they provide valuable peer-support from others in recovery and new social connections and friendships. For example, Liddon et al. (2018) found that significantly more men preferred group interventions than women. Moreover, Compton et al. (2007) note that around 50% of people obtaining treatment for substance abuse (a predominantly male disorder) use 12-step programs, a well-known informal group program used to overcome addictions. Similarly, an emerging literature indicates that ecotherapy programs such as bushcraft or wilderness-type group interventions can help foster recovery in men with mental health issues (Chalquist, 2009; Jordan & Hinds, 2016; McIver et al., 2018). These interventions build on decades of research on Aboriginal mental health, indicating that traditional communal activities such as hunting, fishing, trapping, and sweat lodges can have healing value for troubled Aboriginal men (Kirmayer & Valaskakis, 2009; Schiff & Moore, 2006). Of note, these activities have a wider purpose and meaning beyond the individual (e.g., providing food for the family) and often occur in shoulder-to-shoulder silent fellowship with other men from different generations. In other words, they involve camaraderie, reciprocity, and mentorship; all of which have been identified as critical ingredients in many of the aforementioned studies examining key components of men's mental health interventions.

For example, Addis and Mahalik (2003) reviewed the men's mental health literature, noting that "men are more likely to look for help when they perceive an opportunity to reciprocate." Such reciprocity can fulfill primeval masculine needs to actively protect, provide, and contribute, rather than sit passively and benefit from the labour of others. Indeed, reciprocity is the norm in many male-dominated employment settings including the military, law enforcement, mining, transporting and manufacturing where all men are expected to "pull their weight." An ethos of reciprocity allows men to contribute to others' well-being, which can make it more acceptable to in turn receive benefits from other men in the group. The importance of reciprocity has been found in many different studies but has been shown as particularly important in veterans' mental health, where ex-servicemen often bring the military ethos "never leave a fallen comrade" into the clinic. Such an ethos has been harnessed by innovative peer-support interventions such as the "veteran's transition program," which actively encourages reciprocity, loyalty, and mutual support through action-oriented group work with veterans with PTSD (Shields & Westwood, 2019).

Similarly, the opportunity to give or receive mentorship, or to find or be a role model, has been identified as a key ingredient of male-oriented interventions in several recent studies (Whitley & Zhou, 2020; Sagar-Ouriaghli et al., 2019). Again, this is supported by the very nature of popular activity-oriented interventions such as sports-, adventure-, or craft-based interventions. On the one hand, such interventions allow older or more experienced men to mentor younger or less experienced men, giving these older men meaning and purpose. On the other hand, they allow younger and less experienced men to engage in new activities and learn new skills, which can similarly bring meaning and purpose. It allows men with mental health issues – who may be isolated, lonely, or estranged from their families – a chance to find mentors and role models, while allowing those with skills and life-experience a chance to mentor others. In other words, skill or action-based interventions inherently create a win-win situation for the men involved.

Despite harmful lone wolf stereotypes perpetuated by the aforementioned media, many men are accustomed to successfully completing tasks in the company and support of other men, with men commonly collaborating in a wide range of human activities including team sports, workplace tasks, fishing, hunting, military units, or DIY projects. As stated by Shields and Westwood (2019), men are typically group trained, group ready, and group experienced and are primed to work well in an environment characterized by group camaraderie, reciprocity, peer support, and mentorship. Sadly, these findings have often been lost on formal mental healthcare systems, which still tend to predominantly offer "one-size-fits-all" solutions based on medication and one-on-one talking therapies in formal healthcare settings. This implies a need for reform.

6.5 Making Male-Friendly and Male-Sensitive Services

In surveys, men frequently report a lack of male-friendly options within the formal mental health system, which may suffer from the male gender blindness discussed in Chap. 1 (Seager & Barry, 2019; Liddon et al., 2018). As such, business-as-usual in terms of formal health service delivery and provision is not an option if we are serious about improving men's mental health. Instead, there is a need for reform and innovation within the formal mental health system so that services are better tailored to the above-described male preferences. However, such reform and innovation has been slow to occur. Almost 20 years ago, Addis and Mahalik (2003) stated that there are two options to address men's mental health issues: "change individual men to fit the services or change the services to fit the 'average' man". But the call to change services has not often been heeded in the intervening years, with the aforementioned American Psychological Association (2018) guidelines for psychological practice with men and boys still emphasizing a "change men" rather than "change services" approach. Ashfield and Gouws (2019) note the impotency of such an approach, stating that "trying to change male characteristics does not work, but tailoring approaches to fit male characteristics does…health services responsible for male clients need to have an informed model of manhood and the demands that are made on men." This must involve going with the grain of masculinity, rather than treating masculinity as a pathology.

What does a male-positive and male-friendly service look like? It can integrate many of the aforementioned factors that have been identified as engaging and effective for men's mental health, including group-based and activity-based programs that involve reciprocity, camaraderie and mentorship. Moreover, such male-positive interventions must be underpinned by a nonjudgmental empathic approach that avoids blaming and shaming men for their mental health woes (Whitley, 2018). Englar-Carlson & Kiselica (2013) talk about the importance of adopting a strength-based rather than deficit-based approach in interventions aiming to improve men's mental health. This means focusing on the positive aspects of masculinity and individual men's life experience, rather than focusing on their deficits and alleged pathologies. This can involve respecting and harnessing masculine norms, for example, providing practical services that help men regain or succeed in the provider, protector, or breadwinner role, a role that brings meaning and purpose to many men's lives (Oliffe & Han, 2014; Seager & Barry, 2019). Examples of such programs include psychosocial interventions such as supported employment and vocational rehabilitation, as well as formal therapies such as cognitive behavioral therapies that can help men set and achieve goals related to work, family, and social integration. Such programs offer much promise for men's mental health and are sometimes part of the formal mental healthcare system, meaning they are well-funded and accessible. But these programs must take a male-positive strength-based approach that involves "foregrounding male aptitude not ineptitude" (Ashfield & Gouws, 2019). This means clinicians must view men's typical stoicism and self-help ethos as part of the solution rather than part of the problem and must studiously avoid a "blaming and shaming" approach that attacks masculine norms and preferences.

Indeed, two British reports on men's mental health note the importance of using male-friendly language and concepts in formal and informal clinical interventions (Robertson et al., 2015; Wilkins, 2015). This can involve, for example, reframing therapy and mental health interventions as "programs," "courses," or "workshops" of "mental fitness," "mental training," or "mental coaching," rather than using the nomenclature of mainstream psychiatry, which can be off-putting for many men. This is consistent with other research, with the American Association of Suicidology recommending that suicide prevention activities for men are framed in the context of traditional masculine values such as "competence," "achievement," and "self-reliance" (Berman & McNelis, 2005). Similarly, other studies indicate that framing help-seeking as a demonstration of masculine values such as courage, competence, independence, and control is typically welcomed by men and can often lead to male engagement (Oliffe et al., 2012; Emslie et al., 2006). All of this means that formal and informal services need to assess their marketing and branding to ensure it is male friendly and male positive, while individual clinicians must be careful in their use of language, ensuring that this is male sensitive rather than victim blaming.

Interestingly, the aforementioned British reports note that services and interventions aiming to improve men's mental health may be more effective and attractive if they are available for all men, rather than just for men with a defined and diagnosed mental illness (Robertson et al., 2015; Wilkins, 2015). This is especially feasible for group interventions such as sports, wilderness, or other activity-based programs, in contrast to individual therapies, which often require a diagnosis for professional reimbursement. Making such informal interventions available for all men has a triple benefit inasmuch as:

(i) Use of such services may incur less stigma as they are not targeted specifically at people with mental illness and not advertised as a "mental health" service, thus making them more attractive to men fearful of being stigmatized.
(ii) They can provide a beneficial service for men who are lonely or in despair due to disruptive life events such as divorce (see Chap. 9) or unemployment (see Chap. 8), but lack an official diagnosis.
(iii) The mixing of men with or without mental illness (and in different stages of recovery) can offer beneficial opportunities for mentorship, reciprocity, and camaraderie, also providing potential role models and possibilities for intergenerational learning.

6.6 Men's Sheds: An Innovative and Promising Practice

As stated, formal mental health services have typically preceded on a one-size-fits-all solution, with a blindness to male gender issues. Indeed, there are very few formal services devoted specifically to men's health, even though there are many gender-specific services for women such as post-natal clinics, women's refuges and female-focused eating disorder clinics (Liddon et al., 2019). Indeed, Seager (2019, p. 245) notes that "male friendly services and approaches in the UK and elsewhere remain the exception rather than the rule," while Morison et al. (2014) state that "gender specific has become synonymous with addressing women's issues." In this sense, the lack of provision of formal mental health services for men may reflect the wider societal indifference to the male experience, known as the *gender empathy gap*, an issue discussed in more detail in Chap. 1. Thankfully, nonprofits such as the Samaritans, Movember, and a whole range of smaller bottom-up community organization (e.g., sports clubs, churches, youth clubs and even barbershops) are providing informal supports for men's mental health, valiantly attempting to fill in the large gaps in the provision of formal mental health services (Baker, 2020). These

6.6 Men's Sheds: An Innovative and Promising Practice

informal endeavours often take an explicitly gendered approach, attempting to take account of the male experience and male sensibilities in a male-positive and male-sensitive manner. One intervention that is well known in the men's mental health literature is known as "men's sheds," which are presented in detail next as a paradigmatic case of a promising and innovative practice that incorporates many of the essential elements of a male-friendly service.

Men's Sheds began in Australia in the 1990s as a small bottom-up grassroots intervention and have become a popular service aimed at isolated and lonely older men across the world (Golding et al., 2008). Recent estimates indicate over 2000 men's sheds in a myriad of countries including Canada, the United States, and the United Kingdom, serving over 100,000 men in total (US Men's Shed Association, 2021). This is a phenomenal growth for a bottom-up grassroots intervention that is outside the formal healthcare system and rarely receives financial support from government bodies or official health service funders (Misan & Sergeant, 2009).

The International Men's Sheds Organization (2018) states that "A Men's Shed is a dedicated, friendly and welcoming meeting place where men come together and undertake a variety of mutually agreed activities." These sheds are typically located in a small building composed of a few workshops or rooms, where men can engage in a variety of hands-on activities including woodwork, metalwork, repairs, horticulture, music making, cooking, or simply watching TV together (Golding, 2015). Men's sheds are mainly aimed at older men with one survey showing over 50% of attendees are over 65, but many are open and welcoming to younger men (Golding et al., 2007). Importantly, participation in a men's shed typically involves elements of reciprocity, cooperation, peer support, informal learning, and making a contribution (Kingerlee et al., 2019). Many of the tasks conducted in men's sheds are outward-focused community projects, for example, creating wooden benches for local municipal parks (Golding, 2015; Cordier & Wilson, 2014). Such a process would involve the men working together for a common goal that makes a valuable contribution to their local communities, thus giving wider purpose and meaning to the underlying activities. This process can also involve mentoring and peer-support, with more experienced members helping less experienced members in the required woodwork, giving both mentorship and learning opportunities for all (Cordier et al., 2016).

Importantly, a mental health diagnosis is not required to become a member, and the sheds are not branded and marketed as a mental health service in any way, thus avoiding the nomenclature of mainstream psychiatry. Indeed, participants are known as "volunteers" or "members" rather than "clients" or "patients," and there is no expectation of emotional disclosure or mental health talk (Milligan et al., 2015). Instead, there is a strong emphasis on "doing," with publicity material emphasizing the creative activities and social connections arising from participation, with a focus on fun, laughter, and friendship. While there is no pressure for emotional disclosure or mental health discussion, this is often a by-product of the supportive environment with men learning to trust and respect one another over time. In sum, men's sheds integrate and harness many of the aforementioned critical ingredients of a male-friendly and male-positive intervention. The sheds are informal community-based places, not located within hospitals or healthcare settings. They are goal-directed action-focused group interventions that go with the grain of traditional masculinity, exploiting the male tendency to construct, create, and work together with meaning and purpose. They do not take a finger-pointing, victim-blaming approach and do not shame men for alleged emotional illiteracy or lack of mental health awareness, instead taking an angular "health by stealth" approach to men's mental health. Indeed, the men's sheds' motto "men don't talk face-to-face, they talk shoulder-to-shoulder" contains much wisdom, a wisdom that can be conspicuously absent in formal mental health care.

There have been several studies assessing the social and health benefits of participation in a men's shed. These consistently indicate that men's sheds can have a positive influence on men's mental health. These studies have been assessed in several recent review papers. One of these review papers examined 16 studies on men's sheds, finding that all 16 reported that participation in men's shed increased sense of purpose and meaning, while 10 out of 16 studies found a decrease in depression symptoms, and/or suicidal thoughts (Kelly et al., 2019). Another review paper noted that qualitative and quantitative studies consistently found an improvement in mental health and well-being after participation (Milligan et al., 2015), including two quantitative before and after studies (Pretty et al., 2007; Gleibs et al., 2011). Similarly, several qualitative studies have found that men's sheds reduce loneliness and isolation, creating much needed social connection and friendship with others (Foster et al., 2018; Anstiss et al., 2018; Culph et al., 2015; Crabtree et al., 2018). Other studies indicate that the learning and mentoring inherent in men's sheds plays a key role in enhancing self-esteem and well-being (Misan & Sergeant, 2009; Ballinger et al., 2009). That said, these review papers note that most of the literature on men's sheds are characterized by small sample sizes and low response rates, with a relative absence of longitudinal or randomized designs, meaning that further research is necessary to examine causal pathways and the precise impact on mental health (Kelly et al., 2019; Milligan et al., 2016).

In sum, men's sheds are a promising and innovative intervention that incorporate many of the core factors that have been identified as key ingredients in any men's mental health intervention. They incorporate male-friendly and male-positive approaches, harnessing traditional masculinity as a strength rather than a pathology. This helps explain the growing popularity of men's sheds across the world. There is much that formal mental health care can learn from men's sheds.

6.7 Conclusion and Recommendations

Men tend to underutilize formal mental health care in comparison with women. This has typically been attributed to harmful masculine norms that lead to a dysfunctional silence and stubbornness among men. However, this chapter indicates that this monocausal explanation ignores several pertinent factors related to men's underutilization of mental health services. First, there is a high degree of external stigma that can deter men from using mental health services. Second, the formal mental care system can be unwelcoming for men and typically suffers from *male gender blindness*. Third, there are various modalities of healing with men preferring more informal action-based approaches, but these are not readily available in the formal mental healthcare system, which typically proceeds on a "one-size-fits-all" approach.

What can be done to address these issues? First, the formal mental healthcare system (which is typically funded by the taxpayer) must make strident efforts to become more male friendly. This could mean diversifying the mental health workforce so that there are more male clinicians and ensuring that male-friendly marketing, branding, and language is used by clinics and clinicians. Second, there is a need for more choice in the formal mental healthcare system, moving beyond conventional treatments to provide some of the action-based or group-based modalities of healing that are typically preferred by men. Third, more support and funding should be made available to informal bottom-up interventions that take an angular approach to men's mental health. This could involve "social prescribing," with men encouraged to utilize such services by their clinicians, meaning that the formal healthcare system attempts to work in harmony with the informal mental healthcare system. All this may go some way to address the underlying issues discussed in this chapter.

References

Addis, M. E., & Mahalik, J. R. (2003). Men, masculinity, and the contexts of help seeking. *American Psychologist, 58*(1), 5. https://doi.org/10.1037/0003-066X.58.1.5

Affleck, W., Thamotharampillai, U., Jeyakumar, J., & Whitley, R. (2018). "If one does not fulfil his duties, he must not be a man": Masculinity, mental health and resilience amongst Sri Lankan Tamil refugee men in Canada. *Culture, Medicine, and Psychiatry, 42*(4), 840–861. https://doi.org/10.1007/s11013-018-9592-9

Aldersey, H. M., & Whitley, R. (2015). Family influence in recovery from severe mental illness. *Community Mental Health Journal, 51*(4), 467–476. https://doi.org/10.1007/s10597-014-9783-y

American Psychological Association (APA). (2018, August). *APA guidelines for psychological practice with boys and men*. American Psychological Association. Retrieved January 7, 2021, from https://www.apa.org/about/policy/boys-men-practice-guidelines.pdf

Anstiss, D., Hodgetts, D., & Stolte, O. (2018). Men's re-placement: Social practices in a Men's Shed. *Health & Place, 51*, 217–223. https://doi.org/10.1016/j.healthplace.2018.04.009

Ashfield, J. A., & Gouws, D. S. (2019). Dignifying psychotherapy with men: Developing empathic and evidence-based approaches that suit the real needs of the male gender. In J. A. Barry, R. Kingerlee, M. Seager, & L. Sullivan (Eds.), *The Palgrave handbook of male psychology and mental health* (pp. 623–645). Palgrave Macmillan.

Baker, P. (2020, August 11). Barber shops and male mental health. *Trends in Urology & Men's Health*. Wiley Online Library. Retrieved January 7, 2021, from https://trendsinmenshealth.com/news/barber-shops-and-male-mental-health/

Ballinger, M. L., Talbot, L. A., & Verrinder, G. K. (2009). More than a place to do woodwork: A case study of a community-based Men's Shed. *Journal of Men's Health, 6*(1), 20–27. https://doi.org/10.1016/j.jomh.2008.09.006

Banks, I. (2001). No man's land: Men, illness, and the NHS. *BMJ, 323*(7320), 1058–1060. https://doi.org/10.1136/bmj.323.7320.1058

Barnes, P. M., Powell-Griner, E., McFann, K., & Nahin, R. L. (2004). Complementary and alternative medicine use among adults: United States, 2002. *Seminars in Integrative Medicine, 2*(2), 54–71. https://doi.org/10.1016/j.sigm.2004.07.003

Barry, J. A., Kingerlee, R., Seager, M., & Sullivan, L. (Eds.). (2019). *The Palgrave handbook of male psychology and mental health*. Palgrave Macmillan.

Bengs, C., Johansson, E., Danielsson, U., Lehti, A., & Hammarström, A. (2008). Gendered portraits of depression in Swedish newspapers. *Qualitative Health Research, 18*(7), 962–973. https://doi.org/10.1177/1049732308319825

Berman, L., & McNelis, K. (2005). Help-seeking among men: Implications for suicide prevention. *Pogled. The View, 3*(1–2), 36–51. Retrieved from https://www.suicideinfo.ca/wp-content/uploads/2017/06/Help-seeking-among-Men-Implications-for-Suicide-Prevention_oa.pdf

Bilsker, D., Fogarty, A. S., & Wakefield, M. A. (2018). Critical issues in men's mental health. *The Canadian Journal of Psychiatry, 63*(9), 590–596. https://doi.org/10.1177/0706743718766052

Brown, J. S., Evans-Lacko, S., Aschan, L., Henderson, M. J., Hatch, S. L., & Hotopf, M. (2014). Seeking informal and formal help for mental health problems in the community: A secondary analysis from a psychiatric morbidity survey in South London. *BMC Psychiatry, 14*(1), 275. https://doi.org/10.1186/s12888-014-0275-y

Brown, J. S., Sagar-Ouriaghli, I., & Sullivan, L. (2019). Help-seeking among men for mental health problems. In J. A. Barry, R. Kingerlee, M. Seager, & L. Sullivan (Eds.), *The Palgrave handbook of male psychology and mental health* (pp. 397–415). Palgrave Macmillan.

Bullen, K., & Hughes, J. H. (2016). Achieving representation in psychology. A BPS response. *The Psychologist, 29*, 246–255.

Canetto, S. S., & Sakinofsky, I. (1998). The gender paradox in suicide. *Suicide and Life-threatening Behavior, 28*(1), 1–23. https://doi.org/10.1111/j.1943-278X.1998.tb00622.x

Chalquist, C. (2009). A look at the ecotherapy research evidence. *Ecopsychology, 1*(2), 64–74. https://doi.org/10.1089/eco.2009.0003

Chatmon, B. N. (2020). Males and mental health stigma. *American Journal of Men's Health, 14*(4). https://doi.org/10.1177/1557988320949322

Compton, W. M., Thomas, Y. F., Stinson, F. S., & Grant, B. F. (2007). Prevalence, correlates, disability, and comorbidity of DSM-IV drug abuse and dependence in the United States: Results from the national epidemiologic survey on alcohol and related conditions. *Archives of General Psychiatry, 64*(5), 566–576. https://doi.org/10.1001/archpsyc.64.5.566

Cordier, R., & Wilson, N. J. (2014). Community-based Men's sheds: Promoting male health, wellbeing and social inclusion in an international context. *Health Promotion International, 29*(3), 483–493. https://doi.org/10.1093/heapro/dat033

Cordier, R., Wilson, N. J., Stancliffe, R. J., MacCallum, J., Vaz, S., & Buchanan, A. (2016). Formal intergenerational mentoring at Australian Men's Sheds: A targeted survey about mentees, mentors, programmes and quality. *Health & Social Care in the Community, 24*(6), e131–e143. https://doi.org/10.1111/hsc.12267

Corrigan, P. W., Markowitz, F. E., & Watson, A. C. (2004). Structural levels of mental illness stigma and discrimination. *Schizophrenia Bulletin, 30*(3), 481–491. https://doi.org/10.1093/oxfordjournals.schbul.a007096

Courtenay, W. H. (2000a). Constructions of masculinity and their influence on men's well-being: A theory of gender and health. *Social Science & Medicine, 50*(10), 1385–1401. https://doi.org/10.1016/S0277-9536(99)00390-1

Courtenay, W. H. (2000b). Behavioral factors associated with disease, injury, and death among men: Evidence and implications for prevention. *The Journal of Men's Studies, 9*(1), 81–142. https://doi.org/10.3149/jms.0901.81

Crabtree, L., Tinker, A., & Glaser, K. (2018). Men's sheds: The perceived health and wellbeing benefits. *Working with Older People, 22*(2). https://doi.org/10.1108/WWOP-09-2017-0026

References

Culph, J. S., Wilson, N. J., Cordier, R., & Stancliffe, R. J. (2015). Men's Sheds and the experience of depression in older Australian men. *Australian Occupational Therapy Journal, 62*(5), 306–315. https://doi.org/10.1111/1440-1630.12190

Dallaire, R. (2019). *Waiting for first light: My ongoing battle with PTSD*. Vintage Canada.

Eisenberg, D. M., Davis, R. B., Ettner, S. L., Appel, S., Wilkey, S., Van Rompay, M., & Kessler, R. C. (1998). Trends in alternative medicine use in the United States, 1990–1997: Results of a follow-up national survey. *JAMA, 280*(18), 1569–1575. https://doi.org/10.1001/jama.280.18.1569

Ellis, L. A., Collin, P., Hurley, P. J., Davenport, T. A., Burns, J. M., & Hickie, I. B. (2013). Young men's attitudes and behaviour in relation to mental health and technology: Implications for the development of online mental health services. *BMC Psychiatry, 13*(1), 119. https://doi.org/10.1186/1471-244X-13-119

Emslie, C., Ridge, D., Ziebland, S., & Hunt, K. (2006). Men's accounts of depression: Reconstructing or resisting hegemonic masculinity? *Social Science & Medicine, 62*(9), 2246–2257. https://doi.org/10.1016/j.socscimed.2005.10.017

Emslie, C., Ridge, D., Ziebland, S., & Hunt, K. (2007). Exploring men's and women's experiences of depression and engagement with health professionals: More similarities than differences? A qualitative interview study. *BMC Family Practice, 8*(1), 43. https://doi.org/10.1186/1471-2296-8-43

Englar-Carlson, M. (2019). Foreword. In J. A. Barry, R. Kingerlee, M. Seager, & L. Sullivan (Eds.), *The Palgrave handbook of male psychology and mental health* (pp. vii–xiv). Palgrave Macmillan.

Englar-Carlson, M., & Kiselica, M. S. (2013). Affirming the strengths in men: A positive masculinity approach to assisting male clients. *Journal of Counseling & Development, 91*(4), 399–409. https://doi.org/10.1002/j.1556-6676.2013.00111.x

Foster, E. J., Munoz, S. A., & Leslie, S. J. (2018). The personal and community impact of a Scottish Men's Shed. *Health & Social Care in the Community, 26*(4), 527–537. https://doi.org/10.1111/hsc.12560

Gabbidon, J., Farrelly, S., Hatch, S. L., Henderson, C., Williams, P., Bhugra, D., Dockery, L., Lassman, F., Thornicroft, G., & Clement, S. (2014). Discrimination attributed to mental illness or race-ethnicity by users of community psychiatric services. *Psychiatric Services, 65*(11), 1360–1366. https://doi.org/10.1176/appi.ps.201300302

Gaebel, W., Rössler, W., & Sartorius, N. (Eds.). (2017). *The stigma of mental illness-end of the story?* Springer.

Gleibs, I., Haslam, C., Jones, J. M., Haslam, S. A., McNeill, J., & Connolly, H. (2011). No country for old men? The role of a 'Gentlemen's Club' in promoting social engagement and psychological well-being in residential care. *Aging and Mental Health, 15*(4), 456–466. https://doi.org/10.1080/13607863.2010.536137

Golding, B. (2015). *The Men's shed movement: The company of men*. Common Ground Publishing.

Golding, B., Brown, M., Foley, A., Harvey, J., & Gleeson, L. (2007, May 23). *Men's sheds in Australia: Learning through community contexts*. National Centre for Vocational Education Research (NCVER). Retrieved January 7, 2021, from https://www.ncver.edu.au/research-and-statistics/publications/all-publications/mens-sheds-in-australia-learning-through-community-contexts

Golding, B., Kimberley, H., Foley, A., & Brown, M. (2008). Houses and sheds in Australia: An exploration of the genesis and growth of neighbourhood houses and men's sheds in community settings. *Australian Journal of Adult Learning, 48*(2), 237–262.

Harris, M. G., Diminic, S., Reavley, N., Baxter, A., Pirkis, J., & Whiteford, H. A. (2015). Males' mental health disadvantage: An estimation of gender-specific changes in service utilisation for mental and substance use disorders in Australia. *Australian & New Zealand Journal of Psychiatry, 49*(9), 821–832. https://doi.org/10.1177/0004867415577434

International Men's Sheds Organisation. (2018). *What is a Men's Shed?* International Men's Sheds Organisation. Retrieved January 7, 2021, from https://menshed.com/what-is-a-mens-shed/

Jordan, M., & Hinds, J. (Eds.). (2016). *Ecotherapy: Theory, research and practice*. Macmillan International Higher Education.

Kelly, D., Steiner, A., Mason, H., & Teasdale, S. (2019). Men's Sheds: A conceptual exploration of the causal pathways for health and well-being. *Health & Social Care in the Community, 27*(5), 1147–1157. https://doi.org/10.1111/hsc.12765

Kessler, R. C., Demler, O., Frank, R. G., Olfson, M., Pincus, H. A., Walters, E. E., Wang, P., Wells, K. B., & Zaslavsky, A. M. (2005). Prevalence and treatment of mental disorders, 1990 to 2003. *New England Journal of Medicine, 352*(24), 2515–2523. https://doi.org/10.1056/NEJMsa043266

Kingerlee, R., Abotsie, G., Fisk, A., & Woodley, L. (2019). Reconnection: Designing interventions and services with men in mind. In J. A. Barry, R. Kingerlee, M. Seager, & L. Sullivan (Eds.), *The Palgrave handbook of male psychology and mental health* (pp. 647–669). Palgrave Macmillan.

Kirmayer, L. J., & Valaskakis, G. G. (Eds.). (2009). *Healing traditions: The mental health of Aboriginal peoples in Canada*. UBC Press.

Kleinman, A. (1980). *Patients and healers in the context of culture: An exploration of the borderland between anthropology, medicine, and psychiatry* (Vol. 3). University of California Press.

Klesment, M., & Van Bavel, J. (2015). *The reversal of the gender gap in education and female breadwinners in Europe*. Families and Societies Working Paper, 26.

Liddon, L., Kingerlee, R., & Barry, J. A. (2018). Gender differences in preferences for psychological treatment, coping strategies, and triggers to help-seeking. *British Journal of Clinical Psychology, 57*(1), 42–58. https://doi.org/10.1111/bjc.12147

Liddon, L., Kingerlee, R., Seager, M., & Barry, J. A. (2019). What are the factors that make a male-friendly therapy? In J. A. Barry, R. Kingerlee, M. Seager, & L. Sullivan (Eds.), *The Palgrave handbook of male psychology and mental health* (pp. 671–694). Palgrave Macmillan.

Linford, L. C. (2013). *Warrior rising: A soldier's journey to PTSD and back*. FriesenPress.

Link, B. G., & Phelan, J. C. (2001). Conceptualizing stigma. *Annual Review of Sociology, 27*(1), 363–385. https://doi.org/10.1146/annurev.soc.27.1.363

Lynch, L., Long, M., & Moorhead, A. (2018). Young men, help-seeking, and mental health services: Exploring barriers and solutions. *American Journal of Men's Health, 12*(1), 138–149. https://doi.org/10.1177/1557988315619469

Mackenzie, C. S., Gekoski, W. L., & Knox, V. J. (2006). Age, gender, and the underutilization of mental health services: The influence of help-seeking attitudes. *Aging and Mental Health, 10*(6), 574–582. https://doi.org/10.1080/13607860600641200

McDonald, B., Kulkarni, M., Andkhoie, M., Kendall, J., Gall, S., Chelladurai, S., Yaghoubi, M., McClean, S., Szafron, M., & Farag, M. (2017). Determinants of self-reported mental health and utilization of mental health services in Canada. *International Journal of Mental Health, 46*(4), 299–311. https://doi.org/10.1080/00207411.2017.1345045

McIver, S., Senior, E., & Francis, Z. (2018). Healing fears, conquering challenges: Narrative outcomes from a wilderness therapy program. *Journal of Creativity in Mental Health, 13*(4), 392–404. https://doi.org/10.1080/15401383.2018.1447415

Milligan, C., Neary, D., Payne, S., Hanratty, B., Irwin, P., & Dowrick, C. (2016). Older men and social activity: A scoping review of Men's sheds and other gendered interventions. *Ageing & Society, 36*(5), 895–923. https://doi.org/10.1017/S0144686X14001524

Milligan, C., Payne, S., Bingley, A., & Cockshott, Z. (2015). Place and wellbeing: Shedding light on activity interventions for older men. *Ageing and Society, 35*(1), 124–149. https://doi.org/10.1017/S0144686X13000494

Misan, G., & Sergeant, P. (2009). *Men's sheds – A strategy to improve men's health*. National Rural Health Alliance, 10th National Rural Health Conference, North Queensland. Retrieved January 7, 2021, from https://www.ruralhealth.org.au/10thNRHC/10thnrhc.ruralhealth.org.au/papers/docs/Misan_Gary_D7.pdf

Möller-Leimkühler, A. M. (2003). The gender gap in suicide and premature death or: Why are men so vulnerable? *European Archives of Psychiatry and Clinical Neuroscience, 253*(1), 1–8. https://doi.org/10.1007/s00406-003-0397-6

References

Morison, L., Trigeorgis, C., & John, M. (2014). Are mental health services inherently feminised? *The Psychologist, 27*(6), 414–416.

O'Brien, R., Hunt, K., & Hart, G. (2005). 'It's caveman stuff, but that is to a certain extent how guys still operate': Men's accounts of masculinity and help seeking. *Social Science & Medicine, 61*(3), 503–516. https://doi.org/10.1016/j.socscimed.2004.12.008

Ogrodniczuk, J., Oliffe, J., Kuhl, D., & Gross, P. A. (2016). Men's mental health: Spaces and places that work for men. *Canadian Family Physician, 62*(6), 463–464.

Oliffe, J. L., & Han, C. S. E. (2014). Beyond worker's compensation: Men's mental health in and out of work. *American Journal of Men's Health, 8*, 45–53. https://doi.org/10.1177/1557988313490786

Oliffe, J. L., Ogrodniczuk, J. S., Bottorff, J. L., Johnson, J. L., & Hoyak, K. (2012). "You feel like you can't live anymore": Suicide from the perspectives of Canadian men who experience depression. *Social Science & Medicine, 74*(4), 506–514. https://doi.org/10.1016/j.socscimed.2010.03.057

Oliffe, J. L., & Phillips, M. J. (2008). Men, depression and masculinities: A review and recommendations. *Journal of Men's Health, 5*(3), 194–202. https://doi.org/10.1016/j.jomh.2008.03.016

Patrick, S., & Robertson, S. (2016). Promoting mental health and wellbeing for men. *British Journal of. Nursing, 25*(21), 1163. https://doi.org/10.12968/bjon.2016.25.21.1163

Pretty, J., Peacock, J., Hine, R., Sellens, M., South, N., & Griffin, M. (2007). Green exercise in the UK countryside: Effects on health and psychological well-being, and implications for policy and planning. *Journal of Environmental Planning and Management, 50*(2), 211–231. https://doi.org/10.1080/09640560601156466

Reavley, N. J., & Jorm, A. F. (2011). Stigmatizing attitudes towards people with mental disorders: Findings from an Australian National Survey of Mental Health literacy and stigma. *Australian & New Zealand Journal of Psychiatry, 45*(12), 1086–1093. https://doi.org/10.3109/00048674.2011.621061

Robertson, S., Gough, B., Hanna, E., Raine, G., Robinson, M., Seims, A., & White, A. (2018). Successful mental health promotion with men: The evidence from 'tacit knowledge'. *Health Promotion International, 33*(2), 334–344. https://doi.org/10.1093/heapro/daw067

Robertson, S., White, A., Gough, B., Robinson, M., Seims, A., Raine, G., & Hanna, E. (2015). *Promoting mental health and wellbeing with men and boys: What works?* Centre for Men's Health, Leeds Beckett University. Retrieved January 7, 2021, from http://eprints.leedsbeckett.ac.uk/1508/1/Promoting_MentalHealth__Wellbeing_FINAL.pdf

Sagar-Ouriaghli, I., Godfrey, E., Bridge, L., Meade, L., & Brown, J. S. (2019). Improving mental health service utilization among men: A systematic review and synthesis of behavior change techniques within interventions targeting help-seeking. *American Journal of Men's Health, 13*(3), 1–18. https://doi.org/10.1177/1557988319857009

Scheid, T. L. (2005). Stigma as a barrier to employment: Mental disability and the Americans with Disabilities Act. *International Journal of Law and Psychiatry, 28*(6), 670–690. https://doi.org/10.1016/j.ijlp.2005.04.003

Schiff, J. W., & Moore, K. (2006). The impact of the sweat lodge ceremony on dimensions of well-being. *American Indian and Alaska Native Mental Health Research: The Journal of the National Center, 13*(3), 48–69. https://doi.org/10.5820/aian.1303.2006.48

Seager, M. (2019). From stereotypes to archetypes: An evolutionary perspective on male help-seeking and suicide. In J. A. Barry, R. Kingerlee, M. Seager, & L. Sullivan (Eds.), *The Palgrave handbook of male psychology and mental health* (pp. 227–248). Palgrave Macmillan.

Seager, M., & Barry, J. A. (2019). Positive masculinity: Including masculinity as a valued aspect of humanity. In J. A. Barry, R. Kingerlee, M. Seager, & L. Sullivan (Eds.), *The Palgrave handbook of male psychology and mental health* (pp. 105–122). Palgrave Macmillan.

Seaton, C. L., Bottorff, J. L., Oliffe, J. L., Medhurst, K., & DeLeenheer, D. (2019). Mental health promotion in male-dominated workplaces: Perspectives of male employees and workplace representatives. *Psychology of Men & Masculinities, 20*(4), 541–552. https://doi.org/10.1037/men0000182

Seidler, Z. E., Rice, S. M., Ogrodniczuk, J. S., Oliffe, J. L., Shaw, J. M., & Dhillon, H. M. (2019). Men, masculinities, depression: Implications for mental health services from a Delphi expert consensus study. *Professional Psychology: Research and Practice, 50*(1), 51. https://doi.org/10.1037/pro0000220

Shields, D., & Westwood, M. (2019). Counselling male military personnel and veterans: Addressing challenges and enhancing engagement. In J. A. Barry, R. Kingerlee, M. Seager, & L. Sullivan (Eds.), *The Palgrave handbook of male psychology and mental health* (pp. 417–438). Palgrave Macmillan.

Slade, J., Teesson, W., & Burgess, P. (2009, January). *The mental health of Australians 2: Report on the 2007 National Survey of Mental Health and wellbeing*. Australian Government Department of Health. Retrieved January 7, 2020, from https://www1.health.gov.au/internet/main/publishing.nsf/Content/mental-pubs-m-mhaust2

Smith, K. L., Matheson, F. I., Moineddin, R., Dunn, J. R., Lu, H., Cairney, J., & Glazier, R. H. (2013). Gender differences in mental health service utilization among respondents reporting depression in a national health survey. *Health, 5*(10), 1561–1571. https://doi.org/10.4236/health.2013.510212

Statistics Canada. (2007). *The Canadian labour market at a glance. Average hours usually worked*. Statistics Canada. Retrieved January 7, 2020, from https://www150.statcan.gc.ca/n1/pub/71-222-x/2008001/sectionh/h-hours-heures-eng.htm

Struszczyk, S., Galdas, P. M., & Tiffin, P. A. (2019). Men and suicide prevention: A scoping review. *Journal of Mental Health, 28*(1), 80–88. https://doi.org/10.1080/09638237.2017.1370638

Stuart, H., Chen, S. P., Christie, R., Dobson, K., Kirsh, B., Knaak, S., Koller, M., Krupa, T., Lauria-Horner, B., Luong, D., Modgill, G., Patten, S. B., Pietrus, M., Szeto, A., & Whitley, R. (2014). Opening minds in Canada: Background and rationale. *The Canadian Journal of Psychiatry, 59*(1_suppl), 8–12. https://doi.org/10.1177/070674371405901S04

Substance Abuse and Mental Health Services Administration (SAMHSA). (2019, August). *Key substance use and mental health indicators in the United States: Results from the 2018 National Survey on Drug Use and Health*. Center for Behavioral Health Statistics and Quality, Substance Abuse and Mental Health Services Administration. Retrieved January 7, 2021, from https://www.samhsa.gov/data/sites/default/files/cbhsqreports/NSDUHNationalFindingsReport2018/NSDUHNationalFindingsReport2018.pdf

Unützer, J., Klap, R., Sturm, R., Young, A. S., Marmon, T., Shatkin, J., & Wells, K. B. (2000). Mental disorders and the use of alternative medicine: Results from a national survey. *American Journal of Psychiatry, 157*(11), 1851–1857. https://doi.org/10.1176/appi.ajp.157.11.1851

US Men's Shed Association. (2021). *What we do at Men's Shed*. US Men's Shed Association. Retrieved January 7, 2021, from https://usmenssheds.org/what-we-do/

Wahl, O. F. (2012). Stigma as a barrier to recovery from mental illness. *Trends in Cognitive Sciences, 16*(1), 9–10. https://doi.org/10.1016/j.tics.2011.11.002

Wang, P. S., Berglund, P., Olfson, M., Pincus, H. A., Wells, K. B., & Kessler, R. C. (2005). Failure and delay in initial treatment contact after first onset of mental disorders in the National Comorbidity Survey Replication. *Archives of General Psychiatry, 62*(6), 603–613. https://doi.org/10.1001/archpsyc.62.6.603

Whitley, R. (2013). Fear and loathing in New England: Examining the health-care perspectives of homeless people in rural areas. *Anthropology & Medicine, 20*(3), 232–243. https://doi.org/10.1080/13648470.2013.853597

Whitley, R. (2016). Ethno-racial variation in recovery from severe mental illness: A qualitative comparison. *The Canadian Journal of Psychiatry, 61*(6), 340–347. https://doi.org/10.1177/0706743716643740

Whitley, R. (2018). Men's mental health: Beyond victim-blaming. *The Canadian Journal of Psychiatry, 63*(9), 577–580. https://doi.org/10.1177/0706743718758041

Whitley, R., Adeponle, A., & Miller, A. R. (2015). Comparing gendered and generic representations of mental illness in Canadian newspapers: An exploration of the chivalry hypothesis.

References

Social Psychiatry and Psychiatric Epidemiology, 50(2), 325–333. https://doi.org/10.1007/s00127-014-0902-4

Whitley, R., & Campbell, R. D. (2014). Stigma, agency and recovery amongst people with severe mental illness. *Social Science & Medicine, 107*, 1–8. https://doi.org/10.1016/j.socscimed.2014.02.010

Whitley, R., & Zhou, J. (2020). Clueless: An ethnographic study of young men who participate in the seduction community with a focus on their psychological well-being and mental health. *PLoS One, 15*(2), e0229719. https://doi.org/10.1371/journal.pone.0229719

Wilkins, D. (2015). *How to make mental health services work for men.* Men's Health Forum. Retrieved January 7, 2020, from https://www.menshealthforum.org.uk/sites/default/files/pdf/how_to_mh_v4.1_lrweb_0.pdf

World Health Organization (WHO). (2003). *Organization of services for mental health.* World Health Organization (WHO).

Wyllie, C., Platt, S., Brownlie, J., Chandler, A., Conolly, S., Evans, R., Kennelly, B., Kirtley, O., Moore, G., O'Connor, R., & Scourfield, J. (2012, September). *Men, suicide and society: Why disadvantaged men in mid-life die by suicide.* Samaritans. Retrieved January 7, 2021, from https://media.samaritans.org/documents/Samaritans_MenSuicideSociety_ResearchReport2012.pdf

Part II
Men's Issues and Their Relation to Men's Mental Health

Chapter 7
The Gender Gap in Education: Understanding Educational Underachievement in Young Males and Its Relationship to Adverse Mental Health

Evidence suggests that many young males are facing a number of difficulties within the educational system. In comparison with girls, boys have a higher rate of school dropout, detention, and exclusion, as well as lower scores in high school exams, basic literacy tests, and lower rates of enrollment in tertiary education. Importantly, a large body of research indicates that these educational deficits can contribute toward adverse mental health outcomes with a high prevalence among men, including suicide and substance abuse. This has led some scholars to question whether the nature and formation of the educational system is sensitive to male students, while noting that male underperformance is rarely a policy priority at any level of education. All this is discussed in detail throughout this chapter.

7.1 Background

In most western countries, the national or regional government provides free education to children and adolescents, typically divided into primary (or elementary) school for children from ages 5/6 to 11/12 years and secondary (or high) school for youth from ages 11/12 to 16/18 years (Looney, 2009; Organisation for Economic Co-operation and Development [OECD] 2013). Such education is usually compulsory until a legally defined school-leaving age, which ranges from ages 15 to 18 years depending on jurisdiction (OECD, 2018). At ages 15–18 years, school leavers have the option of taking a variety of exams allowing them to earn a high (secondary) school diploma or equivalent certificates. Alternatively, they can leave school without taking any of these exams (OECD, 2014).

These high school diplomas and certificates are frequently required by employers and can open doors to numerous job opportunities (Council on School Health, 2013; OECD, 2014). Moreover, they are typically required for entry into tertiary education, which consists of universities, colleges, and vocational/trade schools

(Hoareau McGrath et al., 2014). Universities generally require a high level of achievement in high school exams for admission, whereas other postsecondary institutions such as trade schools or vocational colleges have a lower benchmark (Hanford, 2014). This means that recent school leavers typically fall into three categories: (i) those who enter the workforce soon after leaving secondary school; (ii) those who go on to some form of postsecondary education at ages 16–18; and (iii) those who become unemployed, sometimes known as people "not in education, employment nor training" (NEETs) (Statistics Canada, 2019a). Importantly, successful completion of postsecondary education can significantly enhance job prospects and is strongly correlated with lifetime income, quality of life, and other psychosocial outcomes (World Economic Forum, 2020).

Individual performance in the educational system is commonly known by the phrase "educational attainment," which has been defined as "the highest level of education that a person has successfully completed. Successful completion of a level of education refers to the achievement of the learning objectives of that level, typically validated through the assessment of acquired knowledge, skills and competencies" (Statistics Canada, 2016a). This definition is consistent with other definitions used in other jurisdictions and by international organizations and is thus used as a foundation for this chapter (United States Census Bureau, 2021; UNESCO, 2012).

Educational attainment is sometimes measured as a continuous variable, referring to the number of years of completed primary, secondary, and tertiary schooling, with a longer period considered *high educational attainment* and a shorter period *low educational attainment* (e.g., Mezuk et al., 2008). However, this form of measurement has some drawbacks, as it does not account for: (i) successful completion of exams; (ii) grade repetition due to failure; and (iii) academic acceleration (i.e., grade skipping) due to talent and success. As such, educational attainment is more frequently measured as a categorical variable, typically grouping people into four categories representing common endpoints within the educational trajectory (Statistics Canada, 2016b). These are:

(i) People leaving secondary school without a high school diploma or equivalent, sometimes called "high school drop-outs".
(ii) People whose highest level of educational attainment is a high school diploma or equivalent.
(iii) People with some postsecondary education but who did not graduate with a certificate, diploma, or degree.
(iv) People who have attained a postsecondary certificate, diploma, or degree including vocational or trade college, associate degree, bachelor's degree or higher, or equivalent professional diploma.

The phrase *low educational attainment* is a core concept in the social science literature and is often used to refer to categories (i) and (ii) combined, i.e., those who dropped out of secondary school merged with those who left the educational system with no more than a high school diploma or equivalent (van Hek et al., 2016; Hussar et al., 2020). This group is sometimes characterized by cognate terminology such as "12 years education or less," "early school-leaving," or other phraseology idiosyncratic to a jurisdiction. In research studies, people categorized as "low educational attainment" are sometimes compared with those considered to have achieved "high educational attainment," which typically refers to people who have attained a postsecondary degree or equivalent professional diploma or higher, i.e., group (iv) above. In some studies, group (iv) is further divided into: (i) those with a trade or vocational diploma or an associate degree; (ii) those with a bachelor's degree or equivalent; and (iii) those with a postgraduate degree or equivalent.

7.2 Low Educational Attainment: A Mental Health Risk Factor

Importantly, a large corpus of research indicates that low educational attainment is a risk factor for a variety of adverse mental health outcomes, while high educational attainment is a protective factor. For example, a longitudinal analysis of data from the US National Epidemiologic Survey on Alcohol and Related Conditions (NESARC) ($N = 34,653$; 87% response rate) found that those with a graduate, professional, or bachelor's degree had the lowest rates of depression, anxiety, and substance use disorder, while those with a high school diploma or less had the highest rates of these disorders (Erickson et al., 2016). Importantly, this survey controlled for other psychiatric disorders and other indicators of socioeconomic status (e.g., income), making it a particularly powerful study. Similar results were found in a recent systematic review (Esch et al., 2014) and a host of other studies from a variety of jurisdictions, some of which are briefly described next in relation to three specific mental health outcomes: (i) suicide; (ii) substance use disorder; and (iii) depression/anxiety.

7.2.1 Suicide

Evidence suggests that low educational attainment is a risk factor for suicide, particularly among males. For example, in a systematic review and meta-analysis, men with less than a high school diploma were over twice as likely (RR 2.42: 95% CI: 1.03–5.70) to kill themselves when compared with men who had completed tertiary education (Li et al., 2011). In contrast, the risk ratio of women with less than a high school diploma showed they were only 1.48 times more likely (95% CI: 0.94–2.34) to kill themselves when compared with women who had completed tertiary education. This study also found that the population attributable fraction for suicide associated with low educational attainment was 41% for men, but 20% for women. In sum, this study found that low educational attainment significantly increases risk of suicide for both men and women, but risk is considerably higher among men, implying that education is a distal yet modifiable risk factor (especially for men), which should be a focus of suicide prevention efforts.

These findings have been confirmed by several studies focused on single jurisdictions. One US study found that suicide rates among the middle-aged were 2.4 times greater for those with a high school diploma or less compared with those with a college degree (Case & Deaton, 2015). Another study examined over 440,000 suicides in the United States from 2000 to 2014, finding that adults who possessed a college degree or higher had the lowest suicide rates, whereas those whose highest education was a high school diploma had the highest rates of suicide (Phillips & Hempstead, 2017). In terms of gender, this study found that men with only a high school diploma had double the risk of suicide compared with men with a college degree or more. In contrast, the magnitude of difference between women of high and low educational attainment was less marked. These results overlap with earlier US studies finding an inverse dose-response relationship between suicide and education, with less education increasing suicide risk, particularly among men (Abel & Kruger, 2005; Kposowa, 2000).

In Europe, a large-scale comparative study examined suicide mortality in ten different European populations, finding that low educational attainment was a significant risk factor for men in eight out of ten countries, with a pooled rate ratio of 1.43 (range 2.72–1.04) as compared with those with high educational attainment (Lorant et al., 2005). Interestingly, this study found less consistent and less intense associations between low educational attainment and suicide in women, with a pooled rate ratio of 0.92 when comparing women with low educational attainment with those with high educational attainment. Perhaps surprisingly, this study found that lower educational attainment was a protective factor for women in three European countries. Again, these findings are consistent with previous European studies, which found a clear gradient in suicide risk, with higher suicide rates associated with lower educational attainment, particularly among males (e.g., Bjorkenstam et al., 2011).

7.2.2 Substance Abuse

A growing body of research indicates that low educational attainment is correlated with a variety of substance use disorders (SUDs). One of the most insightful surveys contributing to this literature was conducted by Compton and colleagues at the US National Institute on Drug Abuse (Compton et al., 2007). In this study, researchers analyzed data from over 40,000 US adults to assess alcohol and drug abuse. Though almost 20 years old, this is still one of the most rigorous and comprehensive surveys, and the results are consistent with more recent research. This study found that those with lower educational attainment had the highest rate of SUDs, with an odds ratio of 1.4 (99% CI: 1.0–2.1) as compared with those with more than a high school education.

These results were confirmed by the aforementioned analysis of NESARC data, which similarly found a negative association between education and any SUD or substance use dependence, with the lowest rates of dependence/disorder among those with a graduate or professional degree (12.3%) and the highest rates in those with a high school diploma (24.2%) or less than high school (22.7%). Indeed, those with less than high school education were over twice as likely (OR 2.55: 99% CI: 2.01–3.23) to have any SUD or substance dependence than those with a graduate or professional degree (Erickson et al., 2016). But neither the NESARC study nor the Compton et al. (2007) study stratified educational attainment by gender.

Another US study of over 1000 individuals found that the risk of developing a substance use disorder was significantly higher among high school dropouts compared with those with a college degree, with an adjusted odds ratio of 3.50 (95% CI:1.71–7.17) (Fothergill et al., 2008). Similarly, a Mexican study found an elevated risk of substance use disorder among high school dropouts, with an odds ratio of 2.16 (95% CI: 1.49–3.13) compared with current students, but again odds ratios were not differentially specified by gender (Benjet et al., 2009).

One study that intentionally examined gender differences in SUD examined alcohol-use disorders (AUD) in a longitudinal analysis of over 1000 Americans (Crum et al., 2006). This study found that adult men who were high school dropouts had an adjusted OR of 3.37 (95% CI: 1.36–8.34) for AUD, compared with adult men with a college degree or higher. In contrast adult women who were high school dropouts had an adjusted OR of 2.37 (95% CI: 0.79–7.10) for AUD compared with adult women with a college degree or higher. In other words, this study overlaps with the aforementioned suicide studies, indicating that low educational attainment is a stronger risk factor for adverse mental health outcomes in men compared with women, and the longitudinal nature of this (and other) studies accounts for reverse causation.

Many of these findings were summarized in a recent systematic review, noting that a preponderance of studies found that secondary school dropout increased risk of SUD, as well as risk of cannabis use, injecting drug use, and opioid use (Esch et al., 2014). Indeed, opioid misuse is an issue of growing societal concern, prompting several recent research studies on the topic. One cross-sectional analysis of young adults participating in the 2015 National Survey on Drug Use and Health found that opioid misuse and related SUD symptoms were significantly higher among school dropouts, compared with those in tertiary education or employment (Schepis et al., 2018). In this study, 11.4% of high school dropouts had misused opioids in the last year, compared with 6.1% of those in college. Similarly, youth who had dropped out of high school had misused tranquilizers or sedatives at a rate of around 3:1 compared with those still in high school (6.7% vs. 2.7%). The authors did not stratify their results by gender, but a variety of other studies detailed in Chap. 3 indicate that less educated men have particularly high rates of both heroin misuse and prescription opioid/fentanyl misuse (e.g., Marsh et al., 2018; Pouget et al., 2017).

7.2.3 Depression and Anxiety

Several studies have indicated an inverse dose-response relationship between educational attainment and depression/anxiety, with more education protective against both these disorders. Indeed, a large-scale meta-analysis found that 35 out of 51 studies reviewed found a significant association between low socioeconomic status

(SES) and depression, with low SES individuals having an overall odds ratio of 1.8 (95% CI: 1.57–2.10) when compared with high SES individuals (Lorant et al., 2003). Importantly, 37 of the 51 studies used level of education as a proxy for socioeconomic status. This study also found that the odds of being depressed decreased by 3% for each additional year of education.

Similarly, the aforementioned analysis of NESARC data found that mood disorders were lowest in those with a professional or graduate degree (7.3%), or a bachelor's or technical degree (9.1%), while those with less than high school had an elevated prevalence of 11.6%. Similarly, anxiety disorders were also lowest in those who had completed tertiary education, compared with those with some college or less education. Indeed, educational attainment at wave 1 was negatively associated with incident depression and anxiety at wave 2 (thus accounting for reverse causation), and those with less than high school education had a 65%–70% higher rate of depression and anxiety compared with those with a graduate or professional degree (Erickson et al., 2016). These findings are consistent with a systematic review, which found that high school dropouts had higher rates of depression than high school graduates at the age of expected graduation, as well as more anxiety in young adulthood per se (Esch et al., 2014). The authors attributed these elevated rates to various factors, including the lack of vocational opportunities for high school dropouts, as well as more precarious and unstable living conditions due to lower income and fewer resources.

To summarize all this epidemiological literature, evidence suggests that there is an inverse dose-response relationship between educational attainment and mental health. Low educational attainment is a risk factor for a variety of adverse mental health outcomes, while high educational attainment is a protective factor. Importantly, the reviewed studies suggest that low educational attainment is a more powerful risk factor for men compared with women. As previously stated, educational attainment is a distal yet modifiable risk factor, which could be the target for prevention and promotion. This raises a variety of questions pertinent to men's mental health. First, are there gender differences in educational attainment between males and females? Second, are males being well-served and well-treated by the current education system? Third, what can be changed to better engage male students within the different levels of education? The rest of this chapter attempts to answer these questions.

7.3 The Educational Gender Gap

A growing body of evidence indicates that boys are performing significantly worse than girls at all levels of education including primary school, secondary school, and tertiary education. This is manifest by a number of pan-national statistics. For example, an analysis of data from a wide range of cohorts in 32 European countries plus the United States found that female educational attainment significantly surpassed male educational attainment in all 33 countries, with the sole exception of Switzerland (van Hek et al., 2016).

Similarly, figures from a variety of jurisdictions including the United Kingdom, New Zealand, and Canada indicate that boys have more than three times the rate of suspension, exclusion, and expulsion than girls in both primary and secondary education (Government of the United Kingdom School Absence and Exclusions Team, 2021; New Zealand Government Ministry of Education, 2020; Scottish Government Education Analytical Services, 2020; Ontario Ministry of Education, 2019). This can seriously impede learning of basic literacy and numeracy skills and can contribute to school dropout and later unemployment (Perry & Morris, 2014; Fabelo et al., 2011; Flannery, 2015).

Relatedly, boys have almost double the rate of placement in special education compared with girls in both primary and secondary schools. For example, a comprehensive report by the US Department of Education entitled *The Condition of Education 2020* found that 4.13 million (18%) male students ages 6–21 years enrolled in public schools were in special education due to a disability compared with 2.12 million (10%) of similarly aged female students (Hussar et al., 2020). This report indicated considerable gender differences in the reasons for such special education including elevated male rates of autism (M:F 5:1), developmental delay (M:F 2:1), and emotional disturbance (M:F 2.5:1), as well as issues related to attention-deficit hyperactivity disorder, discussed in great detail in Chap. 5.

This state of affairs has led numerous high-profile scholars to describe the educational situation of boys in ominous terminology, in best-selling books with dramatic titles including *The Boy Crisis* (Farrell & Gray, 2018), *The War Against Boys* (Sommers, 2015), and *Boys Adrift* (Sax, 2016). Others have used less dramatic language, simply calling this worrying phenomenon a "gender education gap" (e.g., DiPrete & Buchmann, 2013). The following sections of this chapter will examine data regarding this gender gap, divided into three subsections, namely: (i) primary education; (ii) secondary education; and (iii) tertiary education.

7.3.1 Primary Education

Male underachievement in the education system appears at an early age in the primary school level and is manifested in a number of relevant statistics related to literacy, grade repetition, and expulsions. For example, boys tend to have more difficulty than girls in mastering basic reading skills, with the aforementioned US *Condition of Education* report noting that the average reading score for males (217) was significantly lower than females (224) at Grade 4 (Hussar et al., 2020). Similarly, US Department of Education figures indicate that boys are 33% more likely to be retained in a grade during primary school, with 2% of males retained compared with 1.5% females (National Center for Education Statistics, 2019a). In other words, boys are more likely to fail a grade, even at an early age, which is commonly due to problems in reading, writing, and basic literacy (Jimerson et al., 2006; Cannon & Lipscomb, 2011).

Another serious issue facing boys in primary school is an elevated rate of expulsions, suspensions, and exclusions. For example, figures from Scotland indicate that over 90% of primary school exclusions are male, with 2974 male exclusions in 2018/2019, compared with 271 female exclusions. This translates to a rate of 14.6 per 1000 male pupils and 1.4 per 1000 female pupils (Scottish Government Education Analytical Services, 2020).

Evidence suggests that these gender gaps are caused by a variety of factors. One important factor is that teachers tend to hold more negative stereotypes of boys and more positive biases toward girls, leading to differential treatment in the classroom. In short, some evidence suggests a halo effect for girls at school, where teachers minimize or overlook disruptive behaviors in girls, while overly attending to disruptive behaviors in boys. In other words, girls are perceived to be better behaved and more studious, while boys are perceived to be more disruptive and unruly, regardless of actual behaviors on the ground. This can lead to discipline and negative attention for boys and positive attention and encouragement for girls. Much of this literature was discussed in detail in the previous chapter on ADHD (see Chap. 5), but a quick recap will be given here.

As detailed in Chap. 5, several studies find that teachers typically report that boys with ADHD are more disruptive and impaired than girls with ADHD, even though mothers routinely report that boys and girls have similar levels of impairment and disruptive behaviors (Gaub & Carlson, 1997; Gershon, 2002). Indeed, Bauermeister et al. (2007) found that boys with ADHD were more likely than girls with ADHD to be suspended from school, which could be indicative of a halo effect for girls with ADHD. Indeed, Hartung et al. (2002) averaged teacher and mother reports of disruptive behavior in a sample of US primary school age children diagnosed with ADHD, comparing averages between boys and girls. When averaged, mothers reported no significant difference in observed disruptive behaviors between boys and girls, while teachers reported that boys had almost twice the level of disruptive behaviors compared with girls. In other words, teachers may perceive girls to be less disruptive due to the aforementioned halo effect, while they may perceive boys to be more disruptive due to enduring stereotypes of males as an untamed threat to social harmony and good order – an issue discussed in more detail in Chap. 1.

Research reveals that the operation of these negative gender stereotypes and cognitive biases among teachers can extend to all children, regardless of their ADHD status. For example, one study explored the relationship among strengths, classroom behavior, and academic achievement for a sample of Canadian students in Grades 1 and 2. Results indicated that teachers rated female pupils as having more strengths than male pupils including higher levels of school functioning, peer functioning, personality functioning, and personal/physical care (Whitley et al., 2011). Again, this indicates a halo effect for girls in the school setting and negative stereotypes of boys.

Of relevance to such an argument, statistics from a variety of nations indicate that the primary school teaching staff is overwhelmingly female. For example, the US Department of Education *Condition of Education* report found that only 11% of elementary school teachers are men (Hussar et al., 2020). Similar figures are seen in other jurisdictions. In Canada, only 16% of primary school teachers are men, with men making up only 4% of early childhood educators. Indeed, Professor Jon Bradley notes that many Canadian children never encounter a male teacher during their primary and secondary schooling, while Professor Mike Parr argues that this situation means that boys may be unwittingly socialized to perceive reading, teaching, and learning as activities geared to girls (Abraham, 2010).

Indeed, some have argued that the large gender imbalance among the teaching staff may contribute to a school culture, which is implicitly "feminized," which can manifest itself in female-friendly classroom learning activities that may not be fully engaging to boys (Sommers, 2015; Farrell & Gray, 2018). Moreover, the absence of male teachers at the primary level means that impressionable young boys will lack male role models during this crucial period of their lives, which could contribute to boys' alienation in the classroom, and later issues (Sax, 2016; Farrell & Gray, 2018). This may be particularly significant to the growing number of boys raised in fatherless households, who thus lack male role models at home and at school. All this can interact, leading to bored, unengaged, and marginalized boys at the primary school level, meaning they are not sufficiently learning foundational scholarly skills nor gaining a love of education in the formative years of their lives. The discussion of these issues is elaborated in the next section on secondary education, as there has been much more research on gender differentials in secondary educational attainment.

7.3.2 Secondary Education

The previously described gender gaps in literacy, suspensions, and performance continue into secondary school, at times widening and intensifying to place boys at even greater risk of adverse educational outcomes. For example, a large survey of 64 countries (30 OECD countries and 34 partner countries) found that 14% of boys and 9% of girls perform below basic proficiency in the three core subjects of science, reading and mathematics at age 15 years, meaning that boys are over 50% more likely to be low-achievers than girls (OECD, 2015). In the United Kingdom, females obtained significantly higher General Certificate of Secondary Education (GCSE) exam results at ages 15–16 years than males, and males are more concentrated among students with lower grades, with this gender gap widening from 2005 to 2015 (Bramley et al., 2015). Similar gender gaps are seen in the United States, with a large corpus of research indicating that girls tend to receive higher grades than boys throughout high school (Hussar et al., 2020; Meier et al., 2018; Kleinfeld, 2009).

Similarly, US figures indicate that boys are more likely to be retained in a grade compared with girls, with 3.1% of males retained in grades 9–12, compared with 2.6% of females (National Center for Education Statistics, 2019a). Moreover, a wide range of surveys indicate that boys are more likely to experience detention, suspension, or exclusion than girls (McKinley Research Group, 2016; Finn &

Servoss, 2014; Scottish Government Education Analytical Services, 2020). Figures from the UK indicate that males were around three times more likely to be excluded from secondary schools compared with females, with a male rate of 59 per 1000 pupils, compared with a female rate of 20 per 1000 pupils (Scottish Government Education Analytical Services, 2020). US statistics indicate that boys are around four times more likely to receive any form of discipline than girls (Skiba et al., 2014) and constitute over 70% of total suspensions (Petras et al., 2011). Indeed, one US study of over 8000 tenth grade students found that males were around twice as likely to be suspended than females, with 21.2% of males having received an in-school or out-of-school suspension compared with 12.8% of females (Finn & Servoss, 2014). Importantly, this study found that males had a higher rate of suspension than females even after controlling for student and teacher reported misbehavior, indicating that males are 1.86 times more likely to be suspended for exhibiting "average misbehavior" compared with females displaying the same "average misbehavior." This indicates that teacher decisions on suspensions may be founded upon prevalent gender stereotypes and biases discussed in Chap. 1, particularly stereotypes of boys as disruptive or defiant and in need of discipline, as well as an associated *halo effect* for girls.

Moreover, the large gender gap in literacy continues into high school. In a large international survey of OECD countries, 15-year-old girls performed significantly better than 15-year-old boys in reading in all countries surveyed by an average of 38 points, which is the equivalent of one full year of schooling (OECD, 2015). Similarly, Kleinfeld (2009) reviewed a variety of US data, finding that 26% of 12th grade boys have only basic literacy skills, compared with 11% girls. In contrast, 31% of girls achieve proficient/advanced levels of literacy, compared with only 16% boys. The more recent US *Condition of Education* report (2020) confirms that boys continue to experience much lower rates of literacy through secondary school. At grade 8, the average reading score for male students (258) was lower than female students (269), while at grade 12 the average reading score for males was 282, compared with 292 for females. In contrast, the average maths score for grade 8 was the same among males (282) and females (282) and slightly higher for males in grade 12 (153 male and 150 female). Indeed, the aforementioned OECD survey found few significant differences between boys and girls in math and science, and these differences were much smaller than those observed for reading and literacy (OECD, 2015). Similarly, UK data indicates that females score significantly better on GCSE English exams than males, while there is no significant difference in GCSE maths exam results by gender (Sammons et al., 2014).

It has been argued that the small gap in maths and science disfavoring girls has been the subject of much policy and societal discussion and targeted intervention, while the larger gap in reading and literacy disfavoring boys has been routinely ignored and neglected (Meier & Diefenbach, 2018; Farrell & Gray, 2018; Sommers, 2015; Sax, 2016). This may be a consequence of the *gender empathy gap* or *male gender blindness* discussed in Chap. 1 and policy orientations that typically ignore or neglect social inequalities experienced by males. All this is concerning, as poor reading and writing skills can place boys at a serious disadvantage in their quest for educational and employment opportunities upon leaving secondary school.

Another metric where there is a clear preponderance of males is in the high school dropout rate. The calculation of the high school dropout rate varies between jurisdictions and studies and is the topic of some controversy. For example, some dropout figures are relatively low as the denominator includes all adults ages 16–24 years, thus accounting for late learners who dropout during their teens but return to education later to complete a GED or equivalent high school credential. When the denominator simply includes young school-aged adults in their teens, the dropout rate increases dramatically. But whichever method is used, boys invariably have a significantly higher dropout rate than girls.

For example, the aforementioned US *Condition of Education* report examined high school dropout, defined as the percentage of 16–24 year olds who are not enrolled in school and have not earned a high school diploma or equivalent credential. This found that the high school dropout rate of males (6.2%) was almost 50% higher than females (4.4%) (Hussar et al., 2020). This male preponderance was seen across all US racial groups, with the highest rates among Hispanic males (9.6%) and Black males (7.8%). Figures from Australia indicate a similar gender differential, with 20.4% of teen boys dropping out of high school, compared with 11.4% of teen girls, with high rates among Aboriginal Australians (Australian Bureau of Statistics, 2019).

Other related metrics find a similar male preponderance. For example, Canadian figures indicate that 24% of males do not graduate high school on time, compared with 16% of females (Statistics Canada, 2019b). In Aboriginal communities in northern Canada, around one in two boys does not graduate high school on time, while in the province of Quebec it is one in three (Statistics Canada, 2019b). As stated, some people who drop out of high school in their teens return to school to obtain a high school credential later in life, but there remains a gender differential in this process. In Canada, 2016/2017 figures indicate that 14% of males never graduate high school, almost double the 8% rate of females (Statistics Canada, 2019c). This preponderance of males among high school dropouts is a decades-old problem, with surveys from the 1990s to the present indicating a much higher dropout rate in males than females (Statistics Canada, 2015). These dropout rates are especially concerning given that we now live in a service-based economy. Long gone are the days when unqualified unskilled young men could easily find honorable and well-paid occupations in manufacturing, farming, fishing, or other manual labor. This knock-on effect on employment is explored in Chap. 8.

As in primary schools, statistics indicate that the secondary school workforce is also dominated by women. For example, the US *Condition of Education* report found that only 36% of secondary school teachers are men, a decrease from 41% in 1999/2000 (Hussar et al., 2020). Similarly low numbers of male teachers are seen in Australia (39%), as well as in Canada (41%) (Australian Bureau of Statistics, 2019; Statistics Canada, 2016c). Again, it has been argued that this imbalance can contribute toward a feminized school culture characterized by a relative lack of potential male role models and an unengaging environment for male learners (Farrell & Gray, 2018; Sax, 2016).

Sommers (2015) argues that this can create a male-unfriendly environment, with figures showing a decline in traditional boyhood pursuits such as physical education, sports, woodwork, metalwork, and recess break times across a variety of US schools, combined with an increased aversion to "rough and tumble" activities and zero tolerance policies for boisterous behavior. She argues that this prevents boys from expanding their natural energy and exuberance, leading to fidgety and restless boys in the classroom, who are then disciplined or sanctioned by overstrained teachers. This theory is backed up by data from different jurisdictions, which indicate that teachers tend to have more fractured relationships with male pupils than female pupils in the secondary school setting and often perceive males as more defiant and disruptive (e.g., Newcomb et al., 2002; Wentzel, 2002).

For example, a UK survey found that teachers perceived more pro-social behavior in female year 11 pupils than male year 11 pupils, with teachers perceiving that female pupils were more likely to be considerate of other people's feelings and share readily with others, while males were perceived to engage in more antisocial behavior including lying and cheating (Sammons et al., 2014). Such perceptions may affect the teacher-pupil relationship, with one large-scale Canadian study finding that male pupils are much less likely to report getting along well with teachers, and less likely to be interested in what they were learning in class compared with female pupils (Statistics Canada, 2008). This lack of teacher–pupil engagement can create a harmful vicious circle, negatively affecting boys' motivation to learn. Indeed, an Australian study found that boys have lower levels of motivation than girls at secondary school, with boys scoring lower on a variety of measures such as learning focus, planning, study management, and persistence (Martin, 2011). This lack of engagement and motivation can extend to a male–female differential in homework. In fact, a myriad of studies indicate that secondary school girls spend significantly more time on homework than boys, typically over 1.25 h per week more, again indicating a lack of motivation and engagement with class material in boys (Holt & Gershenson, 2015; Xu, 2011). This gender gap even extends to extracurricular activity, with a US report finding that boys are less likely to participate in extracurricular activities than girls in high school, with 54% of girls now participating in such activities compared with 44% of boys, with male activity focused on sports, while female activity is more varied (Meier et al., 2018). All this indicates problems of engagement, motivation, and inclusion of males in the high school setting, but this is rarely considered a public policy priority and is routinely ignored.

7.3.3 Tertiary Education

Interestingly, the education gender gap also extends into the various sectors of tertiary education, with statistics from a variety of jurisdictions indicating that men are typically underrepresented in universities and colleges. In the United States, the

7.3 The Educational Gender Gap

aforementioned *Condition of Education* report indicates that 38% of males ages 18–24 years were enrolled in tertiary education (including community college, vocational college, and trade schools), compared with 44% of females, continuing a trend going back decades (Hussar et al., 2020). Indeed, this report notes that 56% of all undergraduates are female while 44% are male. This gender differential widens when focusing on postgraduate degrees including masters, doctoral, and professional degrees (e.g., medicine, law, or dentistry), with men accounting for only 40% of postgraduate students, while women account for 60% (Hussar et al., 2020). These gender ratios in postsecondary attendance are not a recent phenomenon and stretch back into the 1970s (OECD, 2015; Statistics Canada, 2008). Of note, the Hussar et al. (2020) report notes that female enrollment in postsecondary education is projected to increase at a higher rate than males, meaning that this gender gap in tertiary enrolment will likely increase over time.

Similar figures are seen elsewhere. An analysis of the demographics of Canadian full-time students in 2018/2019 indicates that 58% of bachelor's students are female, compared with 42% males. For master's students, the gender gap widens even further to 60% female and 40% male, just like the US figures. Interestingly, male underrepresentation in tertiary education is particularly high in Anglo-Caribbean nations such as Barbados and Jamaica where young women are around twice as likely to go to university compared with young men (World Economic Forum, 2020). Importantly, men also tend to have higher rates of university dropout, with US figures noting that 65% of female bachelor's students completed their degree within 6 years at the same institution, compared with 59% of males.

Unsurprisingly, a similar gender gap is observed when examining tertiary graduation rates. For example, the US Department of Education notes that US males were awarded 43% of all bachelor's degrees conferred, compared with 57% for females in 2017/2018. The figures are similar for associate degrees, with females awarded 61% of associate degrees in 2017/2018, compared with 39% awarded to males (Hussar et al., 2020). This report also found that 42% of 25- to 29-year-old women had obtained a bachelor's degree or higher, compared with 36% of men. This gender gap had widened since 2000, where 30% of women and 28% of men had obtained a bachelor's or higher degree. In Canada, 2019 figures indicate a similar female preponderance in completion of some form of tertiary education, with 71% of female ages 25–34 years completing some form of tertiary education, compared with 55% of males (Statistics Canada, 2020).

The reasons for the aforementioned gender differences in postsecondary enrollment, retention, and graduation are not well-established, as these differences have not been a research or policy priority for those working on issues of gender and inclusion. Instead, much of the focus has been on female underrepresentation in a narrow range of STEM subjects, while neglecting the wider and larger issue of male underrepresentation in tertiary education per se. Moreover, male underrepresentation is particularly concentrated in certain academic programs including social work, nursing, counselling psychology, child psychology, and education (i.e., teaching), with men typically making up around 10–25% of students in these programs, with numbers declining in recent years (National League for Nursing, 2019;

National Center for Education Statistics, 2019b; Higher Education Statistics Company, 2021). This is rarely perceived as an inequality in need of attention, nor discussed as an area in need of intervention. This lack of male representation in these programs means that there are fewer and fewer male teachers, nurses, social workers, and counselling psychologists working as healthcare providers or as teachers. As such, some elements of health care and education will continue to lack a "male face" for the foreseeable future and may continue to be perceived as a feminized environment by male students and male patients. This is an important issue, given the literature described in this chapter and Chap. 6 indicating the importance of male teachers and male clinicians in promoting male engagement with education and health services.

Given the previously described situation, it might be expected that universities and colleges would be investing in programs that promote male engagement, especially trying to engage men in academic programs such as teaching and psychology, where there is a proven need for more male students. However, this does not seem to be the case and in fact some have argued that universities and colleges are not only indifferent to male under-enrollment but also have actually become somewhat hostile to men and masculinity (e.g., Kipnis, 2017; Reynolds, 2019; Perry, 2019). For example, it has been noted that there are numerous well-funded groups, programs, and offices on most postsecondary campuses addressing women's issues and advocating for empowerment of female students. These receive official support from various quarters and are rarely seen as controversial (Whitley, 2020).

In contrast, there are very few groups or programs focused on men's issues and the advancement of male students on postsecondary campuses (MacDonald, 2018). In fact, reports indicate that a few informal groups have attempted to organize discussions about some of the men's issues discussed throughout this book, but have faced hostility by other campus groups. For example, a group of male and female students at Ryerson University (Canada) created a men's issues group, with lectures on topics such as male suicide. This group was refused official status by the Ryerson University Student Union on numerous occasions (Collier, 2015). A similar phenomenon occurred at Durham University (UK) where a men's issues group has been denied official recognition for many years (Daubney, 2015). Likewise, the University of Toronto Men's Issues Society invited renowned gender scholar Dr. Warren Farrell to talk about men's mental health, but his lecture was met with demonstration and vandalism by protesters (Smeenk, 2012). While these are isolated incidents, they are perhaps indicative of a wider reluctance to sympathetically discuss men's issues on campus and may also be a manifestation of the *gender empathy gap* discussed in Chap. 1.

Moreover, it has been argued that university professors and university administrators are creating moral panics about male students by routinely using stigmatizing all-encompassing terms such as "toxic masculinity" and "rape culture" to refer to male students en masse (e.g., Kipnis, 2017; Veissière, 2018; MacDonald, 2018). These concepts have been criticized for implicitly portraying male students as inherently toxic or potential rapists, a rendering of the stereotypical female victim/male villain dichotomy discussed in Chap. 1. In these arguments, insistent use of such concepts contributes to a male-unfriendly environment, which may in turn discourage male enrollment, retention, and sense of belonging, ultimately harming the mental health of vulnerable male students. Such speculation has not been the topic of in-depth research, but the wider literature points toward a need for research assessing the influence of institutional ambience and social context on male student mental health.

7.4 Failure to Launch and Male Loneliness

The evidence hitherto reviewed in this chapter indicates that young men and boys are facing serious challenges in completing an education, which consequently increases difficulties in entering the workforce. This means that many young men remain in their parental home and do not fully establish themselves as independent functional adults. This phenomenon is sometimes known as *failure to launch,* an umbrella term typically referring to the situation of young adults who are: (i) unemployed, (ii) living with their parents, and (iii) out of the educational system (Kins & Beyers, 2010; Mykyta, 2012). Again, data indicates that failure to launch is a mostly male problem, with a Canadian study indicating that 47% of men in their 20s still live with their parents, compared with 38% of women (Milan, 2016), while a US study found that 55% of 18- to 29-year-old males and 49% of similarly aged females still lived with their parents (Fry et al., 2020). Men experiencing such failure to launch often lack the social capital that comes with participation in education or employment and may also lack financial capital given their impecunious circumstances, meaning an inability to go out and socialize with other youth (Whitley & Zhou, 2020).

This can contribute toward a life of unemployment, isolation, petty crime, drug use, and wasted potential, leaving the affected young men bereft of existential meaning and purpose in life, while creating disaffection and alienation from wider society (Zimbardo & Coulombe, 2016; Sax, 2016; Case & Deaton, 2020). All this may contribute toward abnormally high rates of loneliness in young men, which is a known risk factor for mental illness (Hawkley & Cacioppo, 2010). For example, a recent US survey found that almost one in three millennial men always or often felt lonely and just over a quarter had no close friends. These rates were almost double the rates of loneliness seen in baby-boomer men and higher than rates for millennial women (YouGov, 2019). Indeed, the results from this survey indicated that 23% of all men always or often feel lonely compared with 20% of all women, signifying elevated rates of loneliness in males per se.

Similarly, another large-scale loneliness survey of over 10,000 Americans indicated that young adults have higher rates of loneliness than older adults (Cigna, 2020). This survey indicated that over 70% of young adults reported sometimes or always feeling alone, shy, or that no one really understands them, a figure significantly higher than that seen in older adults. Again, this survey found higher rates of loneliness in men compared with women, with 63% of men having a high loneliness score (as defined by the UCLA loneliness scale) compared with 58% of women.

In Canada, a recent survey by the Angus Reid Institute (2020) found that 63% of 18- to 34-year-old men experienced considerable loneliness and isolation, compared with 53% of similarly aged women. All these findings are consistent with a recent international survey of loneliness with over 46,000 participants spread over 237 countries, islands, and territories (Barreto et al., 2021). This survey found that young men reported the highest levels of loneliness out of all demographic groups, significantly higher than young women, and that older men reported higher levels than older women too. In sum, young men are more likely to experience failure to launch and higher rates of loneliness compared with young women. This may be a consequence of the aforementioned educational difficulties faced by a growing number of young men leading to social exclusion and disenfranchisement from mainstream society. All this may further contribute toward the previously described mental health difficulties, which are associated with low educational attainment, and may in turn contribute to difficulties in employment discussed in Chap. 8.

7.5 Conclusion

This chapter has summarized a growing literature noting that low-educational attainment is a risk factor for a variety of adverse mental health outcomes including suicide, depression, and substance use disorder. Of note, the literature indicates that low educational attainment has a more severe and intense effect on the mental health of men compared with women and may contribute to high levels of loneliness and failure to launch in young men. Higher educational attainment is also associated with higher median earnings (see Chap. 8), and the employment rate is significantly higher for people with postsecondary education. In other words, education sets a foundation for life and can be a springboard to success and good mental health, or a road to failure and worsened mental health.

Writing in 2009, Judith Kleinfeld stated that "while boys and girls both suffer from characteristic problems, those of boys are neglected and far more serious." This remains the case today, as evidenced by a variety of statistics. As stated, males experience significantly higher levels of school dropout, exclusions, and underachievement. Similarly, males experience significantly lower levels of literacy, graduation, and retention. Males also make up a solid minority of postsecondary students, particularly in fields such as education and psychology, perpetuating male underrepresentation in these professions. As noted, these inequalities are rarely on the public radar, despite the massive cost to the affected males and to their families and society as a whole. As such, there is a need for renewed policies, interventions, and programs to help boys and young men in their educational journey. This will not only improve their educational performance but also can improve their employability and their mental health. A multipronged approach is necessary but may involve action in a variety of domains.

First, there is a need to diversify the educational workforce, which is currently female dominated, especially among primary school teachers. This can help provide role models for troubled young men at an early age and may help in the creation of a school environment that is more male friendly. This must also involve universities and colleges making conscious and meaningful efforts to recruit more male students into teacher-training programs, as well as other related programs currently lacking male representation such as child psychology, nursing, and social work.

Second, there is a need to take targeted action to reduce the male high school dropout rate. This demographic has received little policy or research attention, but one approach can involve the diversification of the curriculum so that meaningful time is devoted to traditional boyhood pursuits such as physical education, sports, woodwork, metalwork, and break-times. This may help retain less academically gifted male pupils, while helping them on the road to vocational or trade qualifications. Another approach could involve social and emotional learning programs for at-risk males focused on social skill acquisition, personal development, and mentoring by other males – with an emphasis on learning positive pro-social solutions to their problems (Whitley & Zhou, 2020). Indeed, one leading researcher concluded that schools "need to develop programs to help boys with ADHD effectively without resorting to suspension or expulsion as the primary mean of handling school problems. This practice can increase the risk of demoralization of boys with the disorder and school dropout" (Bauermeister et al., 2007). Such programs may be necessary for all boys, with or without ADHD.

Third, postsecondary institutions and university administrators should reconsider the use of stigmatizing all-encompassing concepts such as "rape culture" or "toxic masculinity" that tar all male students with the same brush. Any policies or practices reliant on such concepts should similarly be reconsidered, with thought given to renewed policies and practices that encourage better academic engagement of male students. Indeed, postsecondary institutions could encourage the formation and expansion of grassroots groups devoted to discussing and addressing the men's issues discussed throughout this book, including men's mental health peer support groups. Such groups could receive official funding and should have a seat at the table in wider discussions about gender issues and discussions about promoting enrolment and retention of underrepresented students.

References

Abel, E. L., & Kruger, M. L. (2005). Educational attainment and suicide rates in the United States. *Psychological Reports, 97*(1), 25–28. https://doi.org/10.2466/pr0.97.1.25-28

Abraham, C. (2010, October 10). Part 2: The endangered male teacher. *The Globe and Mail*. https://www.theglobeandmail.com/news/national/time-to-lead/part-2-the-endangered-male-teacher/article4330079/

Angus Reid Institute. (2020). *Isolation, loneliness and COVID-19: Pandemic leads to sharp increase in mental health challenges, social woes*. Retrieved June 11, 2021, from https://angusreid.org/wp-content/uploads/2020/10/2020.10.13_Social_Isolation.pdf

Australian Bureau of Statistics. (2019, February 19). *Schools*. Retrieved February 22, 2021, from https://www.abs.gov.au/statistics/people/education/schools/latest-release

Barreto, M., Victor, C., Hammond, C., Eccles, A., Richins, M. T., & Qualter, P. (2021). Loneliness around the world: Age, gender, and cultural differences in loneliness. *Personality & Individual Differences, 169*(3), 110066. https://doi.org/10.1016/j.paid.2020.110066

Bauermeister, J. J., Shrout, P. E., Chavez, L., Rubio-Stipec, M., Ramirez, R., Padilla, L., Anderson, A., Garcia, P., & Canino, G. (2007). ADHD and gender: Are risks and sequela of ADHD the same for boys and girls? *Journal of Child Psychology and Psychiatry, 48*(8), 831–839. https://doi.org/10.1111/j.1469-7610.2007.01750.x

Benjet, C., Borges, G., Medina-Mora, M. E., Zambrano, J., & Aguilar-Gaxiola, S. (2009). Youth mental health in a populous city of the developing world: Results from the Mexican Adolescent Mental Health Survey. *The Journal of Child Psychology and Psychiatry, 50*(4), 386–395. https://doi.org/10.1111/j.1469-7610.2008.01962.x

Bjorkenstam, C., Ringback Weitoft, G., Hjern, A., Nordstrom, P., Hallqvist, J., & Ljung, R. (2011). School grades, parental education and suicide – A national register-based cohort study. *Journal of Epidemiology and Community Health, 65*, 993–998. https://doi.org/10.1136/jech.2010.117226

Bramley, T., Vidal Rodeiro, C., & Vitello, S. (2015, October 20). *Gender differences in GCSE*. Cambridge Assessment Research Report. Retrieved February 22, 2021, from https://www.cambridgeassessment.org.uk/Images/gender-differences-in-gcse.pdf

Cannon, J. S., & Lipscomb, S. (2011, March). *Early grade retention and student success: Evidence from Los Angeles*. Public Policy Institute of California. Retrieved February 22, 2021, from https://www.ppic.org/content/pubs/report/R_311JCR.pdf

Case, A., & Deaton, A. (2015). Rising morbidity and mortality in midlife among white non-Hispanic Americans in the 21st century. *PNAS, 112*(49), 15078–15083. https://doi.org/10.1073/pnas.1518393112

Case, A., & Deaton, A. (2020). *Deaths of despair and the future of capitalism*. Princeton University Press.

Cigna. (2020, January). *Loneliness and the workplace: 2020 U.S. report*. Retrieved February 22, 2021, from https://www.cigna.com/about-us/newsroom/studies-and-reports/combatting-loneliness/research-report

Collier, R. (2015, November 9). Ryerson men's issues group says students' union shutting out male voices. *The Globe and Mail*. https://www.theglobeandmail.com/news/toronto/ryerson-mens-issues-group-says-student-union-shutting-out-male-voices/article27180128/

Compton, W. W., Thomas, Y. F., Stinson, F. S., & Grant, B. F. (2007). Prevalence, correlates, disability, and comorbidity of DSM-IV drug abuse and dependence in the United States: Results from the national epidemiologic survey on alcohol and related conditions. *Archives of General Psychiatry, 64*(5), 566–576. https://doi.org/10.1001/archpsyc.64.7.830

Council on School Health. (2013). Out-of-school suspension and expulsion. *Pediatrics, 131*(3), 1000–1007. https://doi.org/10.1542/peds.2012-3932

Crum, R. M., Juon, H.-S., Green, K. M., Robertson, J., Fothergill, K., & Ensminger, M. (2006). Educational achievement and early school behavior as predictors of alcohol-use disorders: 35-year follow-up of the Woodlawn Study. *Journal of Studies on Alcohol and Drugs, 67*(1), 75–85. https://doi.org/10.15288/jsa.2006.67.75

Daubney, M. (2015, June 16). Why are our universities blocking men's societies? *The Telegraph*. https://www.telegraph.co.uk/men/thinking-man/11670138/Why-are-our-universities-blocking-mens-societies.html

DiPrete, T. A., & Buchmann, C. (2013). *The rise of women: The growing gender gap in education and what it means for American schools*. Russell Sage Foundation.

Erickson, J., El-Gabalawy, R., Palitsky, D., Patten, S., Mackenzie, C. S., Stein, M. B., & Sareen, J. (2016). Educational attainment as a protective factor for psychiatric disorders: Findings from a nationally representative longitudinal study. *Depression and Anxiety, 33*(11), 1013–1022. https://doi.org/10.1002/da.22515

References

Esch, P., Bocquet, V., Pull, C., Couffignal, S., Lehnert, T., Graas, M., Fond-Harmant, L., & Ansseau, M. (2014). The downward spiral of mental disorders and educational attainment: A systematic review on early school leaving. *BMC Psychiatry, 14*(1), 237. https://doi.org/10.1186/s12888-014-0237-4

Fabelo, T., Thompson, M. D., Plotkin, M., Carmichael, D., Marchbanks, M. P. III, & Booth, E. A. (2011, July). *Breaking schools' rules: A statewide study of how school discipline relates to students' success and juvenile justice involvement*. Council of State Governments Justice Center & Public Policy Research Institute. Retrieved February 22, 2021, from https://www.ojp.gov/library/abstracts/breaking-schools-rules-statewide-study-how-school-discipline-relates-students

Farrell, W., & Gray, J. (2018). *The boy crisis: Why our boys are struggling and what we can do about it*. BenBella Books.

Finn, J. D., & Servoss, T. J. (2014). Misbehavior, suspensions, and security measures in high school: Racial/ethnic and gender differences. *Journal of Applied Research on Children, 5*(2), 1–50.

Flannery, M. E. (2015, January 5). *The school-to-prison pipeline: Time to shut it down*. National Education Association (NEA). Retrieved February 22, 2021, from https://www.nea.org/advocating-for-change/new-from-nea/school-prison-pipeline-time-shut-it-down

Fothergill, K. E., Ensminger, M. E., Green, K. M., Crum, R. M., Robertson, J., & Juon, H.-S. (2008). The impact of early school behavior and educational achievement on adult drug use disorders: A prospective study. *Drug and Alcohol Dependence, 92*(1–3), 191–199. https://doi.org/10.1016/j.drugalcdep.2007.08.001

Fry, R., Passel, J. S., & Cohn, D. (2020, September 4). *A majority of young adults in the U.S. live with their parents for the first time since the Great Depression*. Pew Research Center. Retrieved February 22, 2021, from https://www.pewresearch.org/fact-tank/2020/09/04/a-majority-of-young-adults-in-the-u-s-live-with-their-parents-for-the-first-time-since-the-great-depression/

Gaub, M., & Carlson, C. L. (1997). Gender differences in ADHD: A meta-analysis and critical review. *Journal of the American Academy of Child & Adolescent Psychiatry, 36*(8), 1036–1045. https://doi.org/10.1097/00004583-199708000-00011

Gershon, J. (2002). A meta-analytic review of gender differences in ADHD. *Journal of Attention Disorders, 5*(3), 143–154. https://doi.org/10.1177/108705470200500302

Government of the United Kingdom School Absence and Exclusions Team. (2021, February 2). *Permanent and fixed-period exclusions in England*. Retrieved February 22, 2021, from https://explore-education-statistics.service.gov.uk/find-statistics/permanent-and-fixed-period-exclusions-in-england

Hanford, E. (2014, September 11). *A 21st-century vocational high school*. APM Reports. Retrieved February 22, 2021, from https://www.apmreports.org/episode/2014/09/11/a-21st-century-vocational-high-school

Hartung, C. M., Willcutt, E. G., Lahey, B. B., Pelham, W. E., Loney, J., Stein, M. A., & Keenan, K. (2002). Sex differences in young children who meet criteria for attention deficit hyperactivity disorder. *Journal of Clinical Child and Adolescent Psychology, 31*(4), 453–464. https://doi.org/10.1207/S15374424JCCP3104_5

Hawkley, L. C., & Cacioppo, J. T. (2010). Loneliness matters: A theoretical and empirical review of consequences and mechanisms. *Annals of Behavioral Medicine, 40*(2), 218–227. https://doi.org/10.1007/s12160-010-9210-8

Higher Education Statistics Company. (2021). *What do HE students study?* Retrieved February 22, 2021, from https://www.hesa.ac.uk/data-and-analysis/students/what-study

Hoareau McGrath, C., Henham, M. L., Corbett, A., Durazzi, N., Frearson, M. Janta, B., Kamphuis, B. W., Katashiro, E., Brankovic, N., Guerin, B., Manville, C., Schwartz, I., Schweppenstedde, D. (2014, May). *Higher education entrance qualifications and exams in Europe: A comparison*. European Parliament. Retrieved February 22, 2021, from https://www.europarl.europa.eu/RegData/etudes/etudes/join/2014/529057/IPOL-CULT_ET(2014)529057_EN.pdf

Holt, S. B., & Gershenson, S. (2015). Gender gaps in high school students' homework time. *Educational Researcher, 44*(8), 432–441.

Hussar, B., Zhang, J., Hein, S., Wang, K., Roberts, A., Cui, J., Smith, M., Bullock Mann, F., Barmer, A., & Dilig, R. (2020, May). *The condition of education 2020*. Institute of Education Sciences (IES), U.S. Department of Education. Retrieved February 22, 2021, from https://nces.ed.gov/pubs2020/2020144.pdf

Jimerson, S. R., Pletcher, S. M. W., Graydon, K., Schnurr, B. L., Nickerson, A., & Kundert, D. K. (2006). Beyond grade retention and social promotion: Promoting the social and academic competence of students. *Psychology in the Schools, 43*(1), 85–97. https://doi.org/10.1002/pits.20132

Kins, E., & Beyers, W. (2010). Failure to launch, failure to achieve criteria for adulthood? *Journal of Adolescent Research, 25*(5), 743–777. https://doi.org/10.1177/0743558410371126

Kipnis, L. (2017). *Unwanted advances: Sexual paranoia comes to campus*. HarperCollins.

Kleinfeld, J. (2009). The state of American boyhood. *Gender Issues, 26*(2), 113–129. https://doi.org/10.1007/s12147-009-9074-z

Kposowa, A. J. (2000). Marital status and suicide in the national longitudinal mortality study. *Journal of Epidemiology & Community Health, 54*, 254–261. https://doi.org/10.1136/jech.54.4.254

Li, Z., Page, A., Martin, G., & Taylor, R. (2011). Attributable risk of psychiatric and socio-economic factors for suicide from individual-level, population-based studies: A systematic review. *Social Science & Medicine, 72*(4), 608–616. https://doi.org/10.1016/j.socscimed.2010.11.008

Looney, J. (2009, July 19). *Assessment and innovation in education-OECD education working paper No. 24*. Organisation for Economic Co-operation and Development (OECD). Retrieved February 22, 2021, from http://www.oecd.org/education/43338180.pdf

Lorant, V., Deliege, D., Eaton, W., Robert, A., Philippot, P., & Ansseau, M. (2003). Socioeconomic inequalities in depression: A meta-analysis. *American Journal of Epidemiology, 157*(2), 98–112. https://doi.org/10.1093/aje/kwf182

Lorant, V., Kunst, A., Huisman, M., & Costa, G. (2005). Socio-economic inequalities in suicide: A European comparative study. *The British Journal of Psychiatry, 187*(1), 49–54. https://doi.org/10.1192/bjp.187.1.49

MacDonald, H. (2018). *The diversity delusion: How race and gender pandering corrupt the university and undermine our culture*. St. Martin's Press.

Marsh, J. C., Park, K., Lin, Y.-A., & Bersamira, C. (2018). Gender differences in trends for heroin use and nonmedical prescription opioid use, 2007–2014. *Journal of Substance Abuse Treatment, 87*, 79–85. https://doi.org/10.1016/j.jsat.2018.01.001

Martin, A. J. (2011). School motivation of boys and girls: Differences of degree, differences of kind, or both? *Australian Journal of Psychology, 56*(3), 133–146. https://doi.org/10.1080/00049530412331283363

McKinley Research Group. (2016, September). *Detentions, suspensions, & expulsions: Data summary*. Retrieved February 22, 2021, from http://arisepartnership.org/wp-content/uploads/2017/02/Detentions_Suspensions__Expulsions_Data_Summary_FINAL_11.08.pdf

Meier, A., Hartmann, B. S., & Larson, R. (2018). A quarter century of participation in school-based extracurricular activities: Inequalities by race, class, gender and age? *Journal of Youth and Adolescence, 47*(6), 1299–1316. https://doi.org/10.1007/s10964-018-0838-1

Meier, M. D., & Diefenbach, H. (2018). The OECD between political and scientific agendas-a critique of the 2015 PISA gender report. *Gender and Education, 32*(5), 626–645. https://doi.org/10.1080/09540253.2018.1471198

Mezuk, B., Eaton, W. W., Golden, S. H., & Ding, Y. (2008). The influence of educational attainment on depression and risk of type 2 diabetes. *American Journal of Public Health, 98*(8), 1480–1485. https://doi.org/10.2105/AJPH.2007.126441

Milan, A. (2016, June 15). *Diversity of young adults living with their parents*. Statistics Canada. Retrieved February 22, 2021, from https://www150.statcan.gc.ca/n1/en/pub/75-006-x/2016001/article/14639-eng.pdf?st=-u_L8wPO

Mykyta, L. (2012, October 25). *Economic downturns and the failure to launch: The living arrangements of young adults in the U.S. 1995-2011*. U.S. Census Bureau. Retrieved February 22,

2021, from https://www.census.gov/content/dam/Census/library/working-papers/2012/demo/SEHSD-WP2012-24.pdf

National Center for Education Statistics. (2019a). *Table 225.90. Number and percentage of elementary and secondary school students retained in grade, by sex, race/ethnicity, and grade level: 1994 through 2017*. U.S. Department of Education. Retrieved February 22, 2021, from https://nces.ed.gov/programs/digest/d19/tables/dt19_225.90.asp?current=yes

National Center for Education Statistics. (2019b). *Table 325.80. Degrees in psychology conferred by postsecondary institutions, by level of degree and sex of student: Selected years, 1949–50 through 2017–18*. U.S. Department of Education. Retrieved February 22, 2021, from https://nces.ed.gov/ipeds/Search?query=psychology%20gender&query2=psychology%20gender&resultType=all&page=1&sortBy=relevance&overlayDigestTableId=201793

National League for Nursing. (2019). *NLN Biennial Survey of Schools of Nursing Academic Year 2017–2018*. Retrieved February 22, 2021, from http://www.nln.org/docs/default-source/default-document-library/executive-summary-(pdf)86d9c95c78366c709642ff00005f0421.pdf?sfvrsn=0

New Zealand Government Ministry of Education. (2020, July). *Stand-downs, suspensions, exclusions and expulsions from school*. Retrieved February 22, 2021, from https://www.educationcounts.govt.nz/indicators/main/student-engagement-participation/Stand-downs-suspensions-exclusions-expulsions

Newcomb, M. D., Abbott, R. D., Catalano, R. F., Hawkins, J. D., Battin-Pearson, S., & Hill, K. (2002). Mediational and deviance theories of late high school failure: Process roles of structural strains, academic competence, and general versus specific problem behavior. *Journal of Counseling Psychology, 49*(2), 172–186. https://doi.org/10.1037/0022-0167.49.2.172

Ontario Ministry of Education. (2019, July 12). *Suspension and expulsion facts, 2017–2018*. Retrieved February 22, 2021, from http://www.edu.gov.on.ca/eng/safeschools/facts1718.html

Organisation for Economic Co-operation and Development (OECD). (2013, December 3). *PISA 2012 results: What makes schools successful? Resources, policies and practices volume IV*. Retrieved February 22, 2021, from https://www.oecd-ilibrary.org/education/pisa-2012-results-what-makes-a-school-successful-volume-iv_9789264201156-en

Organisation for Economic Co-operation and Development (OECD). (2014). *Education at a glannce 2014: OECD indicators*. Retrieved February 22, 2021, from http://www.oecd.org/education/EAG2014-Indicator%20A2%20(eng).pdf

Organisation for Economic Co-operation and Development (OECD). (2015). *The ABC of gender equality in education: Aptitude, behaviour, confidence*. Retrieved February 22, 2021, from https://www.oecd.org/pisa/keyfindings/pisa-2012-results-gender-eng.pdf

Organisation for Economic Co-operation and Development (OECD). (2018, September 11). *Education at a glance 2018: OECD indicators*. Retrieved February 22, 2021, from https://www.oecd-ilibrary.org/education/education-at-a-glance-2018/starting-and-ending-age-for-students-in-compulsory-education-and-starting-age-for-students-in-primary-education-2016_eag-2018-table221-en

Perry, B. L., & Morris, E. W. (2014). Suspending progress: Collateral consequences of exclusionary punishment in public schools. *American Sociological Review, 79*(6), 1067–1087. https://doi.org/10.1177/0003122414556308

Perry, M. J. (2019, February 13). *Will 2019 be the year that colleges and universities stop openly discriminating against men, 47 years after Title IX?* American Enterprise Institute – AEI. Retrieved February 22, 2021, from https://www.aei.org/carpe-diem/will-2019-be-the-year-that-colleges-and-universities-stop-openly-discriminating-against-male-students-47-years-after-title-ix/

Petras, H., Masyn, K., Buckley, J. A., Ialongo, N., & Kellam, S. G. (2011). Who is most at risk for school removal? A multilevel discrete-time survival analysis of individual- and context-level influences. *Journal of Educational Psychology, 103*(1), 223–237. https://doi.org/10.1037/a0021545

Phillips, J. A., & Hempstead, K. (2017). Differences in U.S. suicide rates by educational attainment, 2000–2014. *American Journal of Preventive Medicine, 53*(4), 123–130. https://doi.org/10.1016/j.amepre.2017.04.010

Pouget, E. R., Fong, C., & Rosenblum, A. (2017). Racial/ethnic differences in prevalence trends for heroin use and non-medical use of prescription opioids among entrants to opioid treatment programs, 2005–2016. *Substance Use & Misuse, 53*(2), 290–300. https://doi.org/10.1080/10826084.2017.1334070

Reynolds, G. H. (2019, February 12). Higher education discriminates against men, but Title IX complaints may change that. *USA Today*. https://www.usatoday.com/story/opinion/2019/02/12/colleges-universities-discriminate-men-title-ix-complaints-toxic-masculinity-column/2831834002/

Sammons, P., Sylva, K., Melhuish, E., Siraj, I., Taggart, B., Toth, K., & Smees, R. (2014, September). *Influences on students' GCSE attainment and progress at age 16*. Retrieved February 22, 2021, from https://dera.ioe.ac.uk/20875/1/RR352_-_Influences_on_Students_GCSE_Attainment_and_Progress_at_Age_16.pdf

Sax, L. (2016). *Boys adrift: The five factors driving the growing epidemic of unmotivated boys and underachieving young men*. Basic Books.

Schepis, T. S., Teter, C. J., & McCabe, S. E. (2018). Prescription drug use, misuse and related substance use disorder symptoms vary by educational status and attainment in U.S. adolescents and young adults. *Drug and Alcohol Dependence, 189*, 172–177. https://doi.org/10.1016/j.drugalcdep.2018.05.017

Scottish Government Education Analytical Services. (2020). *Exclusions from schools 2018/19-supplementary data*. The Scottish Government. Retrieved February 22, 2021, from https://www.gov.scot/publications/school-exclusion-statistics/

Skiba, R. J., Chung, C.-G., Trachok, M., Baker, T. L., Sheya, A., & Hughes, R. L. (2014). Parsing disciplinary disproportionality: Contributions of infraction, student, and school characteristics to out-of-school suspension and expulsion. *American Educational Research Journal, 51*(4), 640–670. https://doi.org/10.3102/0002831214541670

Smeenk, D. (2012, November 17). Arrest, assaults overshadow "men's issues" lecture. *The Varsity*. https://thevarsity.ca/2012/11/17/arrest-assaults-overshadow-mens-issues-lecture/

Sommers, C. H. (2015). *The war against boys: How misguided policies are harming our young men*. Simon & Schuster.

Statistics Canada. (2008, December 1). *The gap in achievement between boys and girls*. Retrieved February 22, 2021, from https://www150.statcan.gc.ca/n1/pub/81-004-x/200410/7423-eng.htm

Statistics Canada. (2015). *Table 6-high school dropout rates, by province, 1990, 2000 and 2009*. Retrieved February 22, 2021, from https://www150.statcan.gc.ca/n1/pub/89-503-x/2010001/article/11542/tbl/tbl006-eng.htm

Statistics Canada. (2016a, April 7). *Educational attainment of person*. Retrieved February 22, 2021, from https://www23.statcan.gc.ca/imdb/p3Var.pl?Function=DEC&Id=85134

Statistics Canada. (2016b, December 12). *Classification of highest educational attainment*. Retrieved February 22, 2021, from https://www23.statcan.gc.ca/imdb/p3VD.pl?Function=getVD&TVD=305734&CVD=305735&CLV=0&MLV=4&D=1

Statistics Canada. (2016c). *Data tables, 2016 Census*. Retrieved February 22, 2021, from https://www12.statcan.gc.ca/census-recensement/2016/dp-pd/dt-td/Rp-eng.cfm?TABID=2&LANG=E&A=R&APATH=3&DETAIL=0&DIM=0&FL=A&FREE=0&GC=01&GL=-1&GID=1341679&GK=1&GRP=1&O=D&PID=110696&PRID=10&PTYPE=109445&S=0&SHOWALL=0&SUB=0&Temporal=2017&THEME=124&VID=0&VNAMEE=&VNAMEF=&D1=0&D2=0&D3=0&D4=0&D5=0&D6=0

Statistics Canada. (2019a, July 5). *The transition from school to work: the NEET (not in employment, education or training) indicator for 20- to 24-year-olds in Canada*. Retrieved February 22, 2021, from https://www150.statcan.gc.ca/n1/pub/81-599-x/81-599-x2019001-eng.htm

References 175

Statistics Canada. (2019b). *Table A.2.1-True cohort high school graduation rate, by gender, Canada, provinces and territories 2013/2014 to 2016/2017.* Retrieved February 22, 2021, from https://www150.statcan.gc.ca/n1/pub/81-604-x/2019001/tbl/tbla2.1-eng.htm

Statistics Canada. (2019c, December 10). *Education indicators in Canada: An international perspective 2019.* Retrieved February 22, 2021, from https://www150.statcan.gc.ca/n1/en/pub/81-604-x/81-604-x2019001-eng.pdf?st=p88_6Xkx

Statistics Canada. (2020). *Table 37-10-0130-01-Educational attainment of the population aged 25 to 64, by age group and sex.* Organisation for Economic Co-operation and Development (OECD), Canada, provinces and territories. Retrieved February 22, 2021, from https://doi.org/10.25318/3710013001-eng.

United Nations Educational, Scientific and Cultural Organization (UNESCO). (2012). *International standard classification of education (ISCED).* Retrieved February 22, 2021, from http://uis.unesco.org/sites/default/files/documents/international-standard-classification-of-education-isced-2011-en.pdf

United States Census Bureau. (2021). *Educational attainment.* Retrieved February 22, 2021, from https://www.census.gov/topics/education/educational-attainment.html

van Hek, M., Kraaykamp, G., & Wolbers, M. H. J. (2016). Comparing the gender gap in educational attainment: The impact of emancipatory contexts in 33 cohorts across 33 countries. *Educational Research and Evaluation, 22*(5–6), 260–282. https://doi.org/10.1080/13803611.2016.1256222

Veissière, S. P. L. (2018). "Toxic masculinity" in the age of # MeToo: Ritual, morality and gender archetypes across cultures. *Society and Business Review, 13*(3), 274–286. https://doi.org/10.1108/SBR-07-2018-0070

Wentzel, K. R. (2002). Are effective teachers like good parents? Teaching styles and student adjustment in early adolescence. *Child Development, 73*(1), 287–301. https://doi.org/10.1111/1467-8624.00406

Whitley, J., Rawana, E. P., Pye, M., & Brownlee, K. (2011). Are strengths the solution? An exploration of the relationships among teacher-rated strengths, classroom behaviour, and academic achievement of young students. *McGill Journal of Education, 45*(3), 495–510. https://doi.org/10.7202/1003574ar

Whitley, R. (2020, July 8). A silent crisis. *The ACU Review.* Retrieved February 22, 2021, from https://www.acu.ac.uk/the-acu-review/a-silent-crisis/

Whitley, R., & Zhou, J. (2020). Clueless: An ethnographic study of young men who participate in the seduction community with a focus on their psychosocial well-being and mental health. *PLoS One, 15*(2), e0229719. https://doi.org/10.1371/journal.pone.0229719

World Economic Forum. (2020). *The global gender gap index 2020.* Retrieved February 22, 2021, from http://www3.weforum.org/docs/WEF_GGGR_2020.pdf

Xu, J. (2011). Homework completion at the secondary school level: A multilevel analysis. *Journal of Educational Research, 104*(3), 171–182. https://doi.org/10.1080/00220671003636752

YouGov. (2019). *Friendship.* Retrieved February 22, 2021, from https://d25d2506sfb94s.cloudfront.net/cumulus_uploads/document/m97e4vdjnu/Results%20for%20YouGov%20RealTime%20%28Friendship%29%20164%205.7.2019.xlsx%20%20%5BGroup%5D.pdf

Zimbardo, P. G., & Coulombe, N. (2016). *Man, interrupted: Why young men are struggling what we can do about it.* Red Wheel.

Chapter 8
Employment, Unemployment, and Workplace Issues in Relation to Men's Mental Health

Paid work is central to the life of most working-age men in western countries, who can spend a significant portion of their waking hours in the workplace. Indeed, paid work provides vital financial resources for food, accommodation, and other life necessities. But paid work also serves several other psychosocial benefits that have been examined in the social science literature. In a classic tome, Jahoda (1982) posits five *latent functions* of paid work beyond the obvious function of providing financial resources, namely:

(i) Imposing a time structure on the day and week.
(ii) Giving positive social contacts and shared social experiences with others.
(iii) Providing a sense of individual and collective purpose.
(iv) Encouraging regular activity.
(v) Increasing personal status and a positive identity.

Others have expanded on this model, with Warr (1987) proposing a similar framework in another seminal book on the topic, positing nine positive factors arising from paid employment, which he labels *vitamins*, namely:

(i) Opportunity for control.
(ii) Opportunity for skill use.
(iii) Externally generated goals.
(iv) Variety.
(v) Environmental clarity.
(vi) Availability of money.
(vii) Physical security.
(viii) Opportunity for interpersonal contact.
(ix) Valued social position.

As can be seen, there is overlap between these two influential frameworks, with both emphasizing that paid work can impart purpose, structure, status, community, and regular activities. As will be explored in detail in this chapter, all of this has been related to men's mental health in a variety of studies.

8.1 Gender Differences in Paid Work

Evidence suggests that there are broad gender variations in objective outcomes and subjective meaning related to paid work and employment, all of which are relevant to mental health. This manifests itself in a myriad of interesting findings that are constant across a variety of western jurisdictions in recent decades.

First, married men are still typically the primary breadwinner for their families, despite an increasing number of women in the workplace. For example, data from the US Bureau of Labor Statistics (2019a) indicate that (on average) husbands contribute 63% to family income while wives contribute 37%, meaning that women are still typically the secondary wage earner. In fact, data from the Organisation for Economic Co-operation and Development (OECD) indicates that wives are much more likely to work part-time, and "one and a half earner households" are the norm in many European countries including the United Kingdom, the Netherlands, and Germany (OECD, 2010). Similarly, these data indicate that men are significantly more likely to be the breadwinner in married single-income families where only one spouse works. This means that married men's income is essential for food, housing, and other costs associated with supporting a household (Klesment & Van Bavel, 2017). Thus, maintaining gainful employment and being considered a productive and reliable employee is typically a key life priority for working-age men.

Second, men tend to experience heavier workloads and more onerous demands in the workplace than women, with research indicating that males work significantly more hours per week on average than females. For example, Canadian figures indicate that men work an average of 39 hours per week, while women work 33.8 hours per week (Statistics Canada, 2020a). In fact, this survey indicated that over one-million Canadian men reported working over 50 hours per week in their main job, compared with around 300,000 Canadian women, meaning that men are around three times more likely to work long hours than women (Statistics Canada, 2020a). This is consistent with earlier Canadian data, with Wang et al., (2008) finding that 44% of men worked more than 41 hours per week, compared with 18% of women. Similarly, another survey found that men work on average 3.7 hours per day (including Saturday and Sunday), while women worked an average of 2.7 hours per day (Statistics Canada, 2016). This means that men tend to have greater exposure to workplace conditions compared with women. As will be discussed in a later section, this is an important variable, as there is a male preponderance in dirty and dangerous occupations.

Third, evidence suggests that male status and identity is more strongly tied to paid work in comparison with women (Strandh et al., 2013). This familiar argument posits that women tend to draw meaning and status from a variety of social roles (e.g., mother, wife, friend, and homemaker), while men often draw primary status and identity from their productive breadwinner social role. Indeed, several studies indicate that men still tend to be more career-oriented, while women tend to be more family-oriented (Kulik, 2000; Hakim, 2000, 2006; Lubinski et al., 2014; Schwartz & Rubel, 2005). This is manifested in a variety of variables, including the aforementioned gender gap in hours spent at work. Similarly, research indicates that unemployed men spend significantly more hours looking for a job compared with unemployed women and also feel more stigmatized than unemployed women, indicating the importance of work to male status and identity (Kulik, 2000). For many men, the link between work and self is inextricable, especially in nations like the United States and the United Kingdom where the protestant work ethic is embedded into society.

8.2 Unemployment

All of the aforementioned gender-differentials mean that unemployment and job loss can pose a significantly greater challenge for men than women. Perhaps most importantly, job loss and unemployment for men may be more intense due to the financial implications. As stated, men remain the primary breadwinners in most households. As such, the loss of income from the primary wage earner can lead to serious financial strain, with the whole family suffering the consequences. In contrast, the loss of income from a secondary wage earner (typically the wife) may be felt less strongly by both the person losing the job, and the greater family unit. Indeed, wives who lose a job can expect more financial support from their husbands due to his greater share of family income, but the reverse situation will pose more financial problems given the tendency for wives to be the secondary wage earner.

Unemployment for men can also mean a loss of all the positive secondary benefits of paid work identified by Jahoda (1982) and Warr (1987), including a loss of purpose, structure, status, social community, and a variety of other regular activities. Indeed, the workplace remains a meaningful community for many men, especially those in more traditional occupations where the workplace can provide camaraderie through work-related social clubs, sports clubs, trade unions, and the like. Indeed, the social integration of adult men in western countries is often provided through meaningful participation in the workforce. As such disintegration of employment can have a particularly pernicious effect on men, leading to loneliness, monotony, boredom, anxiety about the future, and a crisis of identity (Paul & Moser, 2009; Strandh et al., 2013). As will be explored in the next sections, all these factors can intertwine to negatively affect mental health.

8.3 Employment, Unemployment, and Mental Health

Over the last two decades, there have been several meta-analyses and systematic reviews examining the relationship between (un)employment and mental health (Modini et al., 2016; van der Noordt et al., 2014; Paul & Moser 2009; McKee-Ryan et al., 2005; Murphy & Athanasou, 1999). These papers point to a number of common conclusions, namely:

(i) Employment is a protective factor for a range of mental health outcomes.
(ii) Unemployment is a risk factor for a range of adverse mental health outcomes.
(iii) Moving from employment to unemployment can worsen mental health.
(iv) Moving from unemployment to employment can improve mental health.
(v) The negative impact of both job loss and unemployment on mental health appears to be significantly greater for men than women, especially blue-collar manual workers.

For example, a meta-analysis of 16 longitudinal studies from the 1980s and 1990s found that increased levels of psychological distress were associated with unemployment in 14 of the 16 assessed studies (Murphy & Athanasou, 1999). Moreover, this analysis found that moving from unemployment to employment led to a significant decrease in psychological distress in all the studies assessing this change in status. These findings were confirmed by another meta-analysis during a similar time-period, which focused on the effect of unemployment on both physical and mental health (McKee-Ryan et al., 2005). More recent systematic reviews have led to similar findings. For example, van der Noordt et al., (2014) examined 33 prospective studies finding that employed people had lower rates of psychological distress than the unemployed (OR = 0.79; 95% CI 0.72–0.86), as well as lower rates of depression (OR = 0.52; 95% CI 0.33–0.83). Similarly, Modini et al., (2016) conducted a meta-review of eleven relevant reviews, again concluding that employment significantly benefitted mental health, particularly when there are favorable workplace conditions and good-quality supervision. A strength of these analyses is the focus on longitudinal analysis, thus indicating that unemployment plays a causal role on adverse mental health and ruling out reverse causation. However, an acknowledged weakness of these meta-analyses is that they did not focus on gender, often because the included studies in the time-period assessed did not include a sufficient number of women for a valid comparison.

The first large-scale meta-analysis to include a meaningful gender comparison was conducted by Paul & Moser (2009). This involved assessing 237 cross-sectional studies and 87 longitudinal studies consisting of almost half a million people – making it considerably larger than the earlier meta-analyses. This study confirmed previous findings about the negative mental health effects of unemployment, finding that 34% of the unemployed had psychological problems, more than double the 16% rate for the employed, including higher rates of depression and anxiety. Again, this analysis of longitudinal studies also found that unemployment and job loss is a cause rather than a consequence of mental health issues. Importantly, this study found that unemployed men had significantly higher rates of psychological distress than unemployed women and that this is particularly concentrated among blue-collar men. This led the authors to conclude that "male blue-collar workers are probably more vulnerable to the negative mental health effects of unemployment than other social groups…they should not be neglected when public resources are allocated." The link between unemployment and men's mental health is explored in granular-level detail in the following three subsections devoted to separate discussion of: (i) suicide; (ii) substance abuse; and (iii) depression and anxiety.

8.3.1 Suicide

A large corpus of research indicates that unemployed men have a significantly higher rate of suicide than: (i) other men and (ii) unemployed women. Moreover, several studies indicate that men in low-status and low-income occupations have higher rates of suicide than other men, as well as higher rates than women in low-income and low-status occupations. These results have been summarized in a variety of systematic reviews and meta-analyses.

For example, Milner et al., (2014) conducted a meta-analysis of five high-quality population-based cohort studies, finding that unemployment was a risk factor for suicide, with a relative risk of 1.58 (95% CI 1.33–1.83) compared with employment. The pooled risk ratios indicated that relative risk was much higher in unemployed men (RR 1.51: 95% CI 1.19–1.83) compared with unemployed women, where risk was nonsignificant (RR 1.15: 95% CI 0.85–1.45). These results are consistent with an earlier systematic review and meta-analysis of population-based case control and cohort studies, which found that unemployed men had a relative risk of suicide of 1.68 (95% CI 1.11–2.54) when compared with employed men (Li et al., 2011).

Interestingly, a stratified subanalysis within the Li et al., (2011) review found that men in low-status occupations (defined as manual/non-skilled/blue-collar workers) were over twice more likely (RR = 2.67; 95% CI 1.53–4.68) to kill themselves than men in high-status occupations. In contrast, this review found that women in low-status occupations had a nonsignificant risk ratio of killing themselves of only 1.27 (95% CI 0.54–2.94) compared with women in high-status occupations. Moreover, this review found that the population attributable fraction for suicide associated with low occupational status was 33% (range: 18.5%–46.5%) for men, but only 7% (range: −14.2%–34.4%) for women. The possible reasons behind such high rates of suicide among manual blue-collar workers are discussed in later sections of this chapter on workplace conditions and occupational safety.

Another review of 16 studies found that risk of suicide is greatest in the first five years of unemployment, when the pooled relative risk for the unemployed is 2.50 (95% CI 1.83–3.17) compared with the employed population (Milner et al., 2013). In contrast, this review found that the relative risk after 12–16 years of unemployment was only 1.21 (95% CI 1.10–1.33) compared with the employed, implying some level of adjustment among the long-term unemployed. A weakness of this review is that it did not stratify by gender.

In sum, the results from these three reviews found that being unemployed or working in a low-status occupation significantly increases risk of suicide for both men and women, but risk is significantly higher among men, especially those who have recently lost a job.

These trends can be witnessed in large-scale single-nation studies from a variety of jurisdictions across the western world. For example, a large-scale case-control study in Denmark found that unemployment was a significant risk factor for male suicides, but not for female suicides (Qin et al., 2000). This study found that unemployed men had an age-adjusted odds ratio of suicide of 2.21 (95% CI 1.69–2.88) when compared with employed men and were also around twice as likely to kill themselves as compared with unemployed women. Similarly, a New Zealand cohort study of over two million respondents found that unemployment was a significant risk factor for suicide, with an age-adjusted odds ratio of 2.63 (95% CI 1.87–3.70) when comparing unemployed men with employed men. This ratio was higher than the analogous age-adjusted odds ratio (2.46: 95% CI 1.10–5.49) for unemployed women compared with employed women (Blakely et al., 2003). This finding of a higher suicide rate among unemployed men has been replicated in a variety of recent studies examining gender, employment, and suicide (e.g., Gunnell & Chang, 2016).

Of note, several studies indicate that the male suicide rate rose precipitously during and after the Global Financial Crisis (see Chap. 1) and that this increase was greater than that seen for female suicides (Chang et al., 2013; Hedegaard et al., 2018; Stuckler et al., 2011). These studies indicate that this increase was partially fuelled by a dramatic increase in sudden and unexpected male job loss, which also led to a rise in male unemployment in the following years. These findings have led to concerns that the COVID-19 crisis may fuel a similar rise in male suicide, given that reports indicate that over 30 million Americans have applied for unemployment benefits since the start of the pandemic (Crayne, 2020).

Relatedly, unemployment has also been associated with high rates of suicide among vulnerable subgroups of men. For example, employment levels in certain Canadian and Australian Aboriginal communities have been linked to the high rates of suicide observed therein (Kumar & Tjepkema, 2019; Penney et al., 2009; De Leo et al., 2011). Likewise, elevated rates of suicide among veterans has been linked to difficulties finding employment after release from the services (see Chap. 2), which may be particularly difficult for infantrymen and others without specialist skills that transfer well into civilian life (Kline et al., 2011).

As stated, the Li et al., (2011) review found the highest suicide rates among manual blue-collar occupations. This is consistent with a wide body of research noting that the highest occupational suicide rates are seen in male-dominated industries such as blue-collar manual occupations, while the lowest rates are seen in female-dominated industries such as clerical and office occupations (Milner et al., 2013; Tiesman et al., 2015; Kposowa, 1999). For example, Roberts et al., (2013) found that six occupations in the United Kingdom had an alarmingly high suicide rate greater than 40 per 100,000, namely:

(i) Coal miners.
(ii) Merchant seafarers.
(iii) Building laborers.
(iv) Window cleaners.
(v) Artists.
(vi) Plasterers.

All of these (bar artists) are male-dominated blue-collar manual occupations involving dangerous and risky workplace activities. Of note, this study also found that the suicide rate had more than doubled for coal miners, building laborers, and plasterers between the early 1980s and the early 2000s, while a 50% increase in suicide was seen in other male-dominated dangerous and risky manual occupations including dockers, road construction workers, and refuse collectors. In contrast decreases in suicide were seen in female-dominated occupations including veterinarians, domestic workers, and hairdressers. All this suggests that:

(i) Men working in blue-collar manual occupations have an increased risk of suicide.
(ii) Workplace experience for men, especially dangerous and risky conditions, can increase risk of suicide.
(iii) Men working in industries experiencing contraction and restructuring such as coal-mining and the merchant marine are particularly vulnerable.

All of this is further discussed later in this chapter in sections devoted to workplace conditions, occupational safety, and wider economic change.

To close this section, it is worth noting that job loss can cause a cascade of events that have been linked to suicide. For example, unemployment is a risk factor for the onset of mental illnesses such as substance use disorder and depression (see next sections), which are in turn risk factors for suicide. Similarly, unemployment can have financial implications and can sometimes lead to foreclosure and the loss of a family home, which has also been associated with the rising rate of white middle-aged male suicide (Houle & Light, 2017; Kerr et al., 2017). Similarly, other studies have found an association between bankruptcy and suicide (Komoto, 2014; Kidger et al., 2011). In sum, job loss and unemployment are proximal and distal risk factors for male suicide, while working in a low-status manual blue-collar occupation can also increase risk. Importantly, the impact of these employment-related variables appears to be stronger in men than women.

8.3.2 Substance Abuse

There is less research literature on the relationship between substance abuse and unemployment, compared with the literature on suicide and employment. However, the research that exists is clear: unemployment is a risk factor for substance abuse, substance dependence, and substance use disorder (SUD). For example, Henkel (2011) conducted a review of the literature examining over 130 relevant studies, finding that the unemployed are around two to three times more likely to engage in problematic substance use. A sub-analysis of longitudinal data in this review indicates that the unemployed have a higher probability of developing a SUD compared with the employed, thus ruling out reverse causation. This includes higher rates of cannabis abuse, alcohol abuse, and injecting drug abuse. This review notes that only a few studies give prevalence rates by gender, but those that do present such data reveal a clear pattern: unemployed men have significantly higher rates of substance abuse and SUD than employed men and unemployed women. In contrast, differences between unemployed women and employed women were less marked and less consistent. These findings are consistent with a variety of studies across different western jurisdictions that have focused on specific substances and specific substance use disorders.

In terms of alcohol abuse, a Finnish study of over 1000 young adults found that 20.1% of unemployed males engaged in hazardous drinking, compared with 7.1% of employed males (Kestilä et al., 2008). These figures were higher than the analogous figures for women, which were 14.7% for unemployed women and 4.5% for employed women. In other words, the unemployed were around three times more likely to engage in alcohol abuse compared with the employed, with unemployed men having the highest prevalence.

In terms of cannabis abuse, a French study of over 3000 young adults revealed that 19.3% of unemployed males used cannabis at least ten times per month, compared with 12.4% of employed males (Legleye et al., 2008). Again, analogous figures for females were lower, with only 4.4% of unemployed females and 4.3% of employed females engaging in similar levels of cannabis use. This study also found that unemployed males were significantly more likely to use other illegal drugs such as cocaine, heroin, and ecstasy in comparison with employed males and unemployed females. In terms of past year use, 10.4% of unemployed males had used these drugs, compared with 5.2% of employed males and 3.4% of unemployed females.

These results are consistent with an Australian study of over 10,000 adults, which found that 19% of unemployed men engage in harmful use of alcohol, cannabis, opioids, sedatives, or stimulants, compared with 9% of employed men (Andrews et al., 2001). Again these rates were higher than analogous figures for unemployed women (11%) and employed women (4%). In sum, this literature indicates a two- to threefold increased risk for substance abuse in unemployed men compared with employed men and higher rates for unemployed men than unemployed women.

In terms of SUD, the landmark large-scale US Epidemiologic Catchment Area study indicates that job loss can increase the risk of alcohol use disorder more than sixfold, though these studies did not report differential prevalence by gender (Dooley et al., 1992; Catalano et al., 1993). But the aforementioned Henkel (2011) review of the literature assessed a variety of studies including longitudinal research (thus accounting for reverse causation), concluding that men are at greater risk of SUD than women after a job loss and a period of unemployment. This is consistent with earlier reviews, which found that unemployed men had higher rates of alcohol use disorder than unemployed women and employed men (Hammarström, 1994).

Indeed, rates of substance use disorder and associated fentanyl and opioid misuse appear to be higher in certain geographical areas, including areas with high rates of male unemployment and declining industries (Case & Deaton, 2020). This association implies a causal link between small-area deprivation, economic opportunity, and substance abuse. It may also help explain high rates of substance use among Native Americans, Indigenous Canadians, and Aboriginal Australians, who sometimes live in remote and isolated regions with little work or meaningful occupation.

This may contribute toward a wider lack of purpose and meaning, leading some men to misuse substances in a drastic attempt to escape the associated pain and numb their psychological distress, while simultaneously filling a temporal and existential vacuum in their lives. This thesis is explored in more detail in Chap. 2.

8.3.3 Depression and Anxiety

There have been several studies focusing on the link between job loss, unemployment, and depression/anxiety with a focus on gender differentials or men per se. Many of these studies measure depression/anxiety through the use of the GHQ-12 screening questionnaire (Goldberg, 1972). This is one of the most widely used and validated instruments that detects symptoms of depression and anxiety with high specificity and reliability in community samples (Goldberg, 1972; Goldberg et al., 1997). Higher scores on the GHQ-12 indicate higher levels of psychological distress, while lower scores indicate lower levels.

One recent study examined unemployment and mental health in Ireland through a longitudinal analysis of over 5000 households comprising over 8000 individuals (Strandh et al., 2013). This study found that unemployed Irish men have significantly higher GHQ-12 scores than unemployed Irish women, with unemployed men living with a partner and children having particularly high-levels of distress. This indicates that being a "failed breadwinner" for oneself and one's family is a significant risk factor for anxiety and depression among men, which may be particularly acute in more traditional and religious jurisdictions like Ireland, where deviations from conventional gender roles can be stigmatized. Interestingly, this study also found that reemployment led to a significant decrease in psychological distress, with the decrease in reemployed men around double that of reemployed women. In sum, unemployed Irish men in this study tend to have higher rates of depression/anxiety symptoms than unemployed Irish women, and the mental health of Irish men improves much more dramatically on reemployment than Irish women. Again the longitudinal nature of this study overcomes issues of reverse causation.

These findings from Ireland are consistent with many other studies elsewhere. For example, a cross-sectional study of over 4000 individuals in Spain compared GHQ-12 scores by gender and employment status (Artazcoz et al., 2004). The study found that unemployed men had an adjusted odds ratio of 2.98 (95% CI 2.30–3.87) for "poor mental health" (defined as high GHQ-12 scores) compared with employed men, while unemployed women had an adjusted odds ratio of 1.51 (95% CI 1.11–2.06) for "poor mental health" compared with employed women. Similar to the previously described suicide literature, this study found a higher rate of poor mental health in unemployed manual workers, compared with unemployed nonmanual workers. Like the aforementioned study from Ireland, this study found that marriage and living with children significantly increased risk of poor mental health for unemployed men, but significantly decreased risk of poor mental health for unemployed women. In fact, unemployed nonmanual married women with children were around half as likely to have poor mental health than analogous women who are employed. In contrast, unemployed married men with children had over double the odds of poor mental health compared with analogous men who are employed. Again, this study supports the theory that the inability to fulfill expected family responsibilities plays a large role in the onset of poor mental health among unemployed men. Similarly, marriage and presence of children appears to be protective for unemployed women, perhaps because they can rely on their husband's salary for necessities and also because the social roles of wife and mother can bring equivalent meaning and purpose in the absence of paid employment.

Interestingly, a UK cohort study examined outcomes in over 3000 men between ages 24 and 33 years, finding higher rates of poor mental health in the first 12 months of unemployment compared with later months, indicating that the immediate period after a job loss is the most detrimental to mental health (Montgomery et al., 1999). Indeed, this study found that the adjusted relative risk of developing anxiety or depression was 2.10 (95% CI 1.34–3.28) when comparing men who lost a job in the last 12 months to men who remain employed. Again, the longitudinal aspect of this study indicates that unemployment is an upstream risk factor for anxiety and depression symptoms, thus accounting for reverse causation.

Taken in the round, all these findings suggest that being a "failed breadwinner" for one's family is a significant risk factor for poor mental health among men, as this can incur financial problems, which negatively affect the whole family. This may further explain the elevated rates of mental distress among low-status manual workers, who typically receive lower pay and may have less access to savings, investments, and benefits. Moreover, high levels of public stigma are targeted at unemployed men who are considered to be failing in their family duties, which may interact with stigma associated with mental health issues, leading to internalized shame, guilt, and low self-esteem. For example, Kulik (2000) found that unemployed men were significantly more likely to believe that employed people do not respect the unemployed, while other research indicates that unemployed men are commonly stigmatized and shamed by family, friends, and wider society (Affleck et al., 2018). Given that stigma is an important topic in its own right, it is discussed in more detail in Sect. 8.4.5.

To close this section, it is worth noting that research indicates that *employed* low-status manual workers also have higher rates of depression than professionals and people working in high-status occupations. For example, a large-scale meta-analysis found that 35 out of 51 studies found a significant association between low socioeconomic status (SES) and depression, with low SES individuals having an overall odds ratio of 1.81 (95% CI 1.57–2.10) compared with high SES individuals, with the lowest SES group having a 24% increased risk of a new depressive episode compared with the highest group (Lorant et al., 2003). Importantly, 19 of the 51 studies used occupation as a proxy for socioeconomic status, with low-status manual occupations categorized as indicative of low SES. The increased risk of suicide, substance use, depression, and anxiety among low-status manual workers suggests that their work conditions and other workplace issues might be negatively affecting their mental health. This thesis is discussed in detail in the next sections.

8.4 Employment Conditions and Workplace Environment

So far, this chapter has mainly focused on the impact of job loss and unemployment on mental health outcomes but has briefly alluded to some of the literature indicating that manual and low-skilled blue-collar workers tend to have worse mental health than nonmanual and professional workers. This differential implies that employment conditions and workplace environment can also affect mental health. Indeed, considerable research indicates that a variety of workplace-related factors can negatively impinge upon the mental health of workers, namely: (i) precarious employment; (ii) job stress and job strain; (iii) conditions in male-dominated industries; (iv) occupational health and safety; and (v) workplace stigma. All of these are discussed in detail in the following separate subsections, again with a focus on men's mental health.

8.4.1 Precarious Employment

In the last 30 years, there has been a precipitous decline in well-paid, permanent, full-time, "job for life" type employment, with a corresponding increase in temporary, part-time, low-paid, insecure employment (Case & Deaton, 2020). The latter form of employment is referred to in the social science literature as *precarious employment*. Such employment has been characterized as consisting of three overarching dimensions, namely: (i) employment insecurity, (ii) income inadequacy, and (iii) lack of employment rights and protections (Kreshpaj et al., 2020).

Fortunately, there have been a number of systematic reviews and meta-analyses in recent years examining the association between precarious employment and mental health. One of these focused on longitudinal studies in an attempt to synthesize high-quality research and overcome issues of reverse causation (Rönnblad et al., 2019). This resulted in 16 eligible studies, which focused on a variety of outcomes such as depressive symptoms, anxiety symptoms, prescription psychiatric drug use, or poor mental health/high psychological distress (as measured by GHQ-12). The authors separately examined studies that measured precarious employment through the single dimension of "job insecurity" (10 studies) and those that used multidimensional measures of precarious employment (5 studies).

Meta-analyses revealed that those experiencing job insecurity had higher risks of a variety of adverse mental health outcomes compared with those not experiencing job insecurity, with a summary odds ratio of 1.61 (95% CI 1.29–2.00) for depressive symptoms, 1.77 (95% CI 1.18–2.65) for anxiety symptoms, 1.30 (95% CI 1.09–1.56) for prescription psychiatric drug use, and 1.52 (95% CI 1.35–1.70) for all adverse mental health outcomes combined. When using multidimensional measures, the lower number of studies (five) led the authors to conduct a single meta-analysis on all adverse mental health outcomes combined, leading to an odds ratio of 2.01 (95% CI 1.60–2.53) for those experiencing precarious employment compared with those not experiencing precarious employment. These five studies include a well-designed study finding an odds ratio of 3.13 (95% CI 1.28–7.63) for depressive symptoms when comparing people with low education in temporary employment with people with high education and permanent employment (Hammarström et al., 2011).

The aforementioned Rönnblad et al., (2019) meta-analysis did not focus on gender in any way, reflecting the fact that many longitudinal studies on precarious employment do not report differential results for men and women. However, another recent systematic review examined precarious employment and mental health through a "gender sensitive perspective" (Utzet et al., 2020). This resulted in 53 eligible studies, most of which were cross-sectional, but only 22 of these studies included a stratified analysis by sex. The most common measures of precarious employment were "job insecurity" (N = 20), "temporariness" (N = 12), and multi-dimensional measures (N = 10). Again, outcomes measured included depressive symptoms, medication usage, and psychological distress (often using GHQ-12).

In sum, this review indicates that precarious employment is associated with poorer mental health in both sexes, but considerably more studies found that this had a stronger impact on adverse mental health in men compared with women, and some studies found no adverse mental health effects in women at all. For example, Waenerlund et al., (2011) found that the adjusted odds ratio for high psychological distress for precariously employed men was 2.79 (95% CI 1.52–5.14) compared with non-precariously employed men. In contrast, for precariously employed women, the odds ratio was only 1.79 (95% CI 0.98–3.29) compared with non-precariously employed women, indicating a more diluted nonsignificant effect for women. Similar findings of increased risk for men were seen in several other studies in this review (e.g., Muntaner et al., 2010; Wahrendorf et al., 2012; Sousa et al., 2010). As such, precarious employment may have more of an impact on men's mental health than women's mental health, as it does not provide a reliable or adequate form of financial reward for a primary breadwinner, nor a positive status or identity in society.

8.4.2 Job Stress and Job Strain

Related to the concept of precarious employment is the concept of *job stress*, which is sometimes known as *job strain*, and is typically divided into two types: (i) psychosocial job stress and (ii) physical and toxicological job stress. This section will focus on psychosocial job stress, with physical job stress subsumed in Sect. 8.4.4. Of note, there are various forms of psychosocial job stress, which can be experienced by workers including low social support, interpersonal conflict, effort-reward imbalance, and high job insecurity. But one of the most highly researched forms of job stress is the relationship between work demands and worker control: known as the *job strain model* or the *demand/control model* (Karasek, 1979).

This model posits that psychosocial job stress is most severe where workers have high demands and heavy workloads, but low control and decision latitude over how the demands are managed (Karasek & Theorell, 1990). Contrariwise, this model posits that jobs with high demands but high control and decision latitude can promote mental health, as they often involve skill utilization and a degree of challenge that imparts job satisfaction and concomitant self-esteem. According to this dichotomy, workers experiencing *high job strain* (i.e., high demand/low control) typically include manual workers such as miners or factory workers, while workers experiencing *low job strain* (i.e., high demand/high control) includes professionals and nonmanual workers such as lawyers, managers, or physicians.

A large corpus of research has tested the job strain model, while examining other aspects of job stress. This literature has been summarized in a variety of review papers and meta-analyses: all concluding that high demand/low control environments are deleterious to mental health. For example, LaMontagne et al., (2010) conducted a literature review, noting that the vast majority of cross-sectional studies find an association between high levels of job strain and adverse mental health such as depressive symptoms. Importantly, this paper reviewed studies from a variety of countries including France (Neidhammer et al., 1998), New Zealand (Melchior et al., 2007), and Canada (Wang et al., 2008), all indicating that the adverse mental health impact of job strain (i.e., high demand/low control) is significantly greater for men than women. This review included three longitudinal studies, which all found that moving from a low job strain to a high job strain position significantly increased depressive symptoms and/or GHQ scores (de Lange et al., 2002; Stansfeld et al., 1999; Wang et al., 2009). This points to a causal effect, particularly in men.

Similar conclusions arose from a comprehensive meta-analysis, which analyzed 11 high-quality longitudinal studies examining job strain and adverse mental health, again finding that the combination of a high demand/low control environment was a risk factor for common mental disorders (Stansfeld & Candy, 2006). This meta-analysis revealed several key findings related to gender. First, high psychosocial job strain was associated with common mental disorders, with an odds ratio of 1.82 (95% CI 1.06–3.10), but there were not enough studies on job strain per se to stratify by gender. Second, the analysis revealed a positive association between level of psychological demands in the workplace and common mental disorders across all the papers, with a summary odds ratio of 1.39 (95% CI 1.15–1.69). Importantly, a high level of workplace psychological demands appeared to have a greater risk for common mental disorders in men than women, with a summary odds ratio of 1.55 (95% CI 1.29–1.85) for men compared with 1.34 (95% CI 1.16–1.53) for women. Third, low levels of social support and high levels of interpersonal conflict in the workplace were associated with common mental disorders, with an odds ratio of 1.32 (95% CI 1.21–1.44). Again, risk was higher in men, with an odds ratio of 1.38 (95% CI 1.20–1.60) compared with 1.20 (95% CI 1.07–1.35) for women. The longitudinal nature of this meta-analysis points to a causal effect and also indicates larger effects for men than women.

This is consistent with a wider body of research signaling that job satisfaction per se is inversely associated with psychological distress and depression in particular. Indeed, one meta-analysis of almost 500 studies found that low levels of job satisfaction were associated with high psychological distress and higher levels of anxiety and depression scores (Faragher et al., 2005). This converges with other research finding that job satisfaction mediates the positive mental health consequences of employment. For example, a four-wave longitudinal study of over 6000 young adults found that people dissatisfied with their jobs had significantly higher levels of psychological distress (as measured by GHQ-12 scores) than those who were satisfied with their jobs (Graetz, 1993). This study also found that a deterioration in job satisfaction led to a significant increase in levels of psychological distress over time, while an improvement in job satisfaction led to a decrease in psychological distress. Interestingly, one study found that unemployed women are more likely to turn down jobs due to perceived negative conditions compared with men, suggesting that men are more likely to take jobs with low levels of job satisfaction, perhaps because there is greater need, pressure, and expectations for a man to act as primary breadwinner and support himself and his family (Kulik, 2000). In short, many men may not have the luxury to decline such employment.

8.4.3 Male-Dominated Occupations

In terms of proportions of the workforce, some occupations are dominated by men, some are dominated by women, and others have a more even balance of men and women. Some of the most reliable data in this regard comes from the US Bureau of Labor Statistics (2019a), which collects information about the gender composition of the US workforce using broad umbrella categories for different industries and more granular-level categories for specific occupations. Their statistics from 2018 indicate that the following occupational categories are proportionally dominated by males:

(i) Installation, maintenance, and repair occupations: 96.3% male.
(ii) Natural resources, construction, and maintenance occupations: 95% male.
(iii) Construction and extraction occupations: 96.4% male.
(iv) Engineering and architecture occupations: 84.1% male.
(v) Protective service occupations: 77.5% male.
(vi) Production, transportation, and material moving occupations: 76.9% male.

At a more granular level, their statistics indicate that over 90% of workers in the following occupations are male: forestry, fisheries, hunting, logging, construction, roofing, coal mining, iron and steel, quarrying, firefighting, and railway/highway maintenance. In contrast, the following occupations are dominated by females and have much fewer males in the workforce:

(i) Healthcare practitioners and technical occupations: 25% male.
(ii) Education, training, and library occupations: 26.8% male.
(iii) Office and administrative support occupations: 28.4% male.
(iv) Community and social service occupations: 33.5% male.
(v) Sales and office occupations: 39% male.

At a more granular level, figures from the US Bureau of Labor Statistics indicate that over 90% of preschool and kindergarten teachers, speech language pathologists, childcare workers, secretaries, and administrative assistants are female. Of note, these same US Bureau of Labor Statistics data indicate that the following occupations have a more even gender balance:

(i) Management, professional, and related occupations: 48.5% male.
(ii) Legal occupations: 48.4% male.
(iii) Business and financial operations occupations: 47.2% male.
(iv) Professional and related occupations: 43.2% male.
(v) Life, physical, and social science occupations: 53.3% male.
(vi) Arts, design, entertainment, sports, and media occupations: 53.2% male.

In sum, men are overrepresented in manual outdoors occupations that involve dirty, dangerous, and demanding hard labour, which can incur considerable physical and mental strain. These jobs often fall into the aforementioned *high demand/low control* category, which is a risk factor for adverse mental health outcomes, often involving other elements of job stress. For example, many of these male-dominated industries do not follow a predictable 9–5 schedule, but often involve long unsociable hours, shift-work, relocation, and considerable time away from friends and family. All this can contribute to loneliness, isolation, and a lack of social support. Moreover, industries such as fishing and forestry are subject to the whims of a capricious seasonal and economic cycle, which can leave men in a precarious situation, with periods of intense work followed by long periods of no work. This may be especially so in remote rural communities, where work can also be conducted under extremely harsh environmental conditions (Condon et al., 1995). Such punishing conditions have been linked to various adverse health outcomes in men including elevated rates of workplace fatalities, workplace injuries, and high suicide rates in certain occupations (Yur'yev et al., 2012; Alston, 2012). These issues of health and safety and their impact on mental health are discussed in Sect. 8.4.4.

8.4.4 Occupational Health and Safety

Research indicates that men account for the vast majority of workplace injuries and workplace deaths, which is unsurprising given their dominance in dangerous and demanding manual blue-collar labour as described earlier. Indeed, US Bureau of Labor Statistics (2020a) data indicates that men accounted for 92% of workplace fatalities in 2019 (4896 male fatalities compared with 437 female fatalities). In terms of serious workplace injuries, men accounted for 75% of all injuries requiring an overnight stay in a hospital (32,620 men compared with 10,440 women), with men taking 10 days off work on average after such an injury, compared with seven days for women (US Bureau of Labor Statistics, 2020b). This differential in workplace injuries is reflected in disability beneficiaries, with 220,850 American men receiving disability benefits due to injuries, compared with 116,804 women (US

Social Security Administration, 2020). Similar proportions are seen elsewhere, with Canadian figures indicating 1027 workplace fatalities in 2018, of which 997 (97%) were men and 30 (3%) were women (Association of Workers Compensation Boards of Canada, 2020). Both workplace deaths and workplace injuries in North America are concentrated in male-dominated occupations such as construction, extraction, manufacturing, and transport, with common causes of death and injury including "falling from height" and "struck by moving vehicle" (Seager, 2019).

As stated in previous chapters, data indicates that workplace injuries and subsequent disability can be a risk factor for a variety of mental disorders including post-traumatic stress disorder (PTSD), substance use disorder, and suicide (Kleiman & Liu, 2013; Vijayakumar et al., 2011; Russell et al., 2009; Sareen et al., 2007; Monk, 2000). Indeed, workplace injuries commonly occur in male-dominated spaces such as building sites, factories, mines, fishing boats, merchant ships, or on the battlefield (Seager, 2019). These injuries can create a cascade of events leading to intense psychological distress. For example, severe injury is a form of trauma, which by definition can lead to PTSD. Severe injury can also create intense physical pain. This combined psychological and physical distress can lead to the legitimate prescription of pain-killing medication such as opioids. It can also lead to self-medication with substances such as alcohol or cannabis, or the use of opioids obtained from the black market to control the pain. Such substance (ab)use may begin innocently with small doses but can spiral into a more serious issue (see Chap. 3) given the psychophysiological addictive qualities of alcohol, cannabis, and opioids. Such a theory is supported by research, with several studies indicating that a common trajectory is the use of alcohol or cannabis, followed by the legitimate use of prescription opioids, followed by use of black-market opioids, followed by use of heroin (e.g., Marsh et al., 2018). All this can be an effort to control physical or mental pain related to workplace injuries, which are more common in male-dominated professions compared with female-dominated ones. In other words, the high rate of workplace injuries among men should be considered a men's mental health issue, as evidence suggests this can create a cascade of events leading to adverse mental health outcomes.

Similarly, it was previously noted that male-dominated professions tend to have a significantly elevated rate of suicide, with one UK study showing that six occupations had a suicide rate greater than 40 per 100,000, namely: (i) coal miners, (ii) merchant seafarers, (iii) building laborers, (iv) window cleaners, (v) artists, and (vi) plasterers (Roberts et al., 2013). This finding converges with research elsewhere, indicating that other male-dominated occupations have high rates of suicide including law enforcement, the military, fishing, farming, forestry, and transport services (Milner et al., 2013; Tiesman et al., 2015; Kposowa, 1999). In contrast, these studies show that clerical and office occupations had the lowest rates of suicide, perhaps due to better and more pleasant psychosocial and physical conditions therein.

These figures led Warren Farrell (1993) to dub these male-dominated occupations as "the death professions," due to the increased risk of suicide, occupational deaths, life-threatening injuries, and assault occurring therein. Indeed, Farrell's seminal and well-known book *The Myth of Male Power* has a lesser-known subtitle "why males are the disposable sex," with Farrell suggesting that the high death and injury rate in certain male occupations is tacitly accepted by most people as a price worth paying to live in a civilized and functioning society. This may be especially so in relation to manual low-skilled blue-collar labourers at the lower end of the socio-economic spectrum, who can easily be replaced by other low-status men desperate for employment. Indeed Farrell et al., (2016) aptly remark that "working-class men in particular have been expected…to die in tunnels, on tall buildings, down mines and on the high seas, supplying the buildings, transport, food supplies and security that create the comfort of a civilized life for all." These blue-collar working-class manual workers may be the most "disposable" (or "replaceable") of all men, with many such men well-aware of their precarious work status. This again can contribute to worse mental health outcomes in this demographic.

8.4.5 Workplace Stigma

All of the above is compounded by high levels of stigma associated with mental distress in many workplaces. Indeed, some research indicates that certain employers often equate mental illness with malingering, hypochondria, and laziness, meaning that workers with mental health issues may be justifiably worried that raising these issues will affect their income, their reputation, and their career prospects (Ashfield & Gouws, 2019). This is especially the case for those considered "disposable" or "replaceable" in precarious or unskilled employment. All of these factors can lead to a culture of silence about mental health issues in certain workplaces.

This may be particularly so in certain male-dominated workplaces that put a premium on issues of safety such as the police and the military, where people with mental health difficulties may be stereotyped as physically dangerous, unpredictable, a threat to unit morale, and unfit for service (Dallaire, 2019; Linford, 2013). Indeed, a mental health issue in law enforcement or the military will often be noted on an individual's employment file and monitored by superior officers. This can lead to negative outcomes including redeployment to undesired tasks, being overlooked for promotion, general professional stagnation, or even medical discharge. Similar processes may occur to men who reveal mental health issues in other male-dominated occupations where there is access to hazardous materials and a reliance on harmonious teamwork such as mining, oil/gas, transport, security, or manufacturing (Scheid, 2005; Seaton et al., 2019).

In short, some of the negative stereotypes of men with mental health issues discussed in Chap. 1 may prevent men in need from seeking help, which could allow any issues to fester and worsen over time. Indeed, evidence suggests that men are well-aware of these public stereotypes and the potentially negative consequences associated with mental health disclosure in the workplace. For example, an Ipsos MORI survey of over 1000 Canadian men found that 28% believed their job could be at risk if they talked about mental health issues at work, 33% believed they would be overlooked for promotion if they mentioned a mental health problem, and 42% believed it would lead to negative comments from colleagues (Sangar, 2019).

In other words, men in mental distress may have legitimate fears that disclosure of mental health issues will damage their employment status and future job opportunities. Such disclosure could negatively impact various aspects of their employment including job retention, promotion prospects, and career advancement. As such, men may make a calculated cost-benefit analysis, weighing up the socio-occupational costs of disclosure with the potential mental health benefits. For some men, disclosure will be deemed to bring more costs than benefits, especially if the labour market indicates they are easily replaceable (or "disposable"), meaning they will continue to struggle in silence so that they can maintain their employment status and financial income. These processes have been overlooked in much of the men's mental health literature, which has instead taken a narrow individual-level deficit-based approach by focusing on the alleged negative impact of "masculine culture" and the "constraints of masculinity" in the workplace (e.g., O'Brien et al., 2005).

8.5 The Big Picture: Changing Economic Trends and Gender Differentials in Employment

The evidence presented in the previous sections indicates that precarious employment, job strain, and job stress can all contribute to adverse mental health among the workforce. Risk appears to be especially intense among men, particularly blue-collar manual workers.

Importantly, the postwar years have seen massive socioeconomic changes across the western world, which have affected men and women in various ways, especially blue-collar less-educated men. Perhaps the greatest socioeconomic change is the transition from an industrial economy to a knowledge economy. The industrial economy was based on manufacturing, assembly plant production, and other manual industries that offered opportunities for skilled and unskilled men alike. Examples of manpower-heavy industries that flourished in this era include coal mining, car production, ship building, and steel working, which were the foundations for the economic success of a variety of regions including the North American Great Lakes, Northern England, and the Ruhr Valley. These industries provided well-paying and respectable jobs to skilled and unskilled men allowing them to support themselves and their families with a comfortable and respectable lifestyle.

This industrial-based economy has been replaced with a knowledge (or service)-based economy. This knowledge economy places an emphasis on specialized skills and services based on higher education, information technology, and digital innovation. It places a higher demand for cerebral skills and human services rather than traditional manual labor, meaning fewer opportunities for working-class blue-collar men. These wider upstream socioeconomic changes may result in an increased downstream risk of adverse mental health for men of low socioeconomic status.

This socioeconomic shift has led to a massive decline in traditional male industries that do not necessarily require a college degree. For example, figures indicate that the US steel industry employed around 700,000 workers in 1948, compared with 80,000 in 2018 (Bartholomew, 2019). The military also provided work for many less-educated men, but this has also shrunk in many western jurisdictions, with US figures indicating a 40% decline in military manpower from 1986 to 2019. More recently, a comparison of US Bureau of Labor Statistics data from 2013 and 2018 indicates that several male-dominated industries continue to experience a sharp decline in their workforce (US Bureau of Labor Statistics, 2014, 2019b). This includes an 88% decline in aerospace and parts manufacturing, a 35% decline in tire manufacturing, a 32% decline in oil/gas extraction, and a 25% decline in coal mining and mining support activities.

A similar decline is seen in the United Kingdom, where industries such as coal mining, steel making, and ship building have reduced by around 80%–90% in the postwar period (Ritchie, 2019; Stott, 2017). Such shrinking has also been seen in Canada, where the manufacturing sector declined by half between 1961 and 2011. Indeed, the Canadian manufacturing sector accounted for 9.2% of total employment in 2019, compared with 19.1% in 1976, representing a decline of over 50% (Statistics Canada, 2021). This decline has been off-set by an increase in employment opportunities in other sectors including the professional sector, business sector, and digital sector. However, these sectors provide fewer opportunities for unskilled less-educated men.

All this has contributed to a situation where blue-collar and less-educated men are suffering high rates of unemployment and elevated rates of precarious employment. In Canada, the proportion of men who were employed declined from 75% in 1990 to 67% in 2016, while the proportion of men not in the labour market increased from 12% to 22% during the same time period (Statistics Canada, 2017). More recent figures indicate that the unemployment rate is 6.1% for men and 5.3% for women (Statistics Canada, 2020b). Interestingly, several studies indicate particularly high unemployment rates in small towns and rural regions that were once defined by manufacturing, but where factory and plant closures have left little in the way of alternative employment (Watts, 2018; Statistics Canada, 2011; Dolphin, 2009). This can hit the male population particularly hard and may explain the higher rates of male suicide (see Chap. 2) seen in smaller towns and rural regions (Rivera et al., 2017; Browning & Heinesen, 2012; Myles et al., 2017; Alston, 2012; Crawford & Prince, 1999).

Of note, unemployment rates for men are particularly concentrated in those whose highest level of education is a high school diploma or less. A survey of OECD countries indicated a 14% unemployment rate for those with below upper secondary education, compared with 5% for those with tertiary education or higher (OECD, 2015). In 2016, the unemployment rate for Canadian males without a high school diploma was 15%, compared with 5% for males with postsecondary education (Uppal, 2017). This is concerning given the trends of increasing and elevated rates of high school dropout among men noted in Chap. 7 and the higher risk of adverse mental health outcomes among these high school dropouts.

Relatedly, surveys indicate that young men are disproportionately represented in the *Not in Education, Employment nor Training* (NEETs) category. For example, the latest UK statistics document 191,000 male NEETs ages 16–24 years, compared with 124,000 female NEETs ages 16–24 years (Office of National Statistics, 2019). In Canada, the NEET rate for 25–29 year-old men who are actively seeking work is twice that of 25- to 29-year-old women in the same situation (Brunet, 2018). This may contribute to a gender gap in housing arrangements, with 47% of Canadian men in their twenties still living with their parents, compared with 38% of Canadian women (Milan, 2016).

In other words, the shifting economy has created significant challenges to finding a stable, secure, and well-paying job for working-class men lacking postsecondary education. But even these working-class men with a job are facing challenging times. For example, several studies indicate that men are experiencing a decline in median wages compared with their female counterparts, with decreases again concentrated among blue-collar occupations (Statistics Canada, 2020c; Autor et al., 2019; Hernandez, 2018; Miller, 2016). Moreover, unskilled men can no longer hold reasonable expectations of obtaining a job for life, as more and more positions offer temporary contracts or other "flexible" work conditions, which often means lower wages, worse benefits, and fewer rights (Cherlin, 2014; Case & Deaton, 2020). This can increase the aforementioned job insecurity, job strain, and job stress, which have been associated with adverse mental health. Indeed, the three most common occupations among young men without a high school diploma in Canada are construction trade helpers, labourers, and transport truck drivers (Uppal, 2017). Of note, all these jobs are characterized by high demand/low control job environments and occupational health and safety issues, which have been associated with adverse mental health.

Incidentally, such jobs are unlikely to be unionized, and in fact the above-described changing socioeconomic conditions have led to a decline in trade union membership across the western world, with US figures indicating a 50% decline from 1983 to 2018 (Pedersini, 2010; Lafer & Loustaunau, 2020; US Bureau of Labor Statistics, 2019c). This decline may impact various aspects of psychosocial well-being, as trade unions were an important part of civil society that provided workers and their families with social support, meaningful activities, and political clout in the workplace and in wider society.

One of the connecting threads throughout this chapter is that the mental health of blue-collar less-educated men is at particular risk due to their higher risk of unemployment, precarious employment, high job stress/strain, and other adverse working conditions. This conclusion is supported by a recent innovative US study, which found that adult men who stated in their youth that they planned for a working-class job (e.g., manufacturing) were around three times as likely to die by suicide (HR = 2.91; 95% CI 1.07–7.88) or overdose (HR = 2.62; 95% CI 1.15–5.94) in adulthood than those who stated in their youth that they planned to work in a professional job (Muller et al., 2020). The authors of this innovative study attributed these elevated rates to the decline of working-class jobs, meaning that less-educated men are often left unemployed, with few opportunities and thus bereft of all the positive benefits associated with work discussed at the beginning of this chapter. All this can contribute to what have become known as *deaths of despair*, which is an umbrella term for suicide deaths, overdose deaths, and early mortality associated with alcohol and drug abuse (Case & Deaton, 2015, 2017, 2020). As described in Chaps. 2 and 3, such deaths of despair are intensely concentrated among the male population, especially low-skilled men without a college degree. Sadly, these deaths of despair may worsen with the progression of time, given the above-described decline in opportunities for working-class men without a college degree.

8.6 Conclusion

Evidence suggests that unemployment, precarious employment, and job stress/strain are all risk factors for adverse mental health outcomes including depression, substance use disorder, and suicide. These appear to have a stronger impact on the mental health of men than women. This gender differential may be due to three related factors. First, men typically remain the primary breadwinner for their family, and their income is essential to support the household, meaning that unemployment can have serious consequences for their standard of living and quality of life. Second, men tend to work longer unsociable hours meaning absence from family and friends and also tend to work in more dangerous and risky occupations, meaning greater exposure to hazardous psychosocial or physical conditions in the workplace, which can create job stress and job strain. Third, men draw considerable status and positive identity from their role as a productive worker and family breadwinner; this status is respected by wider society, while male unemployment remains highly stigmatized. All of this can interact to create considerable psychological distress in men who are unemployed or precariously employed, while men who are securely employed can reap the many psychosocial benefits of employment. Of note, these risk factors appear to be concentrated in blue-collar men and men lacking a postsecondary education, a demographic left behind by changes in the global economy.

To conclude, unemployment is a tragedy for affected men and women alike and can have nefarious consequences for them and their families including poverty, social exclusion, and alienation. However, unemployment and precarious employment is also an issue of importance to society as a whole. As stated, unemployment can increase risk of substance use and has been implicated as a causal factor in the opioid crisis ravaging many North American cities (Case & Deaton, 2020). Unemployment has also been linked to criminality and antisocial behavior in the United Kingdom (Jawadi et al., 2021; Wu & Wu, 2011) and risky driving and other negative social outcomes that can impact the wider community (Hammarström, 1994). As such, unemployment should be considered a public health issue of societal import and a modifiable risk factor in need of upstream and downstream interventions, some of which are discussed in Chap. 10.

References

Affleck, W., Carmichael, V., & Whitley, R. (2018). Men's mental health: Social determinants and implications for services. *The Canadian Journal of Psychiatry, 63*(9), 581–589. https://doi.org/10.1177/0706743718762388.

Alston, M. (2012). Rural male suicide in Australia. *Social Science & Medicine, 74*(4), 515–522. https://doi.org/10.1016/j.socscimed.2010.04.036.

Andrews, G., Henderson, S., & Hall, W. (2001). Prevalence, comorbidity, disability and service utilisation: Overview of the Australian National Mental Health Survey. *The British Journal of Psychiatry, 178*(2), 145–153.

Artazcoz, L., Benach, J., Borrell, C., & Cortès, I. (2004). Unemployment and mental health: Understanding the interactions among gender, family roles, and social class. *American Journal of Public Health (AJPH), 94*(1), 82–88. https://doi.org/10.2105/AJPH.94.1.82.

Ashfield, J. A., & Gouws, D. S. (2019). Dignifying psychotherapy with men: Developing empathic and evidence-based approaches that suit the real needs of the male gender. In J. A. Barry, R. Kingerlee, M. Seager, & L. Sullivan (Eds.), *The Palgrave handbook of male psychology and mental health* (pp. 623–645). Palgrave Macmillan.

Association of Workers Compensation Boards of Canada. (2020, May). *National work injury, disease and fatality statistics/Statistiques nationales des accidents, maladies et décès professionnels*. Retrieved March 17, 2021, from https://awcbc.org/wp-content/uploads/2020/05/National-Work-Injury-Disease-and-Fatality-Statistics-2016-2018.pdf.

Autor, D., Dorn, D., & Hanson, G. (2019). When work disappears: Manufacturing decline and the falling marriage market value of young men. *American Economic Review: Insights, 1*(2), 161–178. https://doi.org/10.1257/aeri.20180010.

Bartholomew, B. (2019, August). *The steel industry and its place in the American economy*. BDO Global. Retrieved March 12, 2021, from https://www.bdo.com/insights/business-financial-advisory/valuation-business-analytics/the-steel-industry-and-its-place-in-the-american-e.

Blakely, T., Collings, S. C. D., & Atkinson, J. (2003). Unemployment and suicide. Evidence for a causal association? *Journal of Epidemiology & Community Health, 57*(8), 594–600. https://doi.org/10.1136/jech.57.8.594.

Browning, M., & Heinesen, E. (2012). Effect of job loss due to plant closure on mortality and hospitalization. *Journal of Health Economics, 31*(4), 599–616. https://doi.org/10.1016/j.jhealeco.2012.03.001.

Brunet, S. (2018, October 10). *The transition from school to work-the NEET (not in employment, education or training) indicator for 25- to 29-year-old women and men in Canada*. Statistics Canada. Retrieved March 12, 2021, from https://www150.statcan.gc.ca/n1/pub/81-599-x/81-599-x2018013-eng.htm.

Case, A., & Deaton, A. (2015). Rising morbidity and mortality in midlife among white non-Hispanic Americans in the 21st century. *Proceedings of the National Academy of Sciences of the United States of America, 112*(49), 15078–15083. https://doi.org/10.1073/pnas.1518393112.

Case, A., & Deaton, A. (2017). Mortality and morbidity in the 21st century. *Brookings Papers on Economic Activity*, 397–443. https://doi.org/10.1353/eca.2017.0005.

Case, A., & Deaton, A. (2020). *Deaths of despair and the future of capitalism*. Princeton University Press.

Catalano, R., Dooley, D., Wilson, G., & Hough, R. (1993). Job loss and alcohol abuse: A test using data from the epidemiologic catchment area project. *Journal of Health and Social Behavior, 34*(3), 215–225. https://doi.org/10.2307/2137203.

Chang, S.-S., Stuckler, D., Yip, P., & Gunnell, D. (2013). Impact of 2008 global economic crisis on suicide: Time trend study in 54 countries. *BMJ, 347*. https://doi.org/10.1136/bmj.f5239.

Cherlin, A. J. (2014). *Labor's love lost: The rise and fall of the working-class family in America*. Russell Sage Foundation.

Condon, R. G., Collings, P., & Wenzel, G. (1995). The best part of life: Subsistence hunting, ethnicity, and economic adaptation among young adult Inuit males. *Arctic, 48*(1), 31–46.

Crawford, M. J., & Prince, M. (1999). Increasing rates of suicide in young men in England during the 1980s: The importance of social context. *Social Science & Medicine, 49*(10), 1419–1423. https://doi.org/10.1016/S0277-9536(99)00213-0.

Crayne, M. P. (2020). The traumatic impact of job loss and job search in the aftermath of COVID-19. *Psychological Trauma Theory Research Practice and Policy, 12*(S1), S180–S182. https://doi.org/10.1037/tra0000852.

Dallaire, R. (2019). *Waiting for first light: My ongoing battle with PTSD*. Random House Canada.

de Lange, A. H., Taris, T. W., Kompier, M. A. J., Houtman, I. L. D., & Bongers, P. M. (2002). Effects of stable and changing demand-control histories on worker health. *Scandinavian Journal of Work, Environment & Health, 28*(2), 94–108. https://doi.org/10.5271/sjweh.653.

De Leo, D., Sveticic, J., Milner, A., & McKay, K. (2011). *Suicide in indigenous populations of Queensland*. Australian Academic Press.

Dolphin, T. (2009, October). *The impact of the recession on northern city-regions*. The Progressive Policy Think Tank. Retrieved March 18, 2021, from https://www.ippr.org/files/images/media/files/publication/2011/05/impact_recession_north_1731.pdf.

Dooley, D., Catalano, R., & Hough, R. (1992). Unemployment and alcohol disorder in 1910 and 1990: Drift versus social causation. *Journal of Occupational and Organizational Psychology, 65*(40), 277–290. https://doi.org/10.1111/j.2044-8325.1992.tb00505.x.

Faragher, E. B., Cass, M., & Cooper, C. L. (2005). The relationship between job satisfaction and health: A meta-analysis. *Occupational and Environmental Medicine, 62*(2), 105–112. https://doi.org/10.1136/oem.2002.006734.

Farrell, W. (1993). *The myth of male power: Why men are the disposable sex*. Simon & Schuster.

Farrell, W., Seager, M. J., & Barry, J. A. (2016). The male gender empathy gap: Time for psychology to take action. *New Male Studies, 5*(2), 6–16.

Goldberg, D. P. (1972). *The detection of psychiatric illness by questionnaire: A technique for the identification and assessment of non-psychotic psychiatric illness*. Oxford University Press.

Goldberg, D. P., Gater, R., Sartorius, N., Ustun, T. B., Piccinelli, M., Gureje, O., & Rutter, C. (1997). The validity of two versions of the GHQ in the WHO study of mental illness in general health care. *Psychological Medicine, 27*(1), 191–197. https://doi.org/10.1017/S0033291796004242.

Graetz, B. (1993). Health consequences of employment and unemployment: Longitudinal evidence for young men and women. *Social Science & Medicine, 36*(6), 715–724. https://doi.org/10.1016/0277-9536(93)90032-Y.

Gunnell, D., & Chang, S.-S. (2016). Economic recession, unemployment, and suicide. In R. C. O'Connor & J. Pirkis (Eds.), *The international handbook of suicide prevention* (2nd ed., pp. 284–300). John Wiley & Sons.

Hakim, C. (2000). Sex differences in work-life balance goals. In D. M. Houston (Ed.), *Work-life balance in the 21st century* (pp. 55–79). Palgrave Macmillan.

Hakim, C. (2006). Women, careers, and work-life preferences. *British Journal of Guidance & Counselling, 34*(3), 279–294. https://doi.org/10.1080/03069880600769118.

Hammarström, A. (1994). Health consequences of youth unemployment. *Social Science & Medicine, 38*(5), 699–709. https://doi.org/10.1016/S0033-3506(94)80097-9.

Hammarström, A., Virtanen, P., & Janlert, U. (2011). Are the health consequences of temporary employment worse among low educated than among high educated? *European Journal of Public Health, 21*(6), 756–761. https://doi.org/10.1093/eurpub/ckq135.

Hedegaard, H., Curtin, S. C., & Warner, M. (2018, June). *Suicide rates in the United States continue to increase*. CDC National Center for Health Statistics. Retrieved March 12, 2021, from https://www.cdc.gov/nchs/data/databriefs/db309.pdf.

Henkel, D. (2011). Unemployment and substance use: A review of the literature (1990-2010). *Current Drug Abuse Reviews, 4*(1), 4–27. https://doi.org/10.2174/1874473711104010004.

Hernandez, R. (2018, August). *The fall of employment in the manufacturing sector*. US Bureau of Labor Statistics. Retrieved March 19, 2021, from https://www.bls.gov/opub/mlr/2018/beyond-bls/the-fall-of-employment-in-the-manufacturing-sector.htm.

Houle, J. N., & Light, M. T. (2017). The harder they fall? Sex and race/ethnic specific suicide rates in the U.S. foreclosure crisis. *Social Science & Medicine, 180*, 114–124. https://doi.org/10.1016/j.socscimed.2017.03.033.

Jahoda, M. (1982). *Employment and unemployment: A social-psychological analysis.* Cambridge University Press.

Jawadi, F., Mallick, S. K., Idi Cheffou, A., & Augustine, A. (2021). Does higher unemployment lead to greater criminality? Revisiting the debate over the business cycle. *Journal of Economic Behavior and Organization, 182*(1), 448–471. https://doi.org/10.1016/j.jebo.2019.03.025.

Karasek, R. (1979). Job demands, job decision latitude, and mental strain: Implications for job redesign. *Administrative Science Quarterly, 24*(2), 285–308. https://doi.org/10.2307/2392498.

Karasek, R., & Theorell, T. (1990). *Healthy work: Stress, productivity, and the reconstruction of working life.* Basic Books.

Kerr, W. C., Kaplan, M. S., Huguet, N., Caetano, R., Giesbrecht, N., & McFarland, B. H. (2017). Economic recession, alcohol, and suicide rates: Comparative effects of poverty, foreclosure, and job loss. *American Journal of Preventive Medicine, 52*(4), 469–475. https://doi.org/10.1016/j.amepre.2016.09.021.

Kestilä, L., Martelin, T., Rahkonen, O., Joutsenniemi, K., Pirkola, S., Poikolainen, K., & Koskinen, S. (2008). Childhood and current determinants of heavy drinking in early adulthood. *Alcohol and Alcoholism, 43*(4), 460–469. https://doi.org/10.1093/alcalc/agn018.

Kidger, J., Gunnell, D., Jarvik, J. G., Overstreet, K. A., & Hollingworth, W. (2011). The association between bankruptcy and hospital-presenting attempted suicide: A record linkage study. *Suicide & Life-Threatening Behavior, 41*(6), 676–684. https://doi.org/10.1111/j.1943-278X.2011.00063.x.

Kleiman, E. M., & Liu, R. T. (2013). Social support as a protective factor in suicide: Studies from American and English representative samples. *Journal of Affective Disorders, 150*(2), 540–545. https://doi.org/10.1016/j.jad.2013.01.033.

Klesment, M., & Van Bavel, J. (2017). The reversal of the gender gap in education, motherhood, and women as main earners in Europe. *European Sociological Review, 33*(3), 465–481. https://doi.org/10.1093/esr/jcw063.

Kline, A., Ciccone, D. S., Falca-Dodson, M., Black, C. M., & Losonczy, M. (2011). Suicidal ideation among National Guard troops deployed to Iraq: The association with postdeployment readjustment problems. *The Journal of Nervous and Mental Disease, 199*(12), 914–920. https://doi.org/10.1097/NMD.0b013e3182392917.

Komoto, Y. (2014). Factors associated with suicide and bankruptcy in Japanese pathological gamblers. *International Journal of Mental Health and Addiction, 12*(5), 600–606. https://doi.org/10.1007/s11469-014-9492-3.

Kposowa, A. J. (1999). Suicide mortality in the United States: Differentials by industrial and occupational groups. *American Journal of Industrial Medicine, 36*(6), 645–652. https://doi.org/10.1002/(SICI)1097-0274(199912)36:6<645::AID-AJIM7>3.0.CO;2-T.

Kreshpaj, B., Orellana, C., Burström, B., Davis, L., Hemmingsson, T., Johansson, G., Kjellberg, K., Jonsson, J., Wegman, D. H., & Bodin, T. (2020). What is precarious employment? A systematic review of definitions and operationalizations from quantitative and qualitative studies. *Scandinavian Journal of Work, Environment & Health, 46*(3), 235–247. https://doi.org/10.5271/sjweh.3875.

Kulik, L. (2000). Jobless men and women: A comparative analysis of job search intensity, attitudes toward unemployment, and related responses. *Journal of Occupational and Organizational Psychology, 73*(4), 487–500. https://doi.org/10.1348/096317900167173.

Kumar, M. B., & Tjepkema, M. (2019, June 28). *Suicide among First Nations people, Métis and Inuit (2011–2016): Findings from the 2011 Canadian Census Health and Environment Cohort (CanCHEC).* Statistics Canada. Retrieved March 18, 2021, from https://www150.statcan.gc.ca/n1/pub/99-011-x/99-011-x2019001-eng.htm.

Lafer, G., & Loustaunau, L. (2020, July 23). *Fear at work-An inside account of how employers threaten, intimidate, and harass workers to stop them from exercising their right to collective* bargaining. Economic Policy Institute. Retrieved March 19, 2021, from https://files.epi.org/pdf/202305.pdf.

LaMontagne, A. D., Keegel, T., Louie, A. M., & Ostry, A. (2010). Job stress as a preventable upstream determinant of common mental disorders: A review for practitioners and policymakers. *Advances in Mental Health: Promotion, Prevention and Early Intervention, 9*(1), 17–35. https://doi.org/10.5172/jamh.9.1.17.

Legleye, S., Beck, F., Peretti-Watel, P., & Chau, N. (2008). Le rôle du statut scolaire et professionnel dans les usages de drogues des hommes et des femmes de 18 à 25 ans. *Revue d'Épidémiologie et de Santé Publique, 56*(5), 345–355. https://doi.org/10.1016/j.respe.2008.06.262.

Li, Z., Page, A., Martin, G., & Taylor, R. (2011). Attributable risk of psychiatric and socio-economic factors for suicide from individual-level, population-based studies: A systematic review. *Social Science & Medicine, 72*(4), 608–616. https://doi.org/10.1016/j.socscimed.2010.11.008.

Linford, C. (2013). *Warrior rising: A soldier's journey to PTSD and back*. FriesenPress.

Lorant, V., Deliège, D., Eaton, W., Robert, A., Philippot, P., & Ansseau, M. (2003). Socioeconomic inequalities in depression: A meta-analysis. *American Journal of Epidemiology, 157*(2), 98–112. https://doi.org/10.1093/aje/kwf182.

Lubinski, D., Benbow, C. P., & Kell, H. J. (2014). Life paths and accomplishments of mathematically precocious males and females four decades later. *Psychological Science, 25*(12), 2217–2232. https://doi.org/10.1177/0956797614551371.

Marsh, J. C., Park, K., Lin, Y.-A., & Bersamira, C. (2018). Gender differences in trends for heroin use and nonmedical prescription opioid use, 2007-2014. *Journal of Substance Abuse Treatment, 87*, 79–85. https://doi.org/10.1016/j.jsat.2018.01.001.

McKee-Ryan, F. M., Song, Z., Wanberg, C. R., & Kinicki, A. J. (2005). Psychological and physical well-being during unemployment: A meta-analytic study. *Journal of Applied Psychology, 90*(1), 53–76. https://doi.org/10.1037/0021-9010.90.1.53.

Melchior, M., Caspi, A., Milne, B. J., Danese, A., Poulton, R., & Moffitt, T. E. (2007). Work stress precipitates depression and anxiety in young, working women and men. *Psychological Medicine, 37*(8), 1119–1129. https://doi.org/10.1017/S0033291707000414.

Milan, A. (2016, June 15). *Diversity of young adults living with their parents*. Statistics Canada. Retrieved March 12, 2021, from https://www150.statcan.gc.ca/n1/pub/75-006-x/2016001/article/14639-eng.htm.

Miller, C. C. (2016, March 20). As women take over a male-dominated field, the pay drops. *The New York Times*. https://www.nytimes.com/2016/03/20/upshot/as-women-take-over-a-male-dominated-field-the-pay-drops.html.

Milner, A., Page, A., & LaMontagne, A. D. (2013). Long-term unemployment and suicide: A systematic review and meta-analysis. *PLoS One, 8*(1), e51333. https://doi.org/10.1371/journal.pone.0051333.

Milner, A., Page, A., & LaMontagne, A. D. (2014). Cause and effect in studies on unemployment, mental health and suicide: A meta-analytic and conceptual review. *Psychological Medicine, 44*(5), 909–917. https://doi.org/10.1017/S0033291713001621.

Modini, M., Joyce, S., Mykletun, A., Christensen, H., Bryant, R. A., Mitchell, P. B., & Harvey, S. B. (2016). The mental health benefits of employment: Results of a systematic meta-review. *Australasian Psychiatry, 24*(4), 331–336. https://doi.org/10.1177/1039856215618523.

Monk, A. (2000). The influence of isolation on stress and suicide in rural areas: An international comparison. *Rural Society, 10*(3), 393–403. https://doi.org/10.5172/rsj.10.3.393.

Montgomery, S. M., Cook, D. G., Bartley, M. J., & Wadsworth, M. E. J. (1999). Unemployment pre-dates symptoms of depression and anxiety resulting in medical consultation in young men. *International Journal of Epidemiology, 28*(1), 95–100. https://doi.org/10.1093/ije/28.1.95.

Muller, C., Duncombe, A., Carroll, J. M., Mueller, A. S., Warren, J. R., & Grodsky, E. (2020). Association of job expectations among high school students with early death during adulthood. *JAMA Network Open, 3*(12), e2027958. https://doi.org/10.1001/jamanetworkopen.2020.27958.

Muntaner, C., Solar, O., Vanroelen, C., Martínez, J. M., Vergara, M., Santana, V., Castedo, A., Kim, I. H., & Benach, J. (2010). Unemployment, informal work, precarious employment, child labor, slavery, and health inequalities: Pathways and mechanisms. *International Journal of Health Services: Planning, Administration, Evaluation, 40*(2), 281–295. https://doi.org/10.2190/HS.40.2.h.

Murphy, G. C., & Athanasou, J. A. (1999). The effect of unemployment on mental health. *Journal of Occupational and Organizational Psychology, 72*(1), 83–99. https://doi.org/10.1348/096317999166518.

Myles, N., Large, M., Myles, H., Adams, R., Liu, D., & Galletly, C. (2017). Australia's economic transition, unemployment, suicide and mental health needs. *The Australian and New Zealand Journal of Psychiatry, 51*(2), 119–123. https://doi.org/10.1177/0004867416675035.

Niedhammer, I., Goldberg, M., Leclerc, A., Bugel, I., & David, S. (1998). Psychosocial factors at work and subsequent depressive symptoms in the Gazel cohort. *Scandinavian Journal of Work, Environment & Health, 24*(3), 197–205. https://doi.org/10.5271/sjweh.299.

O'Brien, R., Hunt, K., & Hart, G. (2005). 'It's caveman stuff, but that is to a certain extent how guys still operate': Men's accounts of masculinity and help seeking. *Social Science & Medicine, 61*(3), 503–516. https://doi.org/10.1016/j.socscimed.2004.12.008.

Office of National Statistics. (2019, February 28). *Young people not in education, employment or training (NEET), UK: February 2019*. Retrieved March 12, 2021, from https://www.ons.gov.uk/employmentandlabourmarket/peoplenotinwork/unemployment/bulletins/youngpeoplenotineducationemploymentortrainingneet/february2019.

Organisation for Economic Co-operation and Development (OECD). (2010). *OECD employment outlook 2010: moving beyond the jobs crisis*. Organisation for Economic Co-operation and Development. Retrieved March 12, 2021, from http://www.oecd.org/employment/emp/48806664.pdf.

Organisation for Economic Co-operation and Development (OECD). (2015). *Education at a glance interim report: Update of employment and educational attainment indicators*. Organisation for Economic Co-operation and Development. Retrieved March 12, 2021, from http://www.oecd.org/education/EAG-Interim-report-Chapter2.pdf.

Paul, K. I., & Moser, K. (2009). Unemployment impairs mental health: Meta-analyses. *Journal of Vocational Behavior, 74*(3), 264–282. https://doi.org/10.1016/j.jvb.2009.01.001.

Pedersini, R. (2010). *Trade union strategies to recruit new groups of workers*. European Foundation for the Improvement of Living and Working Conditions. Retrieved March 19, 2021, from https://www.eurofound.europa.eu/sites/default/files/ef_files/docs/eiro/tn0901028s/tn0901028s.pdf.

Penney, C., Senécal, S., & Bobet, E. (2009). Mortalité par suicide dans les collectivités inuites au Canada: taux et effets des caractéristiques des collectivités/Suicide mortality in Inuit communities in Canada: Rates and effects of community characteristics. *Cahiers Québécois de Démographie, 38*(2), 311–343. https://doi.org/10.7202/044818ar.

Qin, P., Agerbo, E., Westergård-Nielsen, N., Eriksson, T., & Mortensen, P. B. (2000). Gender differences in risk factors for suicide in Denmark. *The British Journal of Psychiatry, 177*, 546–550. https://doi.org/10.1192/bjp.177.6.546.

Ritchie, H. (2019, January 28). *The death of UK coal in five charts*. Our World in Data. Retrieved March 19, 2021, from https://ourworldindata.org/death-uk-coal.

Rivera, B., Casal, B., & Currais, L. (2017). Crisis, suicide and labour productivity losses in Spain. *The European Journal of Health Economics: Health Economics in Prevention and Care, 18*(1), 83–96. https://doi.org/10.1007/s10198-015-0760-3.

Roberts, S. E., Jaremin, B., & Lloyd, K. (2013). High-risk occupations for suicide. *Psychological Medicine, 43*(6), 1231–1240. https://doi.org/10.1017/S0033291712002024.

Rönnblad, T., Grönholm, E., Jonsson, J., Koranyi, I., Orellana, C., Kreshpaj, B., Chen, L., Stockfelt, L., & Bodin, T. (2019). Precarious employment and mental health: A systematic review and meta-analysis of longitudinal studies. *Scandinavian Journal of Work, Environment & Health, 45*(5), 429–443. https://doi.org/10.5271/sjweh.3797.

Russell, D., Turner, R. J., & Joiner, T. E. (2009). Physical disability and suicidal ideation: A community-based study of risk/protective factors for suicidal thoughts. *Suicide and Life-threatening Behavior, 39*(4), 440–451. https://doi.org/10.1521/suli.2009.39.4.440.

Sangar, R. (2019, October 9). *Mental health in the workplace: Global impact study*. Ipsos MORI. Retrieved March 12, 2021, from https://www.ipsos.com/en-ca/news-polls/mental-health-workplace-global-impact-study.

Sareen, J., Cox, B. J., Stein, M. B., Afifi, T. O., Fleet, C., & Asmundson, G. J. (2007). Physical and mental comorbidity, disability, and suicidal behavior associated with posttraumatic stress disorder in a large community sample. *Psychosomatic Medicine, 69*(3), 242–248. https://doi.org/10.1097/PSY.0b013e31803146d8.

Scheid, T. L. (2005). Stigma as a barrier to employment: Mental disability and the Americans with disabilities act. *International Journal of Law and Psychiatry, 28*(6), 670–690. https://doi.org/10.1016/j.ijlp.2005.04.003.

Schwartz, S. H., & Rubel, T. (2005). Sex differences in value priorities: Cross-cultural and multimethod studies. *Journal of Personality and Social Psychology, 89*(6), 1010–1028. https://doi.org/10.1037/0022-3514.89.6.1010.

Seager, M. (2019). From stereotypes to archetypes: An evolutionary perspective on male help-seeking and suicide. In J. A. Barry, R. Kingerlee, M. Seager, & L. Sullivan (Eds.), *The Palgrave handbook of male psychology and mental health* (pp. 227–248). Palgrave Macmillan.

Seaton, C. L., Bottorff, J. L., Oliffe, J. L., Medhurst, K., & DeLeenheer, D. (2019). Mental health promotion in male-dominated workplaces: Perspectives of male employees and workplace representatives. *Psychology of Men & Masculinities, 20*(4), 541–552. https://doi.org/10.1037/men0000182.

Sousa, E., Agudelo-Suárez, A., Benavides, F. G., Schenker, M., García, A. M., Benach, J., Delclos, C., López-Jacob, M. J., Ruiz-Frutos, C., Ronda-Pérez, E., & Porthé, V. (2010). Immigration, work and health in Spain: The influence of legal status and employment contract on reported health indicators. *International Journal of Public Health, 55*(5), 443–451. https://doi.org/10.1007/s00038-010-0141-8.

Stansfeld, S. A., & Candy, B. (2006). Psychosocial work environment and mental health-A meta-analytic review. *Scandinavian Journal of Work, Environment & Health, 32*(6), 443–462. https://doi.org/10.5271/sjweh.1050.

Stansfeld, S. A., Fuhrer, R., Shipley, M. J., & Marmot, M. G. (1999). Work characteristics predict psychiatric disorder: Prospective results from the Whitehall II Study. *Occupational and Environmental Medicine, 56*(5), 302–307. https://doi.org/10.1136/oem.56.5.302.

Statistics Canada. (2011). *Manufacturing. Canada Year Book, 2011*. Retrieved March 18, 2021, from https://www150.statcan.gc.ca/n1/pub/11-402-x/2011000/chap/man-fab/man-fab-eng.htm.

Statistics Canada. (2016). *Daily average time spent in hours on various activities by age group and sex, 15 years and over, Canada and provinces*. Retrieved March 12, 2021, from https://www150.statcan.gc.ca/t1/tbl1/en/cv.action?pid=4510001401.

Statistics Canada. (2017, May 4). *Study: Young men and women without a high school diploma, 1990 to 2016*. Retrieved March 18, 2021, from https://www150.statcan.gc.ca/n1/daily-quotidien/ 170504/dq170504b-eng.htm.

Statistics Canada. (2020a). *Usual hours worked by job type (main or all jobs), annual*. Retrieved March 12, 2021, from https://www150.statcan.gc.ca/t1/tbl1/en/tv.action?pid=1410003101.

Statistics Canada. (2020b). Labour force characteristics by sex and detailed age group, annual. Retrieved March 18, 2021, from https://www150.statcan.gc.ca/t1/tbl1/en/tv.action?pid=1410032701.

Statistics Canada. (2020c, January 15). *Study: The impact of the manufacturing decline on local labour markets in Canada*. Retrieved March 19, 2021, from https://www150.statcan.gc.ca/n1/daily-quotidien/200115/dq200115a-eng.htm.

Statistics Canada. (2021). Labour force characteristics by industry, annual (x 1,000). Retrieved March 12, 2021, from https://www150.statcan.gc.ca/t1/tbl1/en/cv.action?pid=1410002301.

Stott, P. (2017, November 8). *Shipbuilding in Britain: how to reboot it.* The Conversation. Retrieved March 19, 2021, from https://theconversation.com/shipbuilding-in-britain-how-to-reboot-it-87031.

Strandh, M., Hammarström, A., Nilsson, K., Nordenmark, M., & Russel, H. (2013). Unemployment, gender and mental health: The role of the gender regime. *Sociology of Health & Illness, 35*(5), 649–665. https://doi.org/10.1111/j.1467-9566.2012.01517.x.

Stuckler, D., Basu, S., Suhrcke, M., Coutts, A., & McKee, M. (2011). Effects of the 2008 recession on health: A first look at European data. *The Lancet, 378*(9786), 124–125. https://doi.org/10.1016/S0140-6736(11)61079-9.

Tiesman, H. M., Konda, S., Hartley, D., Chaumont Menéndez, C., Ridenour, M., & Hendricks, S. (2015). Suicide in U.S. workplaces, 2003-2010: A comparison with non-workplace suicides. *American Journal of Preventive Medicine, 48*(6), 674–682. https://doi.org/10.1016/j.amepre.2014.12.011.

Uppal, S. (2017, May 4). *Young men and women without a high school diploma.* Statistics Canada. Retrieved March 12, 2021, from https://files.eric.ed.gov/fulltext/ED585313.pdf.

US Bureau of Labor Statistics. (2014, February 26). Labor force statistics from the current population survey. Retrieved March 12, 2021, from https://www.bls.gov/cps/aa2013/cpsaat18.htm.

US Bureau of Labor Statistics. (2019a, December). *Women in the labor force: A databook.* Retrieved from March 12, 2021, from https://www.bls.gov/opub/reports/womens-databook/2019/home.htm.

US Bureau of Labor Statistics. (2019b, January 18). Labor force statistics from the current population survey. Retrieved March 12, 2021, from https://www.bls.gov/cps/aa2018/cpsaat18.htm.

US Bureau of Labor Statistics. (2019c, January 25). *Union membership rate 10.5 percent in 2018, down from 20.1 percent in 1983.* Retrieved March 12, 2021, from https://www.bls.gov/opub/ted/2019/union-membership-rate-10-point-5-percent-in-2018-down-from-20-point-1-percent-in-1983.htm.

US Bureau of Labor Statistics. (2020a, December 16). Table 1. Fatal occupational injuries by selected demographic characteristics, 2015–19. Retrieved March 12, 2021, from https://www.bls.gov/news.release/cfoi.t01.htm.

US Bureau of Labor Statistics. (2020b, November 4). Table EH1. Number of nonfatal occupational injuries and illnesses involving days away from work by selected worker and case characteristics and medical treatment facility visits, all U.S., private industry, 2019. Retrieved March 12, 2021, from https://www.bls.gov/iif/oshwc/osh/case/cd_eh1_2019.htm.

US Social Security Administration. (2020, October). *Annual statistical report on the social security disability insurance program, 2019.* Retrieved March 12, 2021, from https://www.ssa.gov/policy/docs/statcomps/di_asr/2019/.

Utzet, M., Valero, E., Mosquera, I., & Martin, U. (2020). Employment precariousness and mental health, understanding a complex reality: A systematic review. *International Journal of Occupational Medicine and Environmental Health, 33*(5), 569–598. https://doi.org/10.13075/ijomeh.1896.01553.

van der Noordt, M., Ijzelenberg, H., Droomers, M., & Proper, K. I. (2014). Health effects of employment: A systematic review of prospective studies. *Occupational and Environmental Medicine, 71*(10), 730–736. https://doi.org/10.1136/oemed-2013-101891.

Vijayakumar, L., Kumar, M. S., & Vijayakumar, V. (2011). Substance use and suicide. *Current Opinion in Psychiatry, 24*(3), 197–202. https://doi.org/10.1097/YCO.0b013e3283459242.

Waenerlund, A.-K., Virtanen, P., & Hammarström, A. (2011). Is temporary employment related to health status? Analysis of the Northern Swedish Cohort. *Scandinavian Journal of Public Health, 39*(5), 533–539. https://doi.org/10.1177/1403494810395821.

Wahrendorf, M., Blane, D., Bartley, M., Dragano, N., & Siegrist, J. (2012). Working conditions in mid-life and mental health in older ages. *Advances in Life Course Research, 18*(1), 16–25. https://doi.org/10.1016/j.alcr.2012.10.004.

References

Wang, J. L., Lesage, A. D., Schmitz, N., & Drapeau, A. (2008). The relationship between work stress and mental disorders in men and women: Findings from a population-based study. *Journal of Epidemiology & Community Health, 62*(1), 42–47. https://doi.org/10.1136/jech.2006.050591.

Wang, J. L., Schmitz, N., Dewa, C., & Stansfeld, S. (2009). Changes in perceived job strain and the risk of major depression: Results from a population-based longitudinal study. *American Journal of Epidemiology, 169*(9), 1085–1091. https://doi.org/10.1093/aje/kwp037.

Warr, P. (1987). *Work, unemployment, and mental health*. Clarendon Press.

Watts, C. (2018, June). *Regional inequality in Australia and the future of work*. Australian Council of Trade Unions. Retrieved March 18, 2021, from https://www.actu.org.au/our-work/policies-publications-submissions/2018/regional-inequality-in-australia-and-the-future-of-work.

Wu, D., & Wu, Z. (2011). Crime, inequality and unemployment in England and Wales. *Applied Economics, 44*(29), 3765–3775. https://doi.org/10.1080/00036846.2011.581217.

Yur'yev, A., Värnik, A., Värnik, P., Sisask, M., & Leppik, L. (2012). Employment status influences suicide mortality in Europe. *International Journal of Social Psychiatry, 58*(1), 62–68. https://doi.org/10.1177/0020764010387059.

Chapter 9
Family Ties: Marriage, Divorce, and the Mental Health of Men and Boys

An amassed corpus of research indicates that major unexpected shocks and sudden life events have the potential to negatively impact psychosocial well-being and cause considerable emotional turmoil (Brown & Harris, 1989; Paykel, 2003). This is especially so when such life events involve loss, rupture, and upheaval for the parties involved (Brown et al., 1995).

In the 1960s, two American psychiatrists attempted to quantify the severity of various different severe life events, based on the consultation of medical records of over 5000 psychiatric patients (Holmes & Rahe, 1967). This led them to create a rating scale of 43 life events, which could cause psychological distress, known as the *Social Readjustment Rating Scale*, or more simply as the *Holmes-Rahe Life Stress Inventory*. This scale lists the most severe events at the top and the least severe events at the bottom. The three most severe life events identified on this scale are: (i) death of a spouse, (ii) divorce, and (iii) marital separation. This scale has been validated in many different contexts and is still considered a gold standard in psychological stress research (Harmon et al., 1970; Hobson et al., 1998; Scully et al., 2000), thus indicating that divorce, separation, and widowhood are very serious life events, which can negatively affect mental health, regardless of sociocultural background.

In the 1980s, the British sociologist Mike Bury enriched stress theory by introducing the concept of *biographical disruption* (Bury, 1982, 1991). Bury writes that a biographical disruption is a particular type of serious unexpected event that can:

(i) Disrupt taken-for-granted assumptions and behaviours.
(ii) Lead to a fundamental rethinking of the person's biography and self-concept.
(iii) Instigate a response to the disruption, which can be adaptive or maladaptive.

While Bury originally coined the concept in relation to the onset of a chronic illness, more recent scholars have noted that divorce, separation, and widowhood can cause biographical disruption, raising intense psychosocial issues for affected individuals (Blakeslee & Wallerstein, 2004; Ketokivi, 2008; Mattingly, 2021; Morgan & Burholt, 2020).

Since then, there have been a variety of empirical studies examining the association between marital status and mental health outcomes. These studies cleft into two broad categories:

(i) Those assessing the mental health impact of marriage, divorce, separation, and widowhood on affected adults.
(ii) Those assessing the mental health impact of marriage, divorce, and separation on affected children.

The first part of this chapter concentrates on adults, while the second part concentrates on children, with a focus throughout on the mental health of men and boys.

9.1 Marital Status and Mental Health in Adults

Research studies on marital status and mental health in adults come in various forms. Some studies involve crude comparisons between two broad populations, (i) the married and (ii) the unmarried, while other studies involve granular-level comparisons between the never married, the divorced, the separated, and the widowed. Some studies are propelled by legal definitions of marriage and divorce, while others collapse together the legally married, common-law marriages, and cohabitation relationships into a new unified category to capture cognate family units. Most studies focus on heterosexual marriage, while a few have examined gay marriage. Some studies elicit cross-sectional associations between marital status and mental health, while others examine longitudinal within-person changes when they transition from one marital status to another.

While the methodologies are different, these studies converge on a set of conclusions, namely:

(i) Moving from unmarried status to marriage confers modest mental health benefits.
(ii) Being happily married is modestly beneficial for mental health.
(iii) Widowhood and never-married status are slight risk-factors for adverse mental health.
(iv) Separation and divorce are strong risk factors for adverse mental health outcomes including suicide, substance use, and depression.
(v) Separation and divorce tend to negatively affect the mental health of both men and women but may be particularly detrimental to men's mental health.

Given the large amount of research examining marital status, marital dissolution, and mental health, the literature is reviewed in three separate subsections focusing on different mental health outcomes, which have been the focus of related research. These three subsections are: (i) depression; (ii) substance abuse; and (iii) suicide.

9.1.1 Depression

Evidence suggests that single, divorced, and separated individuals have higher rates of depression than married individuals. For example, a US cohort study of over 2000 midlife individuals found that 22% of individuals who had become separated or divorced had experienced past-year major depressive disorder (MDD), compared with 8.4% of those who had been continuously married. This translates to an adjusted odds ratio of 2.29 (95% CI: 1.41–3.75) of MDD for the separated and divorced, compared with those who were continuously married (Sbarra et al., 2014). However, this study did not stratify outcomes by sex, nor by granular level marital status, but this weakness has been overcome by a variety of other studies from several different jurisdictions.

For example, Remes et al. (2019) conducted a cohort study of over 20,000 participants in the United Kingdom, examining MDD in men and women. This study found MDD in 1.7% of married men, 3.6% of never-married men, and 6.3% of divorced, separated, or widowed men. Analogous figures for females were 2.7% for married women, 2.4% for never-married women, and 5.6% for divorced, separated, or widowed women. This translates to an adjusted odds ratio of 3.66 (95% CI: 2.53–5.28) of MDD for divorced, separated, or widowed men compared with married men. The odds ratio of MDD for never-married men (compared with married men) was less potent, at 1.46 (95% CI: 0.76–2.83). These odds ratios are a stronger magnitude than the analogous MDD odds ratios for women, which are 2.56 (95% CI: 2.00–3.27) for divorced, separated, or widowed women as compared with married women. The odds ratio for never-married women (compared with the married) was 0.93 (95% CI: 0.48–1.78). In other words, this study found the highest rates and risk of MDD in divorced, separated, or widowed men, with never-married men having higher rates of MDD than never-married women, implying that divorce, separation, and unmarried status is a greater risk factor for MDD in men than women.

These findings are consistent with earlier studies. For example, a cross-sectional survey of around 35,000 people from 15 different countries found that depression was significantly associated with divorce, while marriage was a protective factor (Scott et al., 2010). This study found that the adjusted odds ratio for the onset of MDD was 2.8 (95% CI: 1.8–3.0) for divorced men compared with married men. The analogous adjusted odds ratio for the onset of MDD in divorced women was 1.7 (95% CI: 1.5–2.0) as compared with married women. Again, divorce was a significant risk factor for depression for both men and women, but risk was much higher among divorced men. Interestingly, this study also found that the adjusted odds ratio for the onset of MDD was 0.8 (95% CI: 0.6–0.9) for married men compared with never-married men, demonstrating that marriage was protective for men and that never-married men had a slightly increased risk of major depression.

Similarly, a Canadian longitudinal study of over 15,000 adults participating in the National Population Health Survey found that men whose marriages ended were at higher risk of being diagnosed with depression compared with their female peers (Rotermann, 2007). In this study, the adjusted odds ratio for the onset of depression in the past 2 years for divorced and separated men was 3.3 (95% CI: 1.7–6.5) compared with men who remained married. For divorced and separated women, the adjusted odds ratio was 2.4 (95% CI: 1.6–3.5). Interestingly, subanalysis indicated that men who were separated from their children after marital dissolution had a higher risk of depression than men who were not separated (OR 1.9: 95% CI: 0.9–4.2), while men whose social support had decreased also had a higher risk than men whose social support had not decreased (OR = 2.3: 95% CI: 1.3–3.9). In short, this study confirms that divorced and separated men are at particular risk, especially those who are separated from their children and experience a decrease in social support.

Interestingly, some research indicates that single gay men have higher rates of depression than gay men who are legally married. For example, one large-scale study examined differential rates of psychological distress by marital status in California, finding that single gay men had higher rates than married gay men (Wight et al., 2012). This is an important finding, indicating that marriage confers mental health protection regardless of sexual orientation.

9.1.2 Substance Abuse

A growing body of research has examined the relationship between marital status and substance use. Again, this research indicates higher rates of substance use among unmarried men, particularly among divorced men. For example, Edwards et al. (2018) conducted a longitudinal analysis of over 650,000 Swedes finding high rates of drug abuse onset in both sexes after a divorce, with a summary hazard ratio of 7.31 (95% CI: 6.91–7.74). For women, the hazard ratio was 6.80 (95% CI: 6.25–7.39), while for men the hazard ratio was 8.29 (95% CI: 7.65–8.97), indicating that divorce may have a slightly greater mental health impact on men than women. Interestingly, this study also assessed the association between drug abuse onset and widowhood, finding a hazard ratio of 5.27 (95% CI: 3.42–8.14) for women and 4.22 (95% CI: 2.10–8.46) for men, implying that widowhood is a potent risk factor for drug abuse, but is weaker than divorce, and affects women more than men.

These results overlap with a similar Swedish study of over 900,000 individuals, which examined alcohol use disorder onset after a divorce, which found a hazards ratio of 5.98 (95% CI: 5.65–6.33) for men after a divorce, while widowhood in men incurred a hazard ratio of 3.85 (95% CI: 2.81–5.28) (Kendler et al., 2017). Taken in the round, the combined results from these two studies suggest that the loss of a spouse through divorce or widowhood is detrimental to the mental health of both men and women, but divorce is a more powerful risk factor than widowhood, with divorce being particularly egregious for substance abuse in men.

The above-described findings are consistent with studies elsewhere. For example, Compton et al. (2007) found that men had an odds ratio of 2.6 (99% CI: 2.0–3.3) for past year alcohol or drug use disorder compared with women in a large representative sample of over 43,000 US adults. This study also found that the never married had an odds ratio of 2.0 (99% CI: 1.5–2.7) compared with the married for past year alcohol or drug use disorder; while the widowed, separated, and divorced had an odds ratio of 2.6 (99% CI: 1.8–3.7) compared with the married. This suggests that the unmarried per se are at greater risk of substance use disorder than the married, with widowed, separated, and divorced men at particular risk. Similarly, another US study of over 8000 participants examined past year alcohol use disorder, finding that all divorced and separated individuals had an adjusted odds ratio of 1.7 (95% CI: 0.89–3.28) compared with all married individuals, while men per se had an adjusted odds ratio of 5.86 (95% CI: 3.50–9.82) compared with women per se, again signifying that divorced and separated men may be at greater risk than other demographics (Lin et al., 2012).

9.1.3 Suicide

A robust finding across the suicide literature is that divorced and separated men have a greater risk of suicide compared with: (i) divorced and separated women, (ii) married men, and (iii) other categories of unmarried men such as the widowed and the never married (Evans et al., 2016; Payne et al., 2008).

For example, a recent study of data from the large-scale US National Longitudinal Mortality Study consisting of 1.38 million people examined the relationship between suicide and various types of marital status (Kposowa et al., 2020). This study found that divorced individuals had an adjusted relative risk of 1.97 (95% CI: 1.71–2.23) for suicide compared with the married. This was higher than the rate for separated individuals, who had an adjusted relative risk of 1.52 (95% CI: 1.13–2.04), which was higher than the adjusted relative risk of 1.34 (95% CI: 1.17–1.54) for the single/never married. In other words, this study found that all categories of the "unmarried" had a significantly higher suicide risk than the married, but there was a gradient of effect, with the divorced having the highest risk, followed by the separated, then the never married. Importantly, this study stratified by gender, finding that divorced and separated men had a two-fold relative risk (adjusted RR 2.01; 95% CI: 1.73–2.38) of suicide compared with married men, while divorced and separated women had a less marked adjusted relative risk of 1.46 in comparison with married women (95% CI: 1.10–1.95).

These findings are consistent with previous analyses from earlier waves of this longitudinal survey. For example, Kposowa (2000) found that divorced men were over two times more likely to die by suicide in comparison with married men (RR = 2.08; 95% CI: 1.58–2.72), with divorced men also having significantly higher rates than widowed men and the never married. In this study, rates of suicide in widowed and single men were much lower than divorced men and were not significantly different from the rates for married men. In another analysis, Kposowa (2003) directly compared rates between divorced men and divorced women, finding that divorced men had a relative risk of killing themselves that was over eight times higher than divorced women (RR = 8.36; 95% CI: 4.24–16.38). In other words, this series of analyses from a large-scale US longitudinal study found that divorce and separation are risk factors for suicide for both males and females, but risk was dramatically higher among divorced men.

These results converge with other findings from elsewhere. For example, a large-scale national cohort study of completed suicides in Sweden found that unmarried men were almost twice as likely to kill themselves when compared with married men (HR = 1.97; 95% CI: 1.85–2.10) and significantly more likely to kill themselves when compared with unmarried women, with highest rates among divorced men (Crump et al., 2014). This study also found that divorced men had the highest rate of suicide out of all the subgroups of unmarried men, while widowed men had the lowest rate of suicide. Interestingly, European countries with higher rates of divorce tend to have higher rates of male suicide. For example, Lithuania has the highest suicide mortality rate of all EU countries, with males dying by suicide at nearly six times the rate of women in that country (Eurostat, 2020a). It also has one of the highest divorce rates, showing an ecological link between divorce and male suicide (Eurostat, 2020b).

To conclude this section, a range of other studies have made broad comparisons between the two umbrella categories of "married" and "unmarried" indicating that unmarried men per se are at greater risk of suicide compared with married men. For example, a large-scale Danish case-control study found that the age adjusted relative risk of suicide in single men was over double that for married or cohabiting men (OR = 2.59; 95% CI: 2.18–3.09) and significantly higher than the suicide rate for single women (Qin et al., 2000). Likewise, a large-scale US study using data from the National Center for Health Statistics notes that unmarried men ages 40–60 years were 3.5 times more likely to die by suicide compared with married men of the same age, with markedly higher rates for unmarried men compared with unmarried women (Phillips et al., 2010). Similarly, another large-scale US study showed hazard ratios demonstrating that unmarried men ages 40–75 years had a twofold risk of suicide compared with married men of the same age group (Tsai et al., 2014).

In sum, data from various surveys and various countries using various methodologies indicate that unmarried men per se have an elevated risk of suicide compared with married men, and this is more pronounced among men who are divorced and (to a slightly lesser extent) separated.

9.1.4 *The Psychosocial Impact of Divorce for Men*

In sum, a vast number of studies indicate that divorce and separation are associated with substantial declines in mental health. Indeed, a recent overview paper states that the scientific evidence points to "the disadvantageous state of divorce and widowhood or the stressful transitional period from married to unmarried status, rather than the advantageous status of marriage" (Umberson et al., 2013). In other words, relationship dissolution produces its own unique stressors, which can affect mental health, with research indicating that divorce can precipitate a short-term acute crisis and long-term chronic strain (Amato, 2000; Felix et al., 2013).

Of note, several elements of the research literature indicate that the psychosocial experience of divorce can be particularly painful for men, acting as an acute stressor with chronic consequences. This could be related to a number of related factors. First, data indicates that around 70% of divorces are initiated by the wife, meaning that divorce can be the kind of shocking and unwanted life event for the husband that has been identified as a risk factor for adverse mental health (Affleck, Carmichael, & Whitley, 2018a). This means the husband must often scramble to mobilize his psychological, social, and financial resources to deal with this sudden and unplanned biographical disruption. Many men, particularly low-income men lacking a high-school education (see Chap. 7), may lack these resources, which can lead to emotional upheaval, financial strain, and psychological distress (McManus & DiPrete, 2001; Rotermann, 2007). Indeed, an overview paper notes that psychological distress tends to be lower in the spouse who initiated the divorce (Amato, 2000). This can help explain the increased risk of adverse mental health in divorced men compared with divorced women.

Second, women are more likely to maintain larger friendship and extended family networks when married, whereas men tend to rely on their partner (and her networks) for social support (Alexander, 2001; Kalmijn, 2003). This means that men tend to experience a more intense decrease in social support after a divorce, as there can be a significant drop in social interaction with: (i) their spouse; (ii) her family and friends; (iii) neighbours, especially if the man has to relocate; (iv) other parents, as custody tends to go to the mother, thus diminishing "school gate" type interactions; and (v) mutual friends, who may stigmatize and stereotype a newly separated and single older male (see Chap. 1).

Indeed, the aforementioned Rotermann (2007) study found that men reported a 19% drop in social support after a divorce, while women reported an 11% drop, meaning that men experience almost double the social support deficits after divorce compared with women. This lack of a social safety net can leave divorced and separated men lonely and isolated precisely when they need social support the most (Houle et al., 2008; Rotermann, 2007; Wyllie et al., 2012). This loss can also reduce exposure to family and friends who helpfully monitor and promote men's health-related behaviors such as physical exercise, alcohol use, diet, and other variables. Of note, social support has consistently been associated with good mental health, while lack of social support has been associated with poor mental health (Kawachi & Berkman, 2001; Whitley & McKenzie, 2005). This drop in social support helps further explain worse mental health in divorced men compared with divorced women.

Third, fathers are typically separated from their children after a divorce, with over 80% of custodial parents in the United States and Canada being mothers (Department of Justice Canada, 2000; Grall, 2016). In fact, the aforementioned Rotermann (2007) study found that 34% of divorced men experienced a loss of children from their household following a divorce, compared with only 3% of divorced women, while only 16% of divorced men remained with any children, compared with 56% of women. This was also the conclusion of a seminal literature review, noting that "divorce may be particularly devastating for men because they are mainly the ones who lose their home, children and family" (Payne et al., 2008, p. 30). This separation from children can be particularly painful for the affected men, leading to a massive void and sense of loss, which can breed shame, guilt, grief, a sense of failure, and psychological distress (Bartlett, 2004; Blakeslee & Wallerstein, 2004; Stack, 2000). This experience can be a living bereavement for the men involved and a cause of much mental despair.

Fourth, evidence suggests that men tend to report a negative and highly stressful experience within the family court system, with a common perception that these courts marginalize father involvement in child rearing responsibilities, failing to recognize the value of father–child relationships (Barry & Liddon, 2020; Felix et al., 2013). This experience can lead men to experience a loss of faith in society as a whole, especially when such courts fail to ensure that father and children spend significant amounts of time together and instead demand weighty payments to the mother, which can lead to a serious decline in living standards (McManus & DiPrete, 2001; Shiner et al., 2009). Indeed, Struszczyk et al. (2017) note that separation from children has been cited as a primary cause of male suicide in many coroner's inquests, while Kposowa (2003, p. 993) states that "in the end, the father loses not only his marriage but his children…it may well be that the observed association between divorce and suicide in men is the impact of post-divorce (court sanctioned) arrangements." As stated, this can be particularly painful for these typically middle-aged men.

Fifth, feelings of shame and stigma often accompany divorce, which may be especially intense in religious or more traditional jurisdictions or subcultures. In the process of divorce, many men will not only lose their home, savings, and children but also their reputation as a "family man" and competent breadwinner. As stated in the Chap. 8, this status of a "failed breadwinner" can be particularly damaging to men with a family, and divorced or separated men may now have financial responsibility for two households: their own and that of their ex-spouse. This burden may place intolerable limits on a man's financial and psychosocial resources.

In sum, separation and divorce precipitate a chain of events that can lead to short-term and long-term financial, legal, and psychosocial issues that can be damaging to mental health (Sbarra et al., 2019). As noted earlier, these may be particularly severe for men, especially those with children.

9.1.5 The Psychosocial Stress of Single Unmarried Men

The research evidence indubitably shows that divorced and separated men have the highest risk out of all subcategories of "unmarried men." However, the research evidence also shows that single never-married men also tend to have slightly (but significantly) worse mental health than married men. Such a finding can be partially attributed to the protective nature of marriage, inasmuch as marriage tends to provide: (i) emotional support and social integration; (ii) economic stability and greater financial resources; and (iii) a sense of meaning and purpose (Lodge & Umberson, 2014; Umberson et al., 2013). Moreover, married partners typically monitor and moderate each other's mental health-related behaviors including reducing risky behaviors such as substance misuse, while encouraging helpful behaviors such as exercise (Felix et al., 2013).

Never-married single men may not have experienced the pain of divorce and separation but will lack the above-described protective benefits of marriage. This may be particularly intense for young single men, with recent research indicating high rates of loneliness in this demographic. In fact, a recent global survey of over 43,000 participants from 237 jurisdictions found that young men had the highest rates of loneliness out of all demographics surveyed (Barreto et al., 2021). This finding is consistent with single-jurisdiction surveys, with a recent US survey of over 1000 adults finding that one in three young men said they always or often felt lonely and more than a quarter said they had no close friends, which were higher than rates in women (YouGov, 2019). Similarly, a Canadian survey found that 63% of 18- to 34-year-old Canadian men experienced considerable loneliness and isolation, compared with 53% of similarly aged women (Angus Reid Institute (ARI), 2020). Of note, loneliness is a proven risk factor for a range of mental health issues such as suicide, depression, and substance misuse (Alpass & Neville, 2003; Beutel et al., 2017; Wang et al., 2018).

Importantly, this loneliness and isolation does not occur in a social vacuum, with some evidence indicating that single people may face harmful stigmas and stereotypes when trying to integrate into society: a phenomenon known as *singlism* (Morris et al., 2008). This may be particularly prominent for single men, who may experience the male villain/perpetrator stereotype discussed in Chap. 1. Such stereotypes are embodied in archetypal fictional characters such as Svengali, Don Juan, and Lothario, depicting single men as an untamed and corruptive threat to the social order of civilized society (Byrne & Carr, 2005; DePaulo, 2007).

Importantly, these stereotypes can manifest themselves in social policies and procedures, which exclude and demonize single men. One of the most egregious and well-documented examples of this phenomena is a common airline policy that prohibits solo male passengers from sitting next to an unaccompanied minor, with such men being asked to swap seats with a female passenger, due to fears of pedophilia. While very few men experience the humiliation of being asked to swap airline seats, this sexist policy is indicative of the wider societal suspicion targeted at single men. Even the British Prime Minister Boris Johnson has acknowledged the harm of such stereotyping, after being asked to move seats himself in 2006 (Johnson, 2006).

Other examples of such stereotyping were discussed in Chap. 7, noting that some educational institutions sometimes frame all single young men as potential brutes and rapists, thus unfairly tarring all men with the same brush (Whitley, 2020). These stereotypes may also contribute to judicial decisions in family court, which typically disfavour single fathers, who only gain custody in around 20% of cases. This could be related to the negative stereotypes discussed in detail in Chap. 1, which feed suspicion about the intentions and capabilities of single men, which in turn fuel enduring (and sexist) stigmas that single fathers are ill-suited to raise children.

It is difficult to quantify the combined effect of all these stigmas and stereotypes targeted at single men, and this has not been a focus of research. But the general literature indicates that stigma can act to deter involvement in community organizations such as churches, sports clubs, and other institutions of civil society. Single men in particular may be aware that others will frame them in unflattering terms and have concerns about motive and perceived threat. All this can combine to exacerbate loneliness and social exclusion, which can worsen mental health.

9.1.6 A Unifying Theory? Durkheim and Social Integration

Taken in the round, the evidence suggests that unmarried men are at greater risk of psychological distress compared with married men, with divorced and separated men experiencing the highest risk. An underlying factor explaining these elevated rates may be a common experience of *social alienation* in these men, characterized by a diminished sense of meaning and purpose in life, which in turn can weaken primary "reasons for living" (Kleiman & Beaver, 2013; Rodgers, 2011; Stack, 2000). Research on this topic has tended to center upon the sociological concept of *social integration*, or lack thereof.

Importantly, the nuclear family still remains one of the primary venues for the social integration of adult men across the world. As such, disintegration of a nuclear family can have a particularly pernicious effect on men's mental health. Indeed, the key conclusion of Durkheim's famous tome *Suicide: A Study in Sociology* was that social integration was the core underlying factor explaining differential patterns of suicide in nineteenth century Europe. Durkheim noted that groups such as unmarried men and childless women had higher rates of suicide, which were imputed to lack of social integration. Similarly, he noted that Roman Catholics and Jews had lower suicide rates than Protestants, arguing that this was due to Protestantism being a more individualistic and less socially cohesive worldview than Catholicism or Judaism (Durkheim, 1897). This led him to coin terms such as: (i) *egoistic suicide*, referring to suicides by people lacking meaningful social connections and social integration, and (ii) *anomic suicide*, referring to suicides by people discombobulated by dramatic social, economic, or political upheaval.

These conceptualizations have been used by many contemporary researchers. For example, the theory of egoistic suicide has been used to explain higher rates of suicide in divorced men (Rossow, 1993). Central to these Durkheimian understandings of suicide is the role of meaning and purpose. For example, considerable research indicates that men tend to draw a significant amount of existential meaning from their protector and provider family breadwinner roles, as discussed in more detail in Chap. 8 (Alston, 2012; Dyke & Murphy, 2006; Oliffe et al., 2011). This can be a powerful source of pride and purpose, and failure to fulfil these roles can leave men shamed and stigmatized in the eyes of themselves, their family, and wider society, which can negatively affect social, familial, and intrapsychic integration (Affleck, Thamotharampillai, et al., 2018b). This failure can be worsened by a decline in social support from others outside the family upon separation or divorce, which may both signify and deepen social disintegration, which in turn can increase risk of suicide for men.

Similarly, some never-married men may feel socially estranged due to the above-described stigmas and stereotypes associated with single men. Others may consider their single status a failure, especially if they aspire to be part of a nuclear family with a wife and children. This can be especially so in subcultures or communities where marriage and childbearing are the norm in certain age brackets, thereby making single men statistically "abnormal." All this can exacerbate the aforementioned stigma and stereotypes and worsen mental health in these demographics.

9.1.7 The Big Picture: A Worsening Situation?

The aforementioned literature indicates that divorce and separation can damage the mental health of men and women but may be especially injurious to men's mental health. Similarly, this literature indicates that single never-married men tend to experience a modestly increased risk of adverse mental health outcomes compared with married men. These findings beg several questions regarding wider social context. Is the divorce rate increasing? Are marriage rates decreasing? What about the percentage of people living alone? In other words, how common are the risk and protective factors identified above and are they becoming more or less prevalent over time? This requires an analysis of social and demographic trends, which are summarized next.

In sum, a large corpus of research from western jurisdictions examining trends over the last decades indicates: (i) a decline in marriage rates; (ii) an increasing rate of divorce; (iii) an increase in single-person households; (iv) a decline in fertility rates; and (v) later mean age of first marriage and first parity. This is a significant shift from the recent past, which was characterized by nuptial longevity, low rates of divorce, and a lower mean age at marriage and first parity. This shift has been labeled *the second demographic transition* and has been related to various factors including new legislation such as no-fault divorce laws, scientific advances such as the birth control pill, greater women's empowerment, increasing individualization, and other factors related to the ongoing sexual and cultural revolution that began in the 1960s (Lesthaeghe, 1995; Putnam, 2000; van de Kaa, 1987).

In terms of marriage, Organisation for Economic Co-operation and Development (OECD) figures indicate that marriage rates have declined by around 25%–50% between 1970 and 2017 in major OECD countries including the United Kingdom, the United States, and Australia (OECD, 2019a). In Canada, figures indicate that the married population are now the minority of adults, with 46% of the adult population legally married, while 54% were unmarried in 2011 (Milan, 2013). This represents a reverse in proportions from 1981, when 61% of the adult population were married, while 39% were unmarried. Similarly, statistics from the United States indicate that only 49% of adults are living with a spouse in legal marriage (United States Census Bureau, 2019a), while 12% of adults are divorced or separated, and 32% are never married. In other words, there are currently more unmarried adults in Canada than married adults, while in the United States, there are equal numbers of unmarried adults and married adults. This does not mean that 50% of the adult population are single, as adults can be in romantic relationships without being married. Indeed, recent figures from the Pew Research Center indicate that 69% of US adults are partnered in some way, meaning that 31% of US adults are currently single (Brown, 2020). But that still leaves a large proportion of the population leading a more solitary single lifestyle.

Interestingly, the mean age at first marriage has increased, with the OECD average now 32 years for men and 30 years for women, whereas figures from the early 1990s indicate an average of 27 years for men and 25 years for women (OECD, 2019b). Similarly, the average age at parity has also increased across the western world, with UK figures indicating the average age for mothers is 31, while for fathers, it is 34 (Littleboy, 2019). Instead of getting married and having children in their 20s, some research indicates that many young people are embracing "hook-up culture" (facilitated by the widespread use of internet dating apps) or serial monogamy (McAnulty, 2012; Owen et al., 2010). This can mean a merry-go-round of sexual partners, without the ongoing support of a reliable and committed individual. Taken together, these figures indicate that a substantial proportion of adults are choosing not to get married, while those who do tend to get married are doing so later in life, thus having children later in life. These trends are projected to continue, with a recent Pew report estimating that 25% of young adults in the United States will never marry (Wang & Parker, 2014). This may contribute to the observed high rate of loneliness in young people discussed earlier in this chapter.

In terms of divorce, evidence suggests that rates have been rising over the last few decades across the western world, though in recent years they have stabilized and may even be slightly declining in some countries. For example, data from the United Kingdom indicates that only 19% of marriages ended in divorce in the early 1960s, but by the mid-1990s, this had doubled to 38% (Ghosh, 2019). Similar figures are seen in the United States, where the divorce rate doubled from 1950–1990, with data indicating that 48% of US marriages in the 1970s ended in divorce (Stevenson & Wolfers, 2007). However, recent figures show a slight fall in divorce rates for those married in the 2000s, with the exception of couples 50 years of age and over, where the divorce rate has more than doubled (Brown & Lin, 2012). This phenomenon is known as *gray divorce* and is an emerging area of research interest. In Canada, the divorce rate has stably hovered around 35%–40% in recent years, but there has also been an increase in gray divorces (Margolis et al., 2019; Milan, 2013). In sum, divorce is still a frequent event affecting large numbers of people in the population, despite a slight decline in rates in recent years.

In terms of household composition, there has been a precipitous increase in the number of people living alone in recent years. For example, the US Census notes that 28% of households are currently single-person households, over double the figure of 13% from 1960 (United States Census Bureau, 2019b). These figures overlap with other western countries: in the United Kingdom, the Office for National Statistics (ONS) reports that the number of people living alone has increased by 20% in the last two decades from 6.8 million in 1999 to 8.2 million in 2019, with single-person households now making up 30% of all households (Sanders, 2019). This increase is driven mainly by middle-aged and older men living alone, including bachelors choosing not to marry, empty nest men experiencing a "grey divorce," and divorced/separated fathers whose children are living with the mother (Sanders, 2019).

9.1.8   Implications of Trends for Mental Health

What do all these trends mean for men's mental health? One interpretation of these trends is that they signify the positive evolution of society, bringing mental health benefits to men and women alike. For example, modern western societies are no longer defined by traditional cultural, familial, and religious worldviews (Giddens, 1991). This brings commendable freedoms, opportunities, and choices to people whose lives may have been otherwise restricted in times past, such as the freedom not to marry, the opportunity to divorce, and the choice to remain childless (Bauman, 2003; Beck & Beck-Gernsheim, 1995). Indeed, humanistic psychologists such as Rogers (1961) and Gergen (1991) argue that this culture of choice allows humans the scope to develop an authentic and autonomous self, unfettered by the manacles of convention and tradition. This development of the self is realized through the creation of an individualized and tailored lifestyle commensurate with personal goals, individual growth, and internal desires, objectives that may have been unattainable or advanced with difficulty in more traditional times of restricted choice.

In fact, it is worth stating that divorce or separation can mean release from a damaging environment, and for some men and women, this is a better choice for their long-term mental health than staying in a toxic relationship (Blakeslee & Wallerstein, 2004; Giddens, 1992). Similarly, the fact that more men are choosing to remain unmarried (and childless) means that fewer men in the future will get divorced. In turn, this means fewer men will be exposed to some of the harmful aspects of divorce (described earlier in this chapter) including separation from children, negative interactions with family court, and weighty financial responsibilities. Moreover, the increasing number of people living alone could be a manifestation of growing desires to live an autonomous lifestyle free of familial responsibilities rather than a symptom of an alleged "epidemic of loneliness."

Indeed, a loose and informal movement of men known as Men Going Their Own Way (MGTOW) has arisen in recent years, comprising of men who are consciously choosing an unmarried lifestyle free of familial responsibilities, feeling that this is better for their overall well-being and quality of life. MGTOW is not a social movement in the conventional sense, but more a philosophy of living, welded together by websites, writings, and local meetups (Smith, 2013). In her popular book on the topic, author Helen Smith aptly sums up the MGTOW phenomena as "men on strike." In a similar vein, Whitley & Zhou (2020) note an increase in the number of men involved in the "seduction community" (sometimes known as "pick-up artists"), who typically eschew committed relationships in favour of a promiscuous libertine lifestyle. In sum, the aforementioned trends in marriage, divorce, and single-person households may denote an increase in societal opportunities and freedom, which could be considered a positive social good in secular democracies that prize individual liberty.

That said, the research literature discussed in this chapter clearly indicates that (a happy) marriage is protective to the mental health of men. Moreover, divorce and separation are significant risk factors for a range of adverse mental health outcomes including suicide, substance abuse, and depression, with never-married single men also at increased risk of these adverse outcomes. This is contributing to an increasing number of single-occupancy households, which is concentrated among middle-aged and older men. In absolute numbers, a substantial proportion of men are experiencing risk factors such as divorce, and an increasing number of men are shunning protective factors such as marriage. All this can interact, leading to decreased social support and increased loneliness among the growing ranks of unmarried men. Ultimately, this could be considered a public health issue of serious concern. To be sure, these trends are beneficial to the many individual men and women who desire a solitary life or prefer to live a libertine lifestyle. But at a wider population level, these trends may further worsen men's mental health. Furthermore, these trends may have a particularly negative effect on a subpopulation that has hitherto been ignored in this chapter: children, particularly boys.

9.2 The Effects of Divorce and Father Absence on Offspring Mental Health

A large corpus of research indicates that parental divorce and separation are an adverse childhood experience that can have harmful effects on the short- and long-term mental health of children, particularly boys. Moreover, this research suggests that growing up in a single-mother household can be especially harmful for mental health and is associated with a range of other deleterious outcomes including educational underachievement, criminal activity, and substance abuse (McLanahan et al., 2013; Sbarra et al., 2019). In contrast, children living with both biological parents (especially married couples) or in single-father households tend to fare far better, even after adjustment for socioeconomic status (Krueger et al., 2015; Harper & McLanahan, 2004).

In sum, this literature indicates that the experience of parental divorce and separation has acute and chronic mental health sequela for children, and that father absence following a divorce or separation is an important risk factor for a range of mental health issues. Of note, the literature shows that father absence due to death of the father or weighty work commitments has a much more neutral effect on

Table 9.1 Negative outcomes related to father absence

Comparison of outcomes between youth from fatherless households and other families
Sixty-three percent of youth suicides are from fatherless homes.
Ninety percent of all homeless and runaway youths are from fatherless homes.
Eighty-five percent of children who exhibit behavioral disorders are from fatherless homes.
Seventy-one percent of high school dropouts are from fatherless homes.
Seventy percent of youths in state institutions are from fatherless homes.
Seventy-five percent of adolescent patients in substance abuse centers are from fatherless homes.
Eighty-five percent of rapists motivated by displaced anger are from fatherless homes.

Source: US Dept of Justice (1998)

mental health, with children more resilient to this form of absence (East et al., 2006; Spruijt et al., 2001). As such, the rest of this section focuses on father absence due to separation or divorce, driven by a definition that "father absence is defined as existing where the father is not resident in the family home because of parental turmoil, parental relationship instability or breakdown of the parental relationship" (East et al., 2006). The psychosocial impact of father absence has been summarized in an oft-cited US Department of Justice (1998) report, with core statistics regarding mental health and deviant behavior given in Table 9.1.

These oft-cited figures paint a bleak picture about the mental health and well-being of children growing up in fatherless homes. However, this report was published at the end of the 1990s, and the methodology behind the production of the statistics is unclear, meaning that these oft-cited statistics are somewhat out of date and the results should be treated with caution.

Fortunately, several literature reviews have been published in the last decade in an attempt to synthesize more recent evidence regarding the effects of divorce, separation, and father absence on children. The most comprehensive review was published by McLanahan et al. (2013) entitled *The Causal Effects of Father Absence*, which assessed 47 articles with a focus on high-quality longitudinal studies. Similar to the aforementioned US Department of Justice (1998) report, this review revealed that children and adolescents experiencing parental divorce and father absence had higher rates of: (i) delinquency; (ii) externalizing behaviours (e.g., aggression); (iii) drug and alcohol abuse; and (iv) early sexual activity, when compared with children of married parents.

This review also investigated educational outcomes, finding that children experiencing father absence were significantly less likely to graduate high school and had fewer years of schooling compared with children living with two biological parents. Importantly, some studies included in this review indicate that boys were more negatively affected by father absence than girls. This finding overlaps with a synthesis of evidence reported in a more recent review, indicating that boys raised in single-mother households faced more difficulties than girls raised in single-mother households, including higher rates of truancy, behavioural problems, adult unemployment, and social immobility (Golding & Fitzgerald, 2019).

Importantly, the McLanahan et al. (2013) review notes that the experience of parental divorce and father absence in childhood or adolescence has long-term effects across the lifespan, finding that adult children with such experience had: (i) higher rates of unemployment; (ii) lower rates of marriage (in male offspring but not female offspring); (iii) poorer mental health in adulthood; and (iv) increased risk of early sexual activity, all in comparison with adult children raised by their two biological parents. This finding of poorer mental health among adult offspring is consistent with two recent meta-analyses examining the long-term effect of parental divorce on mental health. Autersperg et al. (2019) examined 54 studies with over half a million participants, finding a significant association between parental divorce and offspring adult depression (OR = 1.61, 95% CI: 1.46–1.76), suicide attempts (OR = 1.94, 95% CI: 1.60–2.27), alcohol abuse (OR = 1.66, 95% CI: 1.40–1.92), drug abuse (OR = 1.65, 95% CI: 1.34–1.97), and psychological distress (OR = 1.78, 95% CI: 0.94–2.63). These findings converge with another recent meta-analysis of 18 studies focusing on affective disorders (Sands et al., 2017), which also found a significant association between parental divorce and offspring adult depression (OR = 1.56, 95% CI: 1.31–1.86).

Similarly, another large-scale US study reported a dose-response relationship between father absence and adverse psychosocial outcomes, finding that youth with longer periods of father absence (e.g., from infancy) had significantly increased rates of alcohol use, drug use, smoking, sexual activity, and criminal conviction compared with those with shorter periods of father absence (e.g., from mid-adolescence) (Antecol & Bedard, 2007). In other words, a longer exposure to fathers decreases the risk of deviant behaviors, while a shorter exposure increases the risk. These findings contradict a common narrative that the presence of masculinity is harmful to the mental health of children and adolescents, instead implying that *lack of masculinity* is harmful and that masculinity in the form of a present father is associated with positive mental health.

9.2.1 Single-Father Households

A growing number of studies are examining the psychosocial status of children growing up in single-father motherless households, finding that these children typically have better outcomes than children in single-mother fatherless households. For example, Harper and McLanahan (2004) examined rates of adult incarceration using data from the US National Longitudinal Survey of Youth. This study found that the odds ratio of incarceration for adults who grew up in single-mother households was 3.03, while for adults who grew up in single-father households was 1.27 (both ratios in comparison with intact mother-father families and confidence intervals were not presented). Interestingly, this study also found a threefold risk of incarceration for children living with one biological parent and a stepfather or stepmother, indicating that there is a unique bond between biological parents and children that cannot be sufficiently replaced by stepfathers and stepmothers.

These findings overlap with a subanalysis in the same study, which found that self-reported serious delinquency was significantly higher in children raised by single mothers (OR = 1.4), or raised by a mother–stepfather couple (OR = 1.8), in comparison with children raised by an intact mother–father dyad. Importantly, children raised by single fathers or by father–stepmother dyads did not have a significantly increased risk of serious delinquency compared with children raised by an intact mother–father dyad. The results regarding stepparents are unsurprising, as research indicates that family violence, child abuse, and other negative outcomes are more common in stepparent families (Daly & Wilson, 1985; van IJzendoorn et al., 2009). This can contribute to poor mental health among affected children and youth, particularly boys (Affleck, Carmichael, & Whitley, 2018a).

Similarly, another US study compared a range of psychosocial outcomes according to family structure, finding that children in single-mother families had the worst outcomes, while children in single-father families had the best outcomes, even exceeding children from married couples (Krueger et al., 2015). For example, this study measured seven health outcomes such as headaches, infections, and colds finding that children in single-mother households had higher odds of all seven – compared with children of married couples – while children from single-father households had lower or similar odds to children of married couples. Moreover, this study found children in single-father households were less likely to miss school days (OR = 0.96, 95% CI: 0.87–1.05) compared with children of married couples, while children in single-mother households were significantly more likely to miss school days (OR = 1.48, 95% CI: 1.40–1.57). Relatedly, the results indicated that children from single-mother households were at greatest risk of attention deficit hyperactivity disorder (ADHD) diagnosis (OR = 1.74, 95% CI: 1.63–1.85) compared with children from married couple households, while children from single-father households had an odds ratio of 1.31 (95% CI: 1.15–1.51) compared with children from married couple households. This overlaps with the wider findings on marital status and offspring ADHD discussed in Chap. 5. Taken in the round, all these results overlap with other research noting that children in single-father families tend to have equivalent health to children of intact mother–father families (Coles, 2015; Victorino & Gauthier, 2009).

9.2.2 *Plausible Mechanisms and Pathways to Mental Health*

Much of the previously described literature summarizing the negative impact of divorce on adult men is also applicable to children and adolescents. For example, the experience of divorce can be an unexpected shock for the affected children, causing considerable loss, rupture, and emotional upheaval. For older children, it can create biographical disruption, again contributing to adverse outcomes. In other words, loss of a parent from divorce and separation should be considered a severe life event, in the same manner that loss of spouse is treated as a serious experience.

Moreover, this event can have long-term consequences, particularly related to father absence.

In summarizing the research on father absence, East et al. (2006) accurately state that "the literature fails to articulate clearly the importance of father love, why and how fathers influence their children during childhood development and are essential in psychological health, and why the absence of fathers can cause possible adverse behavioral disturbances." This remains true today, with the mechanisms and pathways explaining the negative impact of father absence still under-researched and under-explored in the scientific literature.

That said, several plausible mechanisms have been suggested to explain the association between divorce, father absence, and mental health. To start, several scholars have noted that the father–child relationship is a unique attachment providing a mixture of love, mentorship, and discipline in equal measure (e.g., East et al., 2006; Farrell & Gray, 2018). Indeed, fathers typically set boundaries and enforce discipline with their children, while offering guidance and support in the transitions from infant to child to adolescent to adult. Sometimes, this involves a form of "tough love" that may be less readily proffered by mothers but offers important life lessons about self-control, personal responsibility, and social awareness. This may be particularly important to growing boys, whose rambunctious energy is often channeled by fathers into positive pro-social outlets such as outdoor activities, sports, competitive games, "rough and tumble" pursuits, and other hobbies that expand physical and intellectual energy. All this can help socialize young boys to be positive members of society, providing pro-social activities for risk, competition, courage, and achievement (Hoff-Sommers, 2015). Such activities may be lacking in single-mother households, with one British study indicating that low father involvement was a significant risk factor for low levels of life satisfaction among teen boys, while high levels of father involvement were associated with higher levels of life satisfaction and also helped protect teenage boys from victimization (Flouri & Buchanan, 2002). This situation led to the coining of a poignant phrase "father hunger," a phrase that encapsulates the void and yearning experienced by children who lack father involvement, supervision, and guidance (Maine, 2004; McGee, 1993; Wilson, 2012).

Indeed, Bowlby (1969) indicated that a strong attachment to both biological parents (including the father) is the foundation of positive mental health, with subsequent research indicating that insecure attachment is associated with negative mental health outcomes such as depression (e.g., Fuhr et al., 2017). As such, the absence of a father can create an existential and psychological void, which may contribute to a cascade of negative events that negatively affect mental health. For example, children lacking fatherly supervision, discipline, or involvement may expand their energy in a dysfunctional manner including externalizing behaviour and delinquency. When this manifests in the school setting, it can lead to punishment and low educational achievement (see Chap. 7). When it manifests in the societal setting, it can lead to criminal justice issues and involvement in delinquent peer groups based on drug and alcohol use. All this can make it difficult to find a job and establish a normal life in the transition to adulthood, which can contribute to higher rates of youth unemployment in children from fatherless families. Hence, the void experienced by a child from a fatherless family can expand with the progression of life; as such individuals are more likely to lack education, work, and involvement in positive pro-social communities. This creates a wider vacuum of meaning and purpose, which can contribute to poor mental health among individuals raised in fatherless families.

This void can also leave young adults scrambling around for alternative mentors, role models, and communities, with some research indicating that these are often found in delinquent peer groups or in other unsavoury communities. For example, one research study showed high rates of father absence among young male "pick-up artists" involved in the "seduction community," with participants commonly stating that they joined this community to find mentors and guides to help them learn social and communication skills they felt were typically imparted by fathers (Whitley & Zhou, 2020). Similarly, the aforementioned Harper and McLanahan (2004) study found that males from fatherless families were three times as likely to be incarcerated than children living with both biological parents, often due to involvement in criminal gangs and delinquent peer groups. Indeed, evidence suggests children from fatherless families are more exposed to negative peer influences and involvement in antisocial peer groups, often revolving around drug and alcohol use (East et al., 2006; Golding & Fitzgerald, 2019).

To close this section, it is worth recapping information presented in detail in Chap. 5 on ADHD, namely, that boys are three times more likely than girls to be diagnosed with ADHD, with a doubling of rates amongst school-aged boys in the last decades, parallel to the increasing rate of divorce and separation. Indeed, increasing numbers of young boys are being medicated with stimulant-based drugs such as Ritalin, with use higher among boys from fatherless families. These high rates of diagnosis and prescription may be directly related to the above-described changes in family structure, with medication being used as a form of social control to dampen boys' natural energy and exuberance in the absence of strong and involved fathers who typically provide discipline and guidance in an intact family unit.

9.2.3 The Big Picture: Trends and Social Context

So far, this chapter has established that divorce and separation is a risk factor for adverse mental health among adult fathers and affected children. Importantly, children raised in single-mother households may be at particular risk, while being raised in a single-father household may confer some protection. This raises the question: what proportions of children are experiencing divorce, separation, father-absence, and other related variables?

Worryingly, evidence suggests that there has been a massive increase in the share of children who were born outside of marriage in recent decades. For example, recent figures from the United Kingdom, the United States, and New Zealand indicate that 40% or more of children are born to unmarried mothers, compared with around 5% in 1960 (OECD, 2020a). Some of these children are born to mothers in cohabiting or romantic relationships with the father, while others are born to uncoupled single mothers. Children born to these uncoupled single mothers can be combined with the children of divorced, separated, and widowed parents to create the category of "single parent household," consisting of one biological parent living with offspring.

Recent figures indicate that the proportion of children growing up in a single parent household has risen dramatically in recent years to around one in five children in western countries: 22% in the United Kingdom, 27% in the United States, and 19% in Canada (OECD, 2020b). Of note, single parent households in western countries are typically single mother households. For example, one Canadian study assessed the primary residence of children after separation and divorce, finding that 70% lived primarily with their mother, 15% primarily with their father, while 9% reported equal living time between the two parents (Sinha, 2014). More recent Canadian data indicate that 81% of children in single parent families lived primarily with their mother, while 19% lived primarily with their father (Statistics Canada, 2017). Similarly, US data shows that 83% of single parent households are headed by the mother (United States Census Bureau, 2016). This gender differential is caused by a variety of factors, but data indicates that family courts dealing with divorce and separation typically award custody to mothers compared with fathers. For examples, Canadian statistics indicate that 79% of court-ordered custody arrangements lead to exclusive custody for the mother and only 7% for the father (Marcil-Gratton & Le Bourdais, 1999). In Australia, the Survey of Separated Parents revealed that the mother has sole or majority responsibility in 83% of cases, while the father has sole or majority responsibility in only 7% of cases, with 9% of cases having equal responsibility (Kaspiew, Carson, Dunstan, et al., 2015a). This survey also found that 45% of court-ordered custody arrangements lead to sole custody for the mother and only 7% for the father, with the remainder having shared time (Kaspiew, Carson, Qu, et al., 2015b).

This has led many to question the wisdom of family law and family courts, which often act to separate children from their fathers, despite the growing evidence that children in single-father households typically fare better than children in single-mother households. Importantly, existing family law and related family court decisions do not appear to be driven by the aforementioned scientific evidence; they instead appear to be propelled by long-standing (and sexist) stereotypes regarding appropriate gender roles, with fathers typically seen as unidimensional providers and breadwinners and mothers typically seen as unidimensional nurturers best suited to the primary caregiving role (East et al., 2006; Rohner & Veneziano, 2001). This mismatch between the scientific evidence and dominant practice has led to calls to reform family law to ensure that boys spend the necessary time with their fathers, for example, by implementing a model known as *shared parenting*, which means children spend approximately 50/50 time with each parent (Deutsch, 2001; Nielsen, 2011). There is a lack of research on this model, but equal exposure to both parents may theoretically boost the mental health of offspring, given the above-described evidence, meaning that "shared parenting" might be a public health intervention with positive mental health consequences for adults and children alike (Kline Pruett & DiFonzo, 2014). More research on this topic is necessary.

9.3 Conclusion

This chapter indicates that unmarried men tend to have worse mental health than married men. Men who are never married have slightly elevated rates of mental health issues compared with married men, but men who are separated or divorced have the highest risk of adverse mental health outcomes compared with married men. Similarly, separation and divorce are severe life events for affected children (particularly boys) that can harm their short- and long-term mental health. Boys raised in fatherless families are at particular risk of adverse psychosocial outcomes, indicating that the absence of masculine influence is harmful to mental health, which is contrary to a common narrative that the presence of masculine influence is harmful to mental health. Worryingly, trends indicate that a substantial and growing number of people are divorcing, separating, or living alone, as well as an increase in single-mother fatherless families.

Of note, unmarried and divorced men are an ignored demographic, and there are few specific services and supports devoted to their well-being. Worse still, they can be stigmatized and demonized in certain sectors of society, which can leave many unmarried and divorced men questioning any notion of an inclusive society. This can have a harmful impact on mental health.

This situation requires concerted action. First, any policies or practices reliant on stereotypes of unmarried men should be dismantled and replaced by nondiscriminatory procedures, with all sectors of society reflecting on their activities to ensure they are truly inclusive and engaging to unmarried men. Second, as mentioned in the Chap. 6, there is a lack of specific support services to help vulnerable single men (young and old alike), especially men undergoing a painful divorce or separation. There is a need to develop, implement, and evaluate interventions, which can help men make this difficult transition. Third, family courts still appear to be driven by gender stereotypes rather than scientific data, and family law reform that accounts for the nefarious consequences of growing up in a fatherless family may positively impact the mental health of both adults and children alike. Fourth, the vacuum being experienced by boys raised in fatherless families is often filled by involvement in delinquent peer networks or by the use of drugs and alcohol. There could be a renewed role for civil society organizations such as churches, trade unions, military cadet formations, and the like in providing mentorship, guidance, and role models for these boys. Fifth, more efforts could be made to support families undergoing issues, such as access to effective forms of marriage counseling and better provision of contraceptives to prevent unplanned pregnancies and unwanted children. All this may help mitigate the nefarious impact of divorce and separation on adults and children alike.

References

Affleck, W., Carmichael, V., & Whitley, R. (2018a). Men's mental health: Social determinants and implications for services. *The Canadian Journal of Psychiatry, 63*(9), 581–589. https://doi.org/10.1177/0706743718762388

Affleck, W., Thamotharampillai, U., Jeyakumar, J., & Whitley, R. (2018b). "If one does not fulfil his duties, he must not be a man": Masculinity, mental health and resilience amongst Sri Lankan Tamil refugee men in Canada. *Culture, Medicine, and Psychiatry, 42*(4), 840–861. https://doi.org/10.1007/s11013-018-9592-9

Alexander, J. (2001). Depressed men: An exploratory study of close relationships. *Journal of Psychiatric and Mental Health Nursing, 8*(1), 67–75. https://doi.org/10.1046/j.1365-2850.2001.00354.x

Alpass, F. M., & Neville, S. J. (2003). Loneliness, health and depression in older males. *Aging and Mental Health, 7*(3), 212–216. https://doi.org/10.1080/1360786031000101193

Alston, M. (2012). Rural male suicide in Australia. *Social Science & Medicine, 74*(4), 515–522. https://doi.org/10.1016/j.socscimed.2010.04.036

Amato, P. R. (2000). The consequences of divorce for adults and children. *Journal of Marriage and the Family, 62*(4), 1269–1287. https://doi.org/10.1111/j.1741-3737.2000.01269.x

Angus Reid Institute (ARI). (2020, October 14). Isolation, loneliness, and COVID-19: Pandemic leads to sharp increase in mental health challenges, social woes. *Angus Reid Institute*. Retrieved April 16, 2021, from https://angusreid.org/isolation-and-loneliness-covid19/.

Antecol, H., & Bedard, K. (2007). Does single parenthood increase the probability of teenage promiscuity, substance use, and crime? *Journal of Population Economics, 20*(1), 55–71.

Autersperg, F., Vlasak, T., Ponocny, I., & Barth, A. (2019). Long-term effects of parental divorce on mental health – A meta-analysis. *Journal of Psychiatric Research, 119*, 107–115. https://doi.org/10.1016/j.jpsychires.2019.09.011

Barreto, M., Victor, C., Hammond, C., Eccles, A., Richins, M. T., & Qualter, P. (2021). Loneliness around the world: Age, gender, and cultural differences in loneliness. *Personality and Individual Differences, 169*(3), 110066. https://doi.org/10.1016/j.paid.2020.110066

Barry, J., & Liddon, L. (2020). Child contact problems and family court issues are related to chronic mental health problems for men following family breakdown. *Psychreg Journal of Psychology, 4*(3). https://doi.org/10.5281/zenodo.4302120

Bartlett, E. E. (2004). The effects of fatherhood on the health of men: A review of the literature. *The Journal of Men's Health and Gender, 1*(2), 159–169. https://doi.org/10.1016/j.jmhg.2004.06.004

Bauman, Z. (2003). *Liquid love: On the frailty of human bonds*. Polity Press.

Beck, U., & Beck-Gernsheim, E. (1995). *The normal chaos of love*. Polity Press.

Beutel, M. E., Klein, E. M., Brähler, E., Reiner, I., Jünger, C., Michal, M., Wiltink, J., Wild, P. S., Münzel, T., Lackner, K. J., & Tibubos, A. N. (2017). Loneliness in the general population: Prevalence, determinants and relations to mental health. *BMC Psychiatry, 17*(97). https://doi.org/10.1186/s12888-017-1262-x

Blakeslee, S., & Wallerstein, J. (2004). *Second chances: Men, women and children a decade after divorce*. Mariner Books.

Bowlby, J. (1969). *Attachment. Attachment and loss: Vol. 1. loss*. Basic Books.

Brown, A. (2020, August 20). A profile of single Americans. *Pew Research Center*. Retrieved April 21, 2021 from https://www.pewresearch.org/social-trends/2020/08/20/a-profile-of-single-americans/.

Brown, G. W., & Harris, T. O. (Eds.). (1989). *Life events and illness*. Guilford Press.

Brown, S. L., & Lin, I.-F. (2012). The gray divorce revolution: Rising divorce among middle-aged and older adults, 1990–2010. *Journals of Gerontology Series B: Psychological Sciences and Social Sciences, 67*(6), 731–741. https://doi.org/10.1093/geronb/gbs089

Brown, G. W., Harris, T. O., & Hepworth, C. (1995). Loss, humiliation and entrapment among women developing depression: A patient and non-patient comparison. *Psychological Medicine, 25*(1), 7–21. https://doi.org/10.1017/S003329170002804X

Bury, M. (1982). Chronic illness as biographical disruption. *Sociology of Health & Illness, 4*(2), 167–182. https://doi.org/10.1111/1467-9566.ep11339939

Bury, M. (1991). The sociology of chronic illness: A review of research and prospects. *Sociology of Health and Illness, 13*, 451–468. https://doi.org/10.1111/j.1467-9566.1991.tb00522.x

Byrne, A., & Carr, D. (2005). Caught in the cultural lag: The stigma of singlehood. *Psychological Inquiry, 16*(2/3), 84–91. https://doi.org/10.1207/s15327965pli162&3_02

Coles, R. L. (2015). Single-father families: A review of the literature. *Journal of Family Theory & Review, 7*(2), 144–166. https://doi.org/10.1111/jftr.12069

Compton, W. M., Thomas, Y. F., Stinson, F. S., & Grant, B. F. (2007). Prevalence, correlates, disability, and comorbidity of DSM-IV drug abuse and dependence in the United States: Results from the National Epidemiologic Survey on Alcohol and Related Conditions. *Archives of General Psychiatry, 64*(5), 566–576. https://doi.org/10.1001/archpsyc.64.5.566

Crump, C., Sundquist, K., Sundquist, J., & Winkleby, M. A. (2014). Sociodemographic, psychiatric and somatic risk factors for suicide: A Swedish national cohort study. *Psychological Medicine, 44*(2), 279–289. https://doi.org/10.1017/S0033291713000810

Daly, M., & Wilson, M. (1985). Child abuse and other risks of not living with both parents. *Ethology and Sociobiology, 6*(4), 197–210. https://doi.org/10.1016/0162-3095(85)90012-3

Department of Justice Canada. (2000). Selected statistics on Canadian families and family law: Second edition. *Department of Justice Canada*. Retrieved April 20, 2021 from https://www.justice.gc.ca/eng/rp-pr/fl-lf/famil/stat2000/pdf/stats.pdf.

DePaulo, B. (2007). *Singled out: How singles are stereotyped, stigmatized, and ignored, and still live happily ever after*. St. Martin's Griffin.

Deutsch, F. M. (2001). Equally shared parenting. *Current Directions in Psychological Science, 10*(1), 25–28. https://doi.org/10.1111/1467-8721.00107

Durkheim, E. (1897). *Suicide: A study in sociology*. Routledge.

Dyke, L. S., & Murphy, S. A. (2006). How we define success: A qualitative study of what matters most to women and men. *Sex Roles, 55*, 357–371. https://doi.org/10.1007/s11199-006-9091-2

East, L., Jackson, D., & O'Brien, L. (2006). Father absence and adolescent development: A review of the literature. *Journal of Child Health Care, 10*(4), 283–295. https://doi.org/10.1177/1367493506067869

Edwards, A. C., Larsson Lönn, S., Sundquist, J., Kendler, K. S., & Sundquist, K. (2018). Associations between divorce and onset of drug abuse in a Swedish National Sample. *American Journal of Epidemiology, 187*(5), 1010–1018. https://doi.org/10.1093/aje/kwx321

Eurostat. (2020a, June). Causes of death statistics. *Eurostat*. Retrieved April 20, 2021, from https://ec.europa.eu/eurostat/statistics-explained/index.php/Causes_of_death_statistics#Causes_of_death_by_sex.

Eurostat. (2020b, October 6). Marriage and divorce statistics. *Eurostat*. Retrieved April 20, 2021, from https://ec.europa.eu/eurostat/statistics-explained/pdfscache/6790.pdf.

Evans, R., Scourfield, J., & Moore, G. (2016). Gender, relationship breakdown, and suicide risk: A review of research in western countries. *Journal of Family Issues, 37*(16), 2239–2264. https://doi.org/10.1177/0192513X14562608

Farrell, W., & Gray, J. (2018). *The boy crisis: Why our boys are struggling and what we can do about it*. BenBella Books.

Felix, D. S., Robinson, W. D., & Jarzynka, K. J. (2013). The influence of divorce on Men's health. *Journal of Men's Health, 10*(10), 3–7. https://doi.org/10.1016/j.jomh.2012.09.002

Flouri, E., & Buchanan, A. (2002). Life satisfaction in teenage boys: The moderating role of father involvement and bullying. *Aggressive Behavior, 28*(2), 126–133. https://doi.org/10.1002/ab.90014

Fuhr, K., Reitenbach, I., Kraemer, J., Hautzinger, M., & Meyer, T. D. (2017). Attachment, dysfunctional attitudes, self-esteem, and association to depressive symptoms in patients with mood disorders. *Journal of Affective Disorders, 212*, 110–116. https://doi.org/10.1016/j.jad.2017.01.021

Gergen, K. J. (1991). *The saturated self*. Basic Books.

Ghosh, K. (2019, November 29). Divorces in England and Wales: 2018. *Office for National Statistics*. Retrieved April 14, 2021, from https://www.ons.gov.uk/peoplepopulationandcommunity/birthsdeathsandmarriages/divorce/bulletins/divorcesinenglandandwales/2018.

Giddens, A. (1991). *Modernity and self-identity: Self and society in the late modern age*. Stanford University Press.

Giddens, A. (1992). *The transformation of intimacy: Sexuality, love, and eroticism in modern societies*. Stanford University Press.

Golding, P., & Fitzgerald, H. (2019). The early biopsychosocial development of boys and the origins of violence in males. *Infant Mental Health Journal, 40*(1), 5–22. https://doi.org/10.1002/imhj.21753

Grall, T. (2016, January). Custodial mothers and fathers and their child support: 2013. *United States Census Bureau*. Retrieved April 20, 2021, from https://www.census.gov/content/dam/Census/library/publications/2016/demo/P60-255.pdf.

Harmon, D. K., Masuda, M., & Holmes, T. H. (1970). The social readjustment rating scale: A cross-cultural study of Western Europeans and Americans. *Journal of Psychosomatic Research, 14*(4), 391–400. https://doi.org/10.1016/0022-3999(70)90007-3

Harper, C. C., & McLanahan, S. S. (2004). Father absence and youth incarceration. *Journal of Research on Adolescence, 14*(3), 369–397. https://doi.org/10.1111/j.1532-7795.2004.00079.x

Hobson, C. J., Kamen, J., Szostek, J., Nethercut, C. M., Tiedmann, J. W., & Wojnarowicz, S. (1998). Stressful life events: A revision and update of the social readjustment rating scale. *International Journal of Stress Management, 5*, 1–23. https://doi.org/10.1023/A:1022978019315

Hoff-Sommers, C. (2015). *The war against boys: How misguided policies are harming our young men*. Simon & Schuster.

Holmes, T. H., & Rahe, R. H. (1967). The social readjustment rating scale. *Journal of Psychosomatic Research, 11*(2), 213–218. https://doi.org/10.1016/0022-3999(67)90010-4

Houle, J., Mishara, B. L., & Chagnon, F. (2008). An empirical test of a mediation model of the impact of the traditional male gender role on suicidal behavior in men. *Journal of Affective Disorders, 107*(1), 37–43. https://doi.org/10.1016/j.jad.2007.07.016

Johnson, B. (2006, November 6). Come off it, folks: How many paedophiles can there be? *The Telegraph*. https://www.telegraph.co.uk/comment/personal-view/3634055/Come-off-it-folks-how-many-paedophiles-can-there-be.html.

Kalmijn, M. (2003). Shared friendship networks and the life course: An analysis of survey data on married and cohabiting couples. *Social Networks, 25*(3), 231–249. https://doi.org/10.1016/S0378-8733(03)00010-8

Kaspiew, R., Carson, R., Dunstan, J., De Maio, J., Moore, S., Moloney, L., Smart, D., Qu, L., Coulson, M., & Tayton, S. (2015a, October). Experiences of separated parents study (evaluation of the 2012 family violence amendments). *Australian Institute of Family Studies*. Retrieved April 15, 2021, from www.aifs.gov.au/publications/experiences-separated-parents-study.

Kaspiew, R., Carson, R., Qu, L., Horsfall, B., Tayton, S., Moore, S., Coulson, M., & Dunstan, J. (2015b, October). Court outcomes project (evaluation of the 2012 family violence amendments). *Australian Institute of Family Studies*. Retrieved April 15, 2021, from www.aifs.gov.au/publications/court-outcomes-project.

Kawachi, I., & Berkman, L. F. (2001). Social ties and mental health. *Journal of Urban Health, 78*, 458–467. https://doi.org/10.1093/jurban/78.3.458

Kendler, K. S., Larsson Lönn, S., Salvatore, J., Sundquist, J., & Sundquist, K. (2017). Divorce and the onset of alcohol use disorder: A Swedish population-based longitudinal cohort and co-relative study. *American Journal of Psychiatry, 174*(5), 451–458. https://doi.org/10.1176/appi.ajp.2016.16050589

Ketokivi, K. (2008). Biographical disruption, the wounded self and the reconfiguration of significant others. In E. Widmer & R. Jallinoja (Eds.), *Beyond the nuclear family: Families in a configurational perspective* (pp. 255–277). Peter Lang.

Kleiman, E. M., & Beaver, J. K. (2013). A meaningful life is worth living: Meaning in life as a suicide resiliency factor. *Psychiatry Research, 210*(3), 934–939. https://doi.org/10.1016/j.psychres.2013.08.002

Kline Pruett, M., & DiFonzo, J. H. (2014). Closing the gap: Research, policy, practice, and shared parenting. *Family Court Review, 52*(2). https://doi.org/10.1111/fcre.12078

Kposowa, A. J. (2000). Marital status and suicide in the National Longitudinal Mortality Study. *Journal of Epidemiology & Community Health, 54*, 254–261. https://doi.org/10.1136/jech.54.4.254

Kposowa, A. J. (2003). Divorce and suicide risk. *Journal of Epidemiology & Community Health, 57*(12), 993. https://doi.org/10.1136/jech.57.12.993

Kposowa, A. J., Ezzat, D. A., & Breault, K. D. (2020). Marital status, sex, and suicide: New longitudinal findings and Durkheim's marital status propositions. *Sociological Spectrum, 40*(2), 81–98. https://doi.org/10.1080/02732173.2020.1758261

Krueger, P. M., Jutte, D. P., Franzini, L., Elo, I., & Hayward, M. D. (2015). Family structure and multiple domains of child well-being in the United States: A cross-sectional study. *Population Health Metrics, 13*(1), 6. https://doi.org/10.1186/s12963-015-0038-0

Lesthaeghe, R. (1995). The second demographic transition in Western countries: An interpretation. In K. O. Mason & A. M. Jensen (Eds.), *Gender and family change in industrialized countries* (pp. 17–62). Clarendon Press.

Lin, J. C., Karno, M. P., Grella, C. E., Warda, U., Liao, D. H., Hu, P., & Moore, A. A. (2012). Alcohol, tobacco, and non-medical drug use disorders in U.S. adults aged 65 and older: Data from the 2001–2002 National Epidemiologic Survey of Alcohol and Related Conditions. *American Journal of Geriatric Psychiatry, 19*(3), 292–299. https://doi.org/10.1097/JGP.0b013e3181e898b4

Littleboy, K. (2019, December 6). Birth characteristics in England and Wales: 2018. *Office for National Statistics (ONS)*. Retrieved April 21, 2021, from https://www.ons.gov.uk/peoplepopulationandcommunity/birthsdeathsandmarriages/livebirths/bulletins/birthcharacteristicsinenglandandwales/2018.

Lodge, A. C., & Umberson, D. (2014). Mental health and family status. In W. C. Cockerham, R. Dingwall, & S. R. Quah (Eds.), *The Wiley Blackwell encyclopedia of health, illness, behavior, and society* (1st ed., pp. 1403–1408) Wiley-Blackwell.

Maine, M. (2004). *Father hunger: Fathers, daughters, and the pursuit of thinness*. Gurze Books.

Marcil-Gratton, N., & Le Bourdais, C. (1999). Custody, access and child support: Findings from The National Longitudinal Survey of Children and Youth. *Department of Justice Canada*. Retrieved April 16, 2021, from https://www.justice.gc.ca/eng/rp-pr/fl-lf/famil/anlsc-elnej/pdf/anlsc-elnej.pdf.

Margolis, R., Choi, Y., Hou, F., & Haan, M. (2019). Capturing trends in Canadian divorce in an era without vital statistics. *Demographic Research, 41*(52), 1453–1478. https://www.demographic-research.org/volumes/vol41/52/41-52.pdf

Mattingly, K. N. (2021). Parental divorce and social support networks in younger and older adults: Extending modes of biographical disruption. In P. N. Claster & S. L. Blair (Eds.), *Aging and the family: Understanding changes in structural and relationship dynamics* (Contemporary perspectives in family research) (Vol. 17, pp. 229–246). Emerald Publishing Limited.

McAnulty, R. (2012). *Sex in college: The things they don't write home about*. Praeger.

McGee, R. S. (1993). *Father hunger*. Vine Books.

McLanahan, S., Tach, L., & Schneider, D. (2013). The causal effects of father absence. *Annual Review of Sociology, 39*, 399–427. https://doi.org/10.1146/annurev-soc-071312-145704

McManus, P., & DiPrete, T. (2001). Losers and winners: The financial consequences of separation and divorce for men. *American Sociological Review, 66*(2), 246–268. https://doi.org/10.2307/2657417

Milan, A. (2013, July). Marital status: Overview, 2011. *Statistics Canada*. Retrieved April 16, 2021, from https://www150.statcan.gc.ca/n1/en/pub/91-209-x/2013001/article/11788-eng.pdf?st=uAatcL79.

Morgan, D. J., & Burholt, V. (2020). Loneliness as a biographical disruption – Theoretical implications for understanding changes in loneliness. *The Journals of Gerontology Series B Psychological Sciences and Social Sciences, 75*(9), 2029–2039. https://doi.org/10.1093/geronb/gbaa097

Morris, W. L., DePaulo, B. M., Hertel, J., & Taylor, L. C. (2008). Singlism—Another problem that has no name: Prejudice, stereotypes and discrimination against singles. In M. A. Morrison & T. G. Morrison (Eds.), *The psychology of modern prejudice* (pp. 165–194). Nova Science Publishers.

Nielsen, L. (2011). Shared parenting after divorce: A review of shared residential parenting research. *Journal of Divorce & Remarriage, 52*, 586–609. https://doi.org/10.1080/10502556.2011.619913

Oliffe, J. L., Han, C. S., Ogrodniczuk, J. S., Phillips, J. C., & Roy, P. (2011). Suicide from the perspectives of older men who experience depression: A gender analysis. *American Journal of Men's Health, 5*(5), 444–454. https://doi.org/10.1177/1557988311408410

Organisation for Economic Co-operation and Development (OECD). (2019a, June 30). SF3.1: Marriage and divorce rates. *Organisation for Economic Co-operation and Development*. Retrieved April 21, 2021, from https://www.oecd.org/els/family/sf_3_1_marriage_and_divorce_rates.pdf.

Organisation for Economic Co-operation and Development (OECD). (2019b). Society at a glance 2019: OECD social indicators. *Organisation for Economic Co-operation and Development*. Retrieved April 14, 2021, from https://www.oecd-ilibrary.org/docserver/1be118b5-en.pdf?expires=1618446022&id=id&accname=guest&checksum=3590CE4C5FA2D4208820AC2642DEFF7F.

Organisation for Economic Co-operation and Development (OECD). (2020a). Share of births outside of marriage. *Organisation for Economic Co-operation and Development*. Retrieved April 14, 2021, from https://www.oecd.org/els/soc/SF_2_4_Share_births_outside_marriage.xlsx.

Organisation for Economic Co-operation and Development (OECD). (2020b). Family database: By indicator – The structure of families. *Organisation for Economic Co-operation and Development*. Retrieved April 21, 2021, from https://stats.oecd.org/Index.aspx?DataSetCode=FAMILY#.

Owen, J. J., Rhoades, G. K., Stanley, S. M., & Fincham, F. D. (2010). "Hooking up" among college students: Demographic and psychosocial correlates. *Archives of Sexual Behavior, 39*(3), 653–663. https://doi.org/10.1007/s10508-008-9414-1

Paykel, E. S. (2003). Life events and affective disorders. *Acta Psychiatrica Scandinavica, 108*(418), 61–66. https://doi.org/10.1034/j.1600-0447.108.s418.13.x

Payne, S., Swami, V., & Stanistreet, D. L. (2008). The social construction of gender and its influence on suicide: A review of the literature. *Journal of Men's Health, 5*(1), 23–35. https://doi.org/10.1016/j.jomh.2007.11.002

Phillips, J. A., Robin, A. V., Nugent, C. N., & Idler, E. L. (2010). Understanding recent changes in suicide rates among the middle-aged: Period or cohort effects? *Public Health Reports, 125*(5), 680–688. https://doi.org/10.1177/003335491012500510

Putnam, R. D. (2000). *Bowling alone: The collapse and revival of American community*. Simon & Schuster.

Qin, P., Agerbo, E., Westergård-Nielsen, N., Eriksson, T., & Mortensen, P. B. (2000). Gender differences in risk factors for suicide in Denmark. *The British Journal of Psychiatry, 177*, 546–550. https://doi.org/10.1192/bjp.177.6.546

Remes, O., Lafortune, L., Wainwright, N., Surtees, P., Khaw, K.-T., & Brayne, C. (2019). Association between area deprivation and major depressive disorder in British men and women: A cohort study. *BMJ Open, 9*(11), e027530. https://doi.org/10.1136/bmjopen-2018-027530

Rodgers, D. T. (2011). *Age of fracture*. Belknap Press of Harvard University Press.

Rogers, C. R. (1961). *On becoming a person: A psychotherapists view of psychotherapy.* Houghton Mifflin.

Rohner, R., & Veneziano, R. A. (2001). The importance of father love: History and contemporary evidence. *Review of General Psychology, 5*(4), 382–405. https://doi.org/10.1037/1089-2680.5.4.382

Rossow, I. (1993). Suicide, alcohol, and divorce; aspects of gender and family integration. *Addiction, 88*(12), 1659–1665. https://doi.org/10.1111/j.1360-0443.1993.tb02041.x

Rotermann, M. (2007). Marital breakdown and subsequent depression. *Health Reports, 18*(2), 33–44.

Sanders, S. (2019, November 15). Families and households in the UK: 2019. *Office for National Statistics (ONS).* Retrieved April 21, 2021, from https://www.ons.gov.uk/peoplepopulationandcommunity/birthsdeathsandmarriages/families/bulletins/familiesandhouseholds/2019.

Sands, A., Thompson, E. J., & Gaysina, D. (2017). Long-term influences of parental divorce on offspring affective disorders: A systematic review and meta-analysis. *Journal of Affective Disorders, 218,* 105–114. https://doi.org/10.1016/j.jad.2017.04.015

Sbarra, D. A., Emery, R. E., Beam, C. R., & Ocker, B. L. (2014). Marital dissolution and major depression in midlife: A propensity score analysis. *Clinical Psychological Science, 2*(3), 249–257. https://doi.org/10.1177/2167702613498727

Sbarra, D. A., Bourassa, K. J., & Manvelian, A. (2019). Marital separation and divorce: Correlates and consequences. In B. H. Fiese, M. Celano, K. Deater-Deckard, E. N. Jouriles, & M. A. Whisman (Eds.), *APA handbook of contemporary family psychology: Foundations, methods, and contemporary issues across the lifespan* (pp. 687–705). American Psychological Association.

Scott, K. M., Wells, J. E., Angermeyer, M., Brugha, T. S., Bromet, E., Demyttenaere, K., de Girolamo, G., Gureie, O., Haro, J. M., Jin, R., Nasser Karam, A., Kovess, V., Lara, C., Levinson, D., Ormel, J., Posada-Villa, J., Sampson, N., Takeshima, T., Zhang, M., & Kessler, R. C. (2010). Gender and the relationship between marital status and first onset of mood, anxiety and substance use disorders. *Psychological Medicine, 40*(9), 1495–1505. https://doi.org/10.1017/S0033291709991942

Scully, J. A., Tosi, H., & Banning, K. (2000). Life event checklists: Revisiting the social readjustment rating scale after 30 years. *Educational and Psychological Measurement, 60*(6), 864–876. https://doi.org/10.1177/00131640021970952

Shiner, M., Scourfield, J., Fincham, B., & Langer, S. (2009). When things fall apart: Gender and suicide across the life-course. *Social Science & Medicine, 69*(5), 738–746. https://doi.org/10.1016/j.socscimed.2009.06.014

Sinha, M. (2014, February). Parenting and child support after separation or divorce. *Statistics Canada.* Retrieved April 16, 2021, from https://www150.statcan.gc.ca/n1/en/pub/89-652-x/89-652-x2014001-eng.pdf?st=LnQ0PX2k.

Smith, H. (2013). *Men on strike: Why men are boycotting marriage, fatherhood, and the American dream – And why it matters.* Encounter Books.

Spruijt, E., DeGoede, M., & Vandervalk, I. (2001). The well being of youngsters coming from six different family types. *Patient Education and Counselling, 45*(4), 285–294. https://doi.org/10.1016/S0738-3991(01)00132-X

Stack, S. (2000). Suicide: A 15-year review of the sociological literature. Part II: Modernization and social integration perspectives. *Suicide and Life-threatening Behavior, 30*(2), 163–176. https://doi.org/10.1111/j.1943-278X.2000.tb01074.x

Statistics Canada. (2017, August 2). *Portrait of children's family life in Canada in 2016.* Statistics Canada. Retrieved April 21, 2021, from https://www12.statcan.gc.ca/census-recensement/2016/as-sa/98-200-x/2016006/98-200-x2016006-eng.cfm.

Stevenson, B., & Wolfers, J. (2007). Marriage and divorce: Changes and their driving forces. *Journal of Economic Perspectives, 21*(2), 27–52. https://doi.org/10.3386/w12944

Struszczyk, S., Galdas, P. M., & Tiffin, P. A. (2017). Men and suicide prevention: A scoping review. *Journal of Mental Health, 28*(1), 80–88. https://doi.org/10.1080/09638237.2017.1370638

Tsai, A. C., Lucas, M., Sania, A., Kim, D., & Kawachi, I. (2014). Social integration and suicide mortality among men: 24-year cohort study of U.S. health professionals. *Annals of Internal Medicine, 161*(2), 85–95. https://doi.org/10.7326/M13-1291

Umberson, D., Thomeer, M. B., & Williams, K. (2013). Family status and mental health: Recent advances and future directions. In C. S. Aneshensel, J. C. Phelan, & A. Bierman (Eds.), *Handbook of the sociology of mental health* (2nd ed., pp. 405–431). Springer Science + Business Media.

United States Census Bureau (2016, November 17). The majority of children live with two parents, Census Bureau reports. *U.S. Census Bureau*. Retrieved April 21, 2021, from https://www.census.gov/newsroom/press-releases/2016/cb16-192.html.

United States Census Bureau (2019a, October 16). America's families and living arrangements: 2019. *U.S. Census Bureau*. Retrieved April 21, 2021, from https://www.census.gov/data/tables/2019/demo/families/cps-2019.html.

United States Census Bureau. (2019b, November 19). One-person households on the rise. *U.S. Census Bureau*. Retrieved April 21, 2021, from https://www.census.gov/library/visualizations/2019/comm/one-person-households.html.

US Department of Justice. (1998, January 5–7). *What can the federal government do to decrease crime and revitalize communities?* U.S. Department of Justice. Retrieved April 16, from https://www.ojp.gov/pdffiles/172210.pdf.

van de Kaa, D. J. (1987). Europe's second demographic transition. *Population Bulletin, 42*(1), 1–59.

van IJzendoorn, M. H., Euser, E. M., Prinzie, P., Juffer, F., & Bakermans-Kranenburg, M. J. (2009). Elevated risk of child maltreatment in families with stepparents but not with adoptive parents. *Child Maltreatment, 14*(4), 369–375. https://doi.org/10.1177/1077559509342125

Victorino, C. C., & Gauthier, A. H. (2009). The social determinants of child health: Variations across health outcomes – A population-based cross-sectional analysis. *BMC Pediatrics, 9*(53). https://doi.org/10.1186/1471-2431-9-53

Wang, W., & Parker, K. (2014, September 24). Record share of Americans have never married. *Pew Research Center*. Retrieved April 21, 2021, from https://www.pewresearch.org/social-trends/2014/09/24/record-share-of-americans-have-never-married/.

Wang, J., Mann, F., Lloyd-Evans, B., Ma, R., & Johnson, S. (2018). Associations between loneliness and perceived social support and outcomes of mental health problems: A systematic review. *BMC Psychiatry, 18*(156). https://doi.org/10.1186/s12888-018-1736-5

Whitley, R. (2020, July 8). A silent crisis. *The ACU Review*. Retrieved April 20, 2021, from https://www.acu.ac.uk/the-acu-review/a-silent-crisis/.

Whitley, R., & McKenzie, K. (2005). Social capital and psychiatry: Review of the literature. *Harvard Review of Psychiatry, 13*(2), 71–84. https://doi.org/10.1080/10673220590956474

Whitley, R., & Zhou, J. (2020). Clueless: An ethnographic study of young men who participate in the seduction community with a focus on their psychosocial well-being and mental health. *PLoS One, 15*(2), e0229719. https://doi.org/10.1371/journal.pone.0229719

Wight, R. G., LeBlanc, A. J., & Badgett, M. V. L. (2012). Same-sex legal marriage and psychological well-being: Findings from the California Health Interview Survey. *American Journal of Public Health, 103*(2), 339–346. https://doi.org/10.2105/AJPH.2012.301113

Wilson, D. (2012). *Father hunger: Why God calls men to love and lead their families*. Thomas Nelson.

Wyllie, C., Platt, S., Brownlie, J., Chandler, A., Conolly, S., Evans, R., Kenelly, B., Kirtley, O., Moore, G., O'Connor, R. C., & Scourfield, J. (2012, October). Men, suicide and society: Why disadvantaged men in mid-life die by suicide. *Samaritans*. Retrieved April 20, 2021, from https://media.samaritans.org/documents/Samaritans_MenSuicideSociety_ResearchReport2012.pdf.

YouGov. (2019). *Friendship*. YouGov. Retrieved April 16, 2021, from https://d25d2506sfb94s.cloudfront.net/cumulus_uploads/document/m97e4vdjnu/Results%20for%20YouGov%20RealTime%20%28Friendship%29%20164%205.7.2019.xlsx%20%20%5BGroup%5D.pdf.

Chapter 10
Men's Mental Health: Time for a Paradigm Shift

The data marshaled in this book points to one inescapable conclusion: we need a paradigm shift in the field of men's mental health. We need to move away from tired and cliched notions that men's mental health woes are caused by factors such as "toxic masculinity" or men's supposed emotional illiteracy, toward a more holistic interdisciplinary perspective that is based on hard scientific evidence rather than soft unscientific ideologies. This paradigm shift must involve five particular elements:

(i) Greater consideration of the sociocultural determinants of men's mental health issues, especially in relation to education, employment, and the family.
(ii) Acknowledging, respecting, and harnessing the helpful role of traditional masculinity in promoting and fostering men's mental health.
(iii) Adopting a positive strengths-based approach to the mental health of men and boys, instead of a negative deficit-based victim-blaming approach.
(iv) Moving away from simplistic dichotomies and harmful stereotypes that frame all men as inherently privileged or villainous and thus unworthy of attention.
(v) Developing gender-based policies, programs, and procedures in health services and beyond that account for the male experience and integrate male-friendly approaches.

10.1 Sociocultural Determinants of Mental Health

In the not-too-distant past, a young man entering adulthood had three reasonable expectations regarding his future life trajectory. First, men expected a stable occupation – or even a job for life – that could provide wealth, purpose, and camaraderie throughout the life course. Second, men expected home ownership or at least security of housing tenure; a small corner of the earth they could call their own, safely housing themselves and their families. Third, men expected to marry, "settle down" and start a family. Indeed, a stable occupation and home ownership were often pursued precisely to lay a strong foundation for a solid and rewarding family life.

A man would often put his life's energy into achieving and consolidating a successful work life, a rewarding family life, and a stable home life. Striving and achieving these goals gave a man a strong sense of pride, purpose, and meaning, positively anchoring his psychological, social, and economic existence. But as discussed in the various chapters of this book, more and more men are finding it more and more difficult to achieve these common male aspirations. The demise of manufacturing, the upsurge in divorce, stock-market crashes, declining safety nets, and spiraling property prices have changed this landscape beyond recognition.

This broad sociocultural change has been accompanied by other rapid social transformations, the scope, and pace of which may be unprecedented in comparison with previous eras. This includes changes in various domains such as education, religion, gender relations, technology, and wider social life. For example, membership of organizations such as churches, trade unions, veterans' legions, sports clubs, and the like has declined precipitously; meaning men typically have fewer opportunities to meet and befriend other like-minded people (Putnam, 2000). Indeed, evidence presented throughout this book suggests that men are becoming increasingly detached from long-standing communal institutions such as extended family, religious congregations, trade unions, and other local communities. These institutions can provide fellowship, identity, and meaning to life, imparting social support and social capital that can protect the mental health of individuals against the pathogenic influence of acute and chronic stress. In the words of Putnam (2000), more and more men are "bowling alone," leading to high rates of loneliness and alienation in men, as discussed in detail in previous chapters.

Rabbi Jonathan Sacks (2003) has cogently argued that an abiding metaphor of the prewar era was Newtonian physics with its order and predictability. In contrast, Sacks argues that an abiding metaphor of the current era is Heisenberg's uncertainty principle, characterized by considerable ambiguity and unpredictability. Of note, Sociologist William Ogburn (1922) argued that rapid sociocultural change typically outpaces the psychosocial ability of humans to adapt, terming this *cultural lag*. This can have a nefarious impact on mental health. Indeed, a key thesis of this book is that rapid cultural change and cultural lag are having a nefarious impact on the mental health and well-being of men and boys and that:

(i) Males have been the forgotten and collateral victims of rapid sociocultural change.
(ii) Many men have had much unrecognized difficulty adapting to these changes.
(iii) There has been little statutory or service response to men's needs in this regard.

In sum, the broad and rapid social transformations in areas such as education, employment, and the family have created an erratic, unpredictable, and troublesome life experience for a growing number of men, with research indicating that this can contribute to mental health difficulties including depression, substance use disorder, and suicide.

As stated in Chap. 1, several scholars have noted that the wider social discourse around men's mental health has often adopted a narrowly focused deficit-based approach that borders on victim blaming, eschewing a contextual-level approach that carefully examines social change and social determinants. It has been noted that this narrow focus often singularly attributes the cause of men's mental health woes to the individual attitudes and behaviours of men, rather than acknowledging a highly complex web of causation. This discourse often centers on the concept of "masculinity," typically arguing that traditional masculinity is detrimental to men's mental health, and that men are the bearers of self-destructive beliefs, behaviors, and attitudes.

For example, the American Psychological Association (APA, 2018) recently released *Guidelines for Psychological Practice with Boys and Men* in a 31-page document aiming to help practicing clinicians better engage males in mental health treatment and foster their recovery. Of note, this document continuously pathologizes "traditional masculinity," stating early on that "conforming to traditional masculinity ideology has been shown to limit males' psychological development …and negatively influence mental health." Listed among the supposed "traditional masculinity" traits that can limit psychological development and adversely influence mental health are "risk," "achievement," "adventure," and "success, power, and competition." These guidelines imply that psychologists need to transform (or emasculate) traditionally masculine men into a new form of man, devoid of masculinity through reeducation and therapy. Such an approach is dangerous for many reasons. First, it implicitly frames men as a psychologically defective version of women, taking a deficit-based approach that simultaneously stigmatizes and blames men for their mental health issues. Second, the proposed therapeutic approach has echoes of conversion therapy, a pseudoscientific, ineffective, and harmful practice, which was used in an attempt to transform gay men into straight men and has recently been outlawed by various jurisdictions. Third, the pathologization of traditional masculinity seems to be based on outdated ideology rather than scientific evidence, as discussed in the next section.

10.2 Traditional Masculinity: Friend or Foe to Mental Health?

The APA is not alone in linking traditional masculinity to poor mental health. Indeed, this link has been made by some scholars working in fields such as "gender studies," where traditional masculinity is routinely pathologized, as well as in other sectors of society such as the media (see Chap. 1). Such pathologization also manifests itself in incessant and insistent discourse about "toxic masculinity." But is traditional masculinity really bad for mental health? Three important pieces of evidence discussed throughout this book indicate that traditional masculinity, in fact, may be very positive for mental health, with a short recap given below.

First, the APA guidelines suggest that "achievement" and "success" are traits of traditional masculinity that can harm mental health. However, many studies indicate that achievement and success are associated with positive mental health. For example, considerable epidemiological evidence reviewed in earlier chapters of this book indicate that people who are successful in life such as graduates, the employed, and the happily married tend to have better mental health than people who are high school dropouts, unemployed, and divorced. Indeed, the copious literature reviewed in this book indicates that success and achievement are directly correlated with positive aspects of mental health, whereas lack of success and achievement is correlated with poor mental health. Such knowledge is the basis for cognitive-behavioral therapy (CBT), one of the most effective evidence-based psychological interventions (Beck et al., 1979). In CBT, clinicians frequently encourage clients to set and achieve goals and successfully acquire new skills. This can result in achievement and success when done correctly, which has consistently been shown to benefit psychological resiliency (Beck, 1997). However, the APA has ignored the considerable evidence that these aspects of traditional masculinity can be beneficial for men's mental health.

Second, the APA guidelines also suggest that "adventure" and "risk" are traits of traditional masculinity that can harm mental health. However, a large corpus of research indicates that men who engage in some form of adventure and risk have better mental health than men whose lives are characterized by idleness and inactivity. For example, research indicates that suicide rates among serving military are lower than the general population, whereas military veterans have higher suicide rates than the general population (US Department of Defense, 2020; US Department of Veterans Affairs, 2020). This has been imputed to various factors, including the relative lack of adventure and sense of mission in civilian life compared with the risky and action-packed life within the various branches of the military (Junger, 2016). Moreover, interventions that involve adventure and taking risk such as bushcraft/outdoor-activity interventions, physical exercise interventions, and men's sheds can be very effective in improving men's mental health, as discussed in detail in Chap. 6. By the same token, Chap. 5 indicates that men whose lives are characterized by inactivity and apathy are prone to depression. Again, this knowledge has been integrated into CBT, where clients are often encouraged to be adventurous and take risks. For example, people with social anxiety are encouraged in CBT to take risk through controlled exposure to anxiety-provoking situations like public speaking, an effective approach consistent with the common male proclivity to deploy agency in the face of difficulty.

Third, considerable literature indicates that an *absence of masculinity* can be detrimental to the mental health of men and boys, while the *presence of masculinity* can lead to positive outcomes. For example, research on attention deficit hyperactivity disorder (see Chap. 4) and other psychosocial variables (see Chap. 7) indicates that boys raised by single mothers have considerably worse outcomes than boys raised by either intact families or by single fathers. By the same token, one theory explaining male under-achievement at school relates to the lack of male teachers (and other male role models per se) for boys. This means that many boys can spend the formative years of their life with little exposure to male mentorship, guidance, or support. To be sure, mothers and female teachers are frequently trying their best, often in the face of difficult circumstances, but the evidence indubitably indicates that this absence of masculinity is hurting the mental health of boys and young men. Similarly, a growing body of research indicates that depleted masculinity can lead to mental health issues in adult men. For example, one study found that refugee men with mental health issues attributed their behavioural and emotional problems to an inability to adequately fulfill the provider and protector role in the host country (Affleck et al., 2018). Interestingly, some men reported that they overcame these feelings of redundancy by taking leadership and mentoring roles in their immigrant community, which helped rebuild their masculine identity, which in turn fostered resiliency and recovery.

In short, evidence suggests that traditional masculinity can be helpful for the mental health of men and boys, implying that clinicians and services that work with the grain of masculinity (rather than against it) will be effective in engaging men and promoting their mental health. This is why some of the interventions reviewed in Chap. 6 are growing in popularity.

10.3 A Strengths-Based Approach

Much of the literature reviewed in this book indicates that men's mental health discourse and practice still frequently adopts a victim-blaming deficit-based approach. An example of this discourse is the undue focus on men "bottling things up," with concomitant encouragements for men to overcome this deficit by "opening-up more" and talking about their feelings. Another example is the pathologization of risk – as seen in the aforementioned APA guidelines – where adventurous men who take risks are berated or stigmatized as the bearers of "toxic masculinity."

This approach not only is victim-blaming but also displays a woeful ignorance of the reality of many men's lives. For example, research indicates that men do take more risks than women, but this is often in the pursuance of their breadwinner and provider role (Byrnes et al., 1999). Men cannot simply abandon inherently risky occupations such as mining, fishing, seafaring, the military, and manufacturing, when such employment benefits the men themselves, their families, and society as a whole. This is especially the case for men who live in small towns and rural areas where there may be few alternative employment options. As Seager (2019, p. 237) notes "it is adaptive to tune out from emotional vulnerability and focus on task performance" when employed in such jobs, and trite calls for men in such occupations to talk more about their mental health negate the fact that this can have negative consequences for job tenure, promotion, and security of employment.

Moreover, many men are socially conditioned to engage in self-sacrifice for the greater good; a process of cultural learning where men are acutely aware of the *women and children first* norm that pervades society. This norm was manifest in the sinking of the Titanic, when men organized the evacuation so that the vast majority of women and children survived. This norm also leads men to engage in risky occupations such as the military to support their wives and children, while defending their country. Of note, military norms across the world expect commissioned and noncommissioned officers alike to put the success of the mission first, the welfare of their men second, and their own well-being last when deployed in theatre. This norm also permeates the everyday health behaviours of civilian men, with one study showing that men were unwilling to access health services with putatively minor complaints because they did not want to waste a physician's time or "make a fuss about nothing" (O'Brien et al., 2005). All this means that glib, trite, and deficit-based calls for men to simply "talk more," "open-up," or "seek help" ignores social realities and may also violate deeply rooted societal norms and masculine instincts.

As described in Chap. 6, this negative deficit-based approach can be deeply off-putting to men with mental health difficulties, meaning that we must move away from a discourse that berates and blames men for their mental health issues. Instead, clinicians and service providers must adopt a positive strengths-based approach to the mental health of men and boys, working with the grain of masculinity that taps into traditional male activities and virtues. This means moving away from an approach that pathologizes masculinity and demands male reeducation, toward an approach that harnesses masculinity to promote men's mental health. Ashfield and Gouws (2019) aptly state that this approach must involve "foregrounding male aptitude not ineptitude." Indeed, this is the main message of Chap. 6, which indicates that successful male-focused interventions typically take advantage of common male proclivities such as tendencies to be practical, active, creative, generative, productive, and supportive. As explained in Chap. 5, some research indicates that harnessing such traditional male virtues can mitigate mental health issues such as depression (Krumm et al., 2017). Such research must be taken seriously.

In sum, a strengths-based approach must be the starting point for any clinical interaction, health promotion initiative, or health services intervention that attempts to improve the mental health of men or boys. This approach is both ethically sound and male-friendly, and a recent review notes that utilization of a strengths-based approach improves outcomes including sense of hope, self-efficacy, educational attainment, and employment, while reducing rates of hospitalization (Tse et al., 2016). In other words, it can address many of the functional issues identified in this book such as unemployment and school dropout, while improving internal psychological well-being. As such, widespread adoption of this approach must be an important part of any paradigm shift.

10.4 Stereotypes and Biases

As argued in Chap. 1, the word "gender" is typically used euphemistically to refer to "women" in public policy and health research, meaning that issues disproportionately affecting men and boys are overlooked or ignored. This phenomenon is labeled *male gender blindness* and was discussed in detail in Chap. 1, with many examples given in later chapters. Moreover, when men and boys are discussed, it is often done in a punitive or unempathic manner, a manifestation of the *gender empathy gap*, also discussed in detail in Chap. 1. This can involve the frequent use of stigmatizing all-encompassing concepts such as describing masculinity as "toxic," an adjective that is not used to refer to any group in society beyond men. Such discourse can also stereotype men as benefiting from an amorphous "male privilege," a stereotype based on faulty inferences and erroneous extrapolations, sometimes known as *the apex fallacy*.

The apex fallacy refers to the tendency to assume that all men are privileged, based on well-founded knowledge that men dominate the upper echelons of society in terms of representation among heads of state, parliamentarians, judges, chief executive officers, and other senior positions. However, these men make up a negligible proportion of the male population, and as argued throughout this book, men also dominate the lower echelons of society. For example, men make up the vast majority of people who are homeless, incarcerated, or injured on the job (see Chaps. 1 and 8), and men have much higher rates of suicide and substance use disorder. Moreover, there are few specific health services or clinics devoted to men's health, and men's issues receive short shrift in society as a whole.

This situation is summed up well by Seager et al. (2014), writing that "most powerful people may still be men, but most men are not powerful people…gender inequality is seen as only affecting women." The sinking of the Titanic illustrates this point, with figures indicating that 97% of first-class female passengers survived, compared with 8% of men travelling second class (Seager et al., 2016). A core argument of this book is that large groups of men lack any power and privilege; however their issues are typically ignored or overlooked – partially due to the previously described biases and stereotypes that deem all men as privileged and thus unworthy of attention.

Additionally, some scholars have argued that men as a group can be demonized in particular contexts, for example, on college campuses (see Chap. 7), where sexual paranoia and related campaigns can send a subtle message that all young men are potential rapists and a threat to communal safety (MacDonald, 2018; Kipnis, 2017). Moreover, there have been many well-documented cases where men and women have attempted to organize discussions about issues affecting men's mental health on campus, but these are met with hostility and vandalism. For example, a group of male and female students at Ryerson University (Canada) created a men's issues group, where men's mental health was a core theme. This group was regularly refused official status by the Ryerson University Student Union (Csanady, 2016). A similar phenomenon occurred at Durham University (the United Kingdom) where a men's issue group has been denied official recognition for many years (Daubney, 2015). Likewise, the University of Toronto Men's Issues Society invited renowned scholar Dr. Warren Farrell to talk about men's mental health, but his lecture was met with protests and vandalism by demonstrators (Smeenk, 2012).

This creates a paradoxical situation, which has been labeled *the men's mental health double-bind* (Whitley, 2019). It is often said that silence is detrimental to men's mental health, and there are frequent calls on social media and elsewhere for men to "talk more" and "open-up" about their mental health (see Chap. 1). But attempts to discuss men's issues can face obstruction and hostility, and men are often facing local situations where they are being implicitly told to shut-up, "check their privilege," and talk less.

An example of the men's mental health double-bind comes (somewhat paradoxically) from the world of academic psychology. In the United Kingdom, several leading psychologists recently formed a male psychology group offering public lectures, a website, a newsletter, and a social space to discuss men's mental health. As the group grew, the leadership applied for the group to be recognized as an official section of the British Psychological Society (BPS), which would require a vote from the whole BPS membership. Bizarrely, this application was opposed by an organized group with its own dedicated website entitled "no to male psychology," which campaigned for a no vote. In the resultant ballot, over 4000 BPS members voted, with two-thirds voting in favour of the new section (Male Psychology Network, 2019). This was welcome news for all who care about men's mental health, but it cannot go unnoticed that around one in three BPS members (who voted) did not want a male psychology section. The negative messages underlying this double-bind are reliant on the biases and stereotypes discussed in Chapt. 1 and throughout this book and must be addressed as part of any paradigm shift in men's mental health.

10.5 Male-Friendly Policies, Programs, and Procedures

It has been argued throughout this book that there is a lack of male-friendly programs, policies, and procedures within various sectors of society including educational institutions, healthcare clinics, health promotion initiatives, the legal system, and law enforcement. In some situations, these lacunae can be addressed by adopting the aforementioned strengths-based model, while also taking heed of social determinants of health. However, institutions can take other measures to address this situation, with three particular measures outlined next.

First, many have argued that it is important to have more men working in services where there is currently an observable lack of males (Johal et al., 2012; Wilkins & Kemple, 2010). This might make such services more appealing and engaging to males. For example, there are very few male teachers at the primary level (see Chap. 7), with Sax (2016) aptly remarking that the only male present in some elementary schools is the janitor. Similarly, professions like clinical psychology and social work are dominated by women, making it very difficult for male clients who may prefer a male therapist or support worker. Of note, there are well-funded efforts to encourage women to enter the STEM fields at universities across the world, but there are few equivalent efforts that encourage men to enter female-dominated fields such as primary education or social work. This could be addressed through local, national, or institutional initiatives, drawing their inspiration from the aforementioned efforts to encourage women (and other underrepresented groups) to

10.5 Male-Friendly Policies, Programs, and Procedures

enter STEM fields. Increasing proportions of men in such fields may have a beneficial effect in various ways. First, it will provide young males and vulnerable male adults with useful male role models and concomitant guidance from accomplished males. Second, it can contribute toward the introduction of male perspective within institutions such as primary schools, which have been hitherto dominated by women, perhaps leading to more male-friendly activities. Third, males working in these professions can combine their lived and professional experience to help create new male-friendly interventions and programs therein.

Second, there is a pressing need for institutional reflection, innovation, and reform to ensure that programs, policies, and procedures are male-friendly. This can occur in schools and workplaces, as well as larger systems such as law enforcement agencies and legal systems. For example, many men report adverse experiences within the legal system, with common perceptions that a double-standard is at play. Data reviewed in Chap. 1 indicates that men experience domestic violence at similar rates to women, but often report that their complaints are treated with ridicule, laughter, or indifference. But when accused of such abuse, men can find the full resources of the state mobilized against them, even in the face of flimsy evidence. Similarly, many men have reported adverse experiences within family court, with data presented in Chap. 9 suggesting that less than 20% of men receive full custody of their children. This can be a living bereavement for the affected men and has been implicated in high suicide rates among divorced and separated men (see Chap. 2). This differential treatment at the hands of the state means that for many men, there is a legal system but not a justice system, implying an urgent need for reform. This could take the form of education and training to help reduce biases and stereotypes for key stakeholders such as the police, the judiciary, healthcare providers, teachers, and others who serve society. Such efforts should aim to enlighten stakeholders about male experiences, while disabusing attendees of the common biases and gendered stereotypes outlined in Chap. 1.

Third, there is a need for local, regional, and national strategies to target and address some of the core issues identified in this book. These strategies should be developed after consultation of the relevant research literature, with input from key stakeholders including service providers, nonprofit organizations, community associations, and anyone else who cares about the well-being of men and boys. Once developed, a dedicated bureau can be tasked with implementing the strategy and monitoring progress. There are some precedents in this regard. In Canada, the government contains a dedicated Minister for Women in charge of a government "Department for Women and Gender Equality," which (inter alia) funds projects in areas such as "ending violence against women and girls; improving the economic security and prosperity of women and girls; and encouraging women and girls in leadership roles" (Department for Women and Gender Equality, 2020). Similarly, the President of the United States is advised by a newly created "White House Gender Policy Council," which (despite its generic name) has an exclusive focus on women and girls (The White House, 2021). The council was created by a lengthy executive order and is tasked with "developing a government wide strategy to advance gender equity and equality… in developing the strategy, the Council shall consider the unique experiences and needs of women and girls." Of note, there is not a single mention of men or boys anywhere in this 2000-word executive order, thus displaying the *male gender blindness* and *gender empathy gap* discussed in Chap. 1. Given the gravity of the many issues discussed in this book, perhaps it is time to create and fund analogous bureaus, strategies, and government ministries tasked with furthering the mental health and well-being of men and boys.

10.6 Conclusion

The evidence is clear: it is time for a paradigm shift in the field of men's mental health. We must move away from simplistic and sophomoric explanations of men's mental health that focus on alleged psychological deficits, toward a discussion of social context and the complex web of causation. To be sure, evidence suggests that individual men may need to change to improve their own mental health; however, health service providers, educational institutions, and society as a whole also need to change. This means more empathy for men and boys and less male gender blindness, as well as policies and programs driven by scientific evidence rather than biases, stereotypes, and harmful ideologies. Importantly, the various sectors of government and civil society need to recognize that males also experience gendered issues that can impact mental health and these issues must be comprehensively addressed as an essential part of an inclusive and empathic public policy. Otherwise, more and more men will become alienated and isolated from society, leading to wasted potential, wrecked families, and ruined lives. This is a deadly serious issue in need of concerted action. We need a paradigm shift. Now.

References

Affleck, W., Thamotharampillai, U., Jeyakumar, J., & Whitley, R. (2018). "If one does not fulfil his duties, he must not be a man": Masculinity, mental health and resilience amongst Sri Lankan Tamil refugee men in Canada. *Culture, Medicine and Psychiatry, 42*(4), 840–861. https://doi.org/10.1007/s11013-018-9592-9

American Psychological Association (APA). (2018, August). *APA guidelines for psychological practice with boys and men*. American Psychological Association. Retrieved May 11, 2021, from https://www.apa.org/about/policy/boys-men-practice-guidelines.pdf

Ashfield, J. A., & Gouws, D. S. (2019). Dignifying psychotherapy with men: Developing empathic and evidence-based approaches that suit the real needs of the male gender. In J. A. Barry, R. Kingerlee, M. Seager, & L. Sullivan (Eds.), *The Palgrave handbook of male psychology and mental health* (pp. 623–645). Palgrave Macmillan.

Beck, A. T. (1997). The past and future of cognitive therapy. *Journal of Psychotherapy Practice & Research, 6*(4), 276–284.

Beck, A. T., Rush, A. J., Shaw, B. F., & Emery, G. (Eds.). (1979). *Cognitive therapy of depression*. The Guilford Press.

References

Byrnes, J. P., Miller, D. C., & Schafer, W. D. (1999). Gender differences in risk taking: A meta-analysis. *Psychological Bulletin, 125*(3), 367–383. https://doi.org/10.1037/0033-2909.125.3.367

Csanady, A. (2016, April 12). Men's issues group taking Ryerson University's student union to court over club status. *The National Post*. https://nationalpost.com/news/canada/mens-issues-group-taking-ryerson-universitys-student-union-to-court-over-club-status

Daubney, M. (2015, June 16). Why are our universities blocking men's societies? *The Telegraph*. https://www.telegraph.co.uk/men/thinking-man/11670138/Why-are-our-universities-blocking-mens-societies.html

Department for Women and Gender Equality. (2020, November 26). *Department for Women and Gender Equality – Women's Program*. Government of Canada. Retrieved May 12, 2021, from https://www.canada.ca/en/women-gender-equality/news/2019/03/department-for-women-and-gender-equality%2D%2Dwomens-program.html

Johal, A., Shelupanov, A., & Norman, W. (2012, October). *Invisible men: Engaging more men in social projects*. The Young Foundation. Retrieved May 12, 2021, from https://youngfoundation.org/wp-content/uploads/2012/10/INVISIBLE_MEN_-_FINAL.pdf

Junger, S. (2016). *Tribe: On homecoming and belonging*. Twelve.

Kipnis, L. (2017). *Unwanted advances: Sexual paranoia comes to campus*. Harper Collins.

Krumm, S., Checchia, C., Koesters, M., Kilian, R., & Becker, T. (2017). Men's views on depression: A systematic review and metasynthesis of qualitative research. *Psychopathology, 50*(2), 107–124. https://doi.org/10.1159/000455256

MacDonald, H. (2018). *The diversity delusion: How race and gender pandering corrupt the university and undermine our culture*. St. Martin's Press.

Male Psychology Network. (2019, August). *Male psychology network*. Retrieved May 11, 2021, from https://malepsychology.org.uk/male-psychology-network/vote-for-a-male-psychology-section/

O'Brien, R., Hunt, K., & Hart, G. (2005). 'It's cavemen stuff, but that is to a certain extent how guys still operate': Men's accounts of masculinity and help seeking. *Social Science and Medicine, 64*, 503–526. https://doi.org/10.1016/j.socscimed.2004.12.008

Ogburn, W. (1922). *Social change with respect to nature and original cult*. Viking.

Putnam, R. D. (2000). *Bowling alone: The collapse and revival of American community*. Simon & Schuster.

Sacks, J. (2003). *The dignity of difference: how to avoid the clash of civilizations*. Continuum.

Sax, L. (2016). *Boys adrift: The five factors driving the growing epidemic of unmotivated boys and underachieving young men*. Basic Books.

Seager, M. (2019). From stereotypes to archetypes: An evolutionary perspective on male help-seeking and suicide. In J. A. Barry, R. Kingerlee, M. Seager, & L. Sullivan (Eds.), *The Palgrave handbook of male psychology and mental health* (pp. 227–248). Palgrave Macmillan.

Seager, M., Barry, J. A., & Sullivan, L. (2016). Challenging male gender blindness: Why psychologists should be leading the way. *Clinical Psychology Forum, 285*, 35–40.

Seager, M., Sullivan, L., & Barry, J. (2014). The male psychology conference, University College London, June 2014. *New Male Studies: An International Journal, 3*(2), 41–68.

Smeenk, D. (2012, November 17). Arrest, assaults overshadow "men's issues" lecture. *The Varsity*. https://thevarsity.ca/2012/11/17/arrest-assaults-overshadow-mens-issues-lecture/

The White House. (2021, March 8). *Executive order on establishment of the white house gender policy council*. The White House. Retrieved May 11, 2021, from https://www.whitehouse.gov/briefing-room/presidential-actions/2021/03/08/executive-order-on-establishment-of-the-white-house-gender-policy-council/

Tse, S., Tsoi, E. W., Hamilton, B., O'Hagan, M., Shepherd, G., Slade, M., Whitley, R., & Petrakis, M. (2016). Uses of strength-based interventions for people with serious mental illness: A critical review. *The International Journal of Social Psychiatry, 62*(3), 281–291. https://doi.org/10.1177/0020764015623970

US Department of Defense. (2020, August 20). *Annual suicide report: Calendar year 2019*. Defense Suicide Prevention Office. Retrieved May 11, 2021, from https://www.dspo.mil/Portals/113/Documents/CY2019%20Suicide%20Report/DoD%20Calendar%20Year%20CY%202019%20Annual%20Suicide%20Report.pdf?ver=YOA4IZVcVA9mzwtsfdO5Ew%3D%3D#:~:text=The%20CY%202019%20suicide%20rate,100%2C000%20Active%20Component%20Service%20members

US Department of Veterans Affairs. (2020). *2020 national veteran suicide prevention annual report*. US Department of Veterans Affairs. Retrieved May 11, 2021, from https://www.mentalhealth.va.gov/docs/data-sheets/2020/2020-National-Veteran-Suicide-Prevention-Annual-Report-11-2020-508.pdf

Whitley, R. (2019, June 10). *The men's mental health double-bind*. Psychology Today. Retrieved May 11, 2021, from https://www.psychologytoday.com/us/blog/talking-about-men/201906/the-men-s-mental-health-double-bind

Wilkins, D., & Kemple, M. (2010). The mental health of men and boys. *Mental Health Today*, 20–25.

Index

A
Aboriginal communities, 163
Absence of masculinity, 238
Addictions, 45–47, 59–61
Adulthood, 196
Adverse behavioral disturbances, 224
Adverse childhood experience, 220
Adverse mental health, 189, 213, 220, 224
Adverse psychosocial outcomes, 227
Aetiology
    addictions, 53
    alcohol and drug abuse, 54
    alcohol-related problems, 54
    divorce, separation and loneliness, 58, 59
    educational failure and subsequent failure, 54–56
    low socio-economic status, 54
    pain/distress, 54
    substance misuse, 53
    substance use disorder, 53
    unemployment and employment issues, 56, 57
Age, 25
Age-adjusted relative risk of suicide, 32
Alcohol-related disorders, 47, 48
Alcohol use, 47, 48
Alcohol-use disorders (AUD), 55, 157
Alleged psychological deficits, 244
Alternative employment, 195, 239
American Academy of Child and Adolescent Psychiatry (2007), 82
American Academy of Pediatrics (2019), 82
American Association of Suicidology, 139
American Psychiatric Association (APA), 46, 88, 105, 237, 239
American psychiatrists, 207
Americans with Disabilities Act, 94
Amphetamine-based psychostimulants, 83
Anomic suicide, 36, 216
Antisocial behavior, 164
Apex fallacy, 241
Attention deficit hyperactivity disorder (ADHD), 159, 223, 225
    adolescence, 72
    childhood, 72
    complexity, 71
    daily functioning and psychosocial development, 71
    DSM-5, 72
    epidemiological characteristics, 71
    epidemiology, 73, 74
    formal diagnosis, 73
    hyperactivity-impulsivity sub-type symptoms, 72, 73
    inattentive sub-type symptoms, 72, 73
    the medicalization of childhood, 96
    medicalization of misbehaviour, 96
    medicalization of underperformance, 96
    mental disorder, 71
    neurodevelopmental disorders, 71
    neurological basis, 71
    process of diagnosis, 72
    psychiatric industry, 96
    psychopathology, 73
    psychosocial impairment, 96
    psychostimulant medication, 97
    risk factors, 71
        absolute gender differences, 83, 84
        adulthood, 81
        childhood maltreatment, 77

Attention deficit hyperactivity disorder (ADHD) (*cont.*)
　educational impact, 80, 81
　low family income, 78
　low parental education, 78
　medication issues, 82
　middle-childhood years, 77
　misuse, 82, 83
　neglect, 77
　relative gender differences, 84, 85
　side effects, 82, 83
　single-mother families, 78, 79
　social control, 95, 96
　sub-types, 73
　US Studies, 75, 76
Australian mental health charity, 3
Average misbehavior, 162

B
Benevolent sexism, 8
Biographical disruption, 207, 223
Black-market opioids, 192
Blue-collar less-educated men, 194, 196
Blue-collar manual occupations, 182
Blue-collar occupations, 196
Blue-collar working-class manual workers, 193
Boys Adrift (book), 159
British Psychological Society (BPS), 242
British sociologist Mike Bury enriched stress theory, 207
Bushcraft/outdoor-activity interventions, 238

C
Canadian and Australian Aboriginal communities, 182
Canadian Chronic Disease Surveillance System, 108
Canadian Community Health Survey, 106, 107
Canadian Indigenous males, 26
Canadian longitudinal study, 209
Canadian manufacturing sector, 195
Canadian statistics, 226
Cannabis-related disorders, 48, 49
Cannabis use disorders, 48, 49
Catholicism/Judaism, 216
Centers for Disease Control and Prevention (CDC), 50, 75
Child custody, 215
Chronic illness, 207
Civil society organizations, 227
Clinical psychology, 242
Coal mining, 195
Cognitive-behavioral therapy (CBT), 61, 238

Common conclusions, 179
Communal safety, 241
Community organizations, 216
Comprehensive meta-analysis, 189
Computerized Diagnostic Interview Schedule for Children, 76
Constraints of masculinity, 194
Conventional gender roles, 185
Court-ordered custody arrangements, 226
COVID-19, 12–13, 36, 182
Criminal activity, 220
Criminal justice system, 27
Cross-sectional analysis, 157
Cross-sectional survey, 209
Cultural change, 236
Cultural lag, 236

D
Danish case-control study, 212
Deaths of despair, 197
Deficit-based approach, 237
Deficit-based calls, 240
Demand/control model, 188
Demand/low control environments, 189
Department for Women and Gender Equality, 10, 243
Depression, 33, 34
Depressive symptoms, 187
Diagnostic and Statistical Manual of Mental Disorders (2013) Fifth Edition (DSM-5), 46, 71, 105
Disruptive behaviors, 160
Divorce, 31–33, 35, 37, 213, 218, 227
Divorce and father absence effects, offspring mental health
　acute and chronic mental health, 220
　adult children experience, 222
　adverse childhood experience, 220
　educational outcomes, 221
　literature reviews, 221
　meta-analysis, 222
　parental relationship instability, 221
　plausible mechanisms and pathways, 223–225
　single-father motherless households, 222, 223

E
Educational achievement, 224
Educational attainment
　categorical variable, 154
　continuous variable, 154
　United States, 158

Educational deficits, 153
Educational institutions, 242
Educational system
    difficulties, 153
    individual performance, 154
    male underperformance, 153
Educational trajectory, 154
Educational underachievement, 220
Educational workforce, 169
Education gender gap
    tertiary education, 164–167
Egoistic suicide, 36, 216
Emotional turmoil, 207
Emotional vulnerability, 239
Empathic public policy, 244
Employed low-status manual workers, 186
Employment conditions and workplace environment
    job strain, 188
    job stress, 188
    longitudinal studies, 188
    mental health impacts, 187
    precarious employment, 187, 188
Employment issues, male suicide
    dangerous and demanding industries, 30
    financial impact, 29
    financial loss, 29
    GFC, 28
    industries, 31
    job loss, 28, 29
    loss of income, 29
    lower socio-economic status, 29
    low status occupations, 29
    male-dominated professions, 30, 31
    mental disorders, 30
    socio-economic status, 30
    traditional industries, 30
    unemployment, 28, 29
Epidemic of loneliness, 219
Epidemiological Catchment Area study, 105
Epidemiological evidence, 238
Epidemiological literature, 158
Ethnicity, 25
Evolutionary psychology, 8, 9

F
Failed breadwinner, 185, 186, 214
Failure to launch, 167
Family responsibilities, 186
Father absence, 220–222, 224
Father–child relationship, 33, 214, 224
Father hunger, 224
Female-dominated occupations, 183
Fentanyl, 50, 51, 55, 57

Financial responsibilities, 219
Financial strain, 179
Formal sector, 127
Free education, 153

G
Gambling addiction, 51
Gambling disorder, 46, 51, 52
Gender, 62, 63, 74, 240
Gender differences, paid work
    Canadian data, 178
    heavier workloads, 178
    male status and identity, 178
    married men, 178
    married single-income families, 178
    objective outcomes, 178
    subjective meaning, 178
    unemployed women, 179
Gender differential, 197
Gender education gap
    primary school education, 159, 160
    secondary education, 161–164
    worrying phenomenon, 159
Gender empathy gap, 140, 166, 241, 244
    biological basis, 8
    biology, 8
    COVID-19, 13
    decision-making, 9
    evidence-based policy, 9
    evolutionary psychology, 8, 9
    favouritism, 8
    gender-based moral typecasting, 7, 8
    in-group favouritism, 8
    inequities, school system, 7
    men and women in distress, 7
    neotenous features, 8
    public and private empathy, men and women, 7
    social norms, 8–9
    statistics, 7
    stereotypes of men, 7
    workplace deaths and injuries, 7
Gender equity, 9
Gender inequality, 241
Gender paradox, 110
Gender pay gap, 1
Gender sensitive perspective, 188
Gender stereotypes of men
    biased gender stereotypes, 5
    the chivalry hypothesis, 6
    COVID-19, 13
    emotional distress, 5
    men's mental health, 5
    negative stereotypes, 6

Gender stereotypes of men (*cont.*)
   social harm., 5
   Syrian refugee resettlement program, 6
   villain and a female victim, 11
   women are wonderful effect, 5
Gendered stereotypes, 243
General Certificate of Secondary Education (GCSE), 161
GHQ-12 screening questionnaire, 185
Global FINANCIAL Crisis (GFC), 23, 24, 28, 36
Good-quality supervision, 180
Gray divorce, 218
Group interventions, 140
Guidelines for Psychological Practice with Boys and Men, 109

H
Halo effect, 85
Hazard ratios, 212
Hazardous drinking, 184
Hazardous materials, 193
Hazardous psychosocial/physical conditions, 197
Health by stealth approach, 137
Health care, 127
Healthcare clinics, 242
Healthcare system, 34
Health gap, 1
Health promotion initiatives, 242
Health service utilization, 108
High demand/low control category, 191
High educational attainment, 154, 155, 168
High job strain, 189
High-quality population-based cohort studies, 181
Holistic interdisciplinary perspective, 235
Holmes-Rahe Life Stress Inventory, 207
Homosexual orientation, 116
Hook-up culture, 218
Household composition, 218
Housing arrangements, 196
Hydrocodone, 50

I
Indigenous and aboriginal men, 26
Individualized and tailored lifestyle, 219
Industrial-based economy, 194
Informal action-based/community-based interventions, 137
Informal sector, 127
Innovation, 243

Institutional reflection, 243
Intense psychological distress, 192
International Classification of Disease (ICD-11), 52
International Men's Sheds Organization, 141
Internet gaming, 45
Internet Gaming Disorder (IGD), 52, 53
Interpersonal conflict, 189
Intimate Partner Violence (IPV), 11
Intrapsychic integration, 217
Ipsos MORI survey, 193
Isolation, 215

J
Job insecurity, 187, 188, 196
Job loss, 25, 28, 29, 34, 35, 187
Job satisfaction, 189, 190
Job strain, 188, 189, 196, 197
Job stress, 188, 196, 197
Justice gap, 1

K
Knowledge economy, 194

L
Lack of masculinity, 222
Large-scale comparative study, 156
Large-scale loneliness survey, 167
Large-scale US Epidemiologic Catchment Area study, 184
Large-scale US study, 222
Latent functions, 177
Law enforcement, 242
Law enforcement agencies and legal systems, 243
Legal marriage, 218
Legal system, 242
Lithuania, 212
Loneliness, 167, 168, 215
Loneliness score, 168
Longitudinal analysis, 210
Longitudinal survey, 211
Long-standing communal institutions, 236
Long-term mental health, 219
Low educational attainment, 54
   adverse mental health outcomes, 155, 168
   depression and anxiety risk factor, 157, 158
   drawbacks, 154
   research studies, 155

Index

social science literature, 154
SUDs risk factor, 156, 157
suicide risk factor, 155, 156
Low job strain, 189
Low socioeconomic status (SES), 157–158

M

Major depressive disorder (MDD), 105, 106, 209
Male depressive syndrome
    aggression, 112
    chronic disorder, 105
    clinical depression, 105
    depressive equivalents, 111, 112
    emotions, 105
    epidemiological instruments, 112
    epidemiological surveys, 110–112
    experience, 112
    feelings, 112
    gender differences, 107, 108, 110
    gender paradox, 110
    impression, 110
    low mood, 105
    masked depression, 111–113
    medical literature, 110
    moods, 105
    prevalence, 106–108, 120
    process, 111
    psychological distress, 111
    qualitative research, 111
    resilience, 108–110
    risk factors
        disability, 115, 116
        divorce, 117, 118
        ethno-racial status, 118
        homosexual orientation, 116
        low educational attainment, 113, 114
        paternal postpartum depression, 118–120
        unemployment and financial strain, 114, 115
    sadness, 105
    service utilization, 111
    societal stereotypes, 111
    socio-cultural framing, 111
    statistics, 110
    treatment, 107, 108
Male dominated occupations
    health and safety impacts, 191
    high demand/low control category, 191
    PTSD, 192
    socio-economic spectrum, 193
    suicide rate, 192
    umbrella categories, 190
    US Bureau of Labor Statistics, 191
    workers, 190
    workplace injuries, 192
Male gender blindness, 9–13, 244
Male perspective, 243
Male privilege, 241
Male suicide
    age-adjusted male suicide rates, USA, 23
    Americas, 23
    Canada, 23
    criminal justice system, 27
    employment issues, 28–31
    Europe, 23
    GFC, 23, 24
    indigenous and aboriginal men, 26
    middle-aged men, 25
    military veterans, 27
    rates, 23, 37
    risk factors
        childhood experiences, 28
        cultural context, 37
        divorce, 31–33
        family issues, 31–33
        individual-level, 28
        marital status, 31–33
        mental disorders, 33–35
        substance use issues, 33–35
    risk of, 24
    rural and remote regions, 25
    social connection, 35–36
    social integration, 35–36
    white men, 25, 26
Male villain/perpetrator stereotype, 215
Manpower-heavy industries, 194
Manual blue-collar workers, 181
Marital dissolution, 208
Marital status, 31–33, 208
Marital status and mental health in adults
    comparisons, 208
    cross-sectional associations, 208
    depression, 209, 210
    divorce, 212–214
    literature review, 208
    psychosocial stress, 214–216
    social integration, 216
    substance abuse, 210, 211
    suicide, 211, 212
Marriage, 214
Masculine culture, 194
Masculine influence, 227
Masculinity, 2, 3, 237
Masked depression, 108, 111–113

Medicalization hypothesis
  ADHD diagnosis, 94, 95
  adolescence, 87
  big pharma, 89, 90
  boisterous and spirited behaviour, 85
  childhood, 87
  cosmetic issues, 86
  depression, 86
  diagnosis, 85, 86
  education, 92–94
  educational institutions, 87
  energy-intensive activities, 87
  factors, 86
  gambling, 86
  Internet-gaming usage, 86
  literature, 86
  modern families, 87
  mothers, 90–92
  psychiatric disorders, 86
  psychiatric industry, 88, 89
  schools, 92–94
  sex steroids, 87
  social phobia, 86
  sociological analysis, 87
Men Going Their Own Way (MGTOW), 219, 220
Men's health-related behaviors, 213
Men's mental health, 220
  academic psychology, 242
  COVID-19, 12–13
  definitions, 3
  depression, 4
  discourse and practice, 239
  education gap, 1, 4
  educational system, 4
  epidemiological research, 4
  failure to launch, 4
  gender empathy gap, 7–9
  gender gaps, 1
  gender stereotypes of men, 5–6
  justice gap, 1
  legacy media, 14
  loneliness, 4
  male gender blindness, 9–12
  masculinity, 2, 3
  paradigm shift, 235, 244
  psychosocial issues, 1
  public health approach, 2
  scientific field, 13
  social determinants, 2, 3, 14
  social media, 14
  social support deficits, 4
  social trends, 4
  sociocultural determinants, 235–237
  suicide (*see* Male suicide)
  toxic masculinity, 235
  unemployment, 4
  victim blaming, 2
Mental disorders, 30, 33–35, 189, 192
Mental distress, 186, 194
Mental health, 179, 186
Mental health benefits, 219
Mental health difficulties, 168
Mental health impact, 210
Mental health issues, 186, 193
Mental health outcomes, 208
Mental health service utilization
  common mental disorders, 127
  depression, 128
  different modalities of healing, 136–138
  environment, 134, 135
  general practitioners/family doctors, 127
  health care, 127
  large-scale US study, 128
  male-friendly options, 138–140
  male-sensitive services, 138–140
  masculinity, 129, 130
  men's formal service, 129, 130
  men's sheds, 140–142
  mental disorder, 128
  professionals, 127
  recommendations, 142, 143
  severe mental illnesses, 127
  spiritual activities, 127
  stigma
    external, 130
    family, 133
    health services, 133, 134
    influential sectors, 131
    internal, 130
    media, 131
    self-stigma, 130
    workplace, 132
  SUD, 129
Mental health services, 35
Mental health treatment, 34
Mental illness, 25, 35–37, 46
Meta-analysis, 180
Methadone, 50, 61
Military veterans, 27
Millennial men, 167
Motivational interviewing, 61
Multidimensional measures, 187
Multipronged approach, 168

N
Naltrexone, 61
National Center for Health Statistics, 212

National Epidemiologic Survey on Alcohol and Related Conditions (NESARC), 55, 156, 158
National Health Interview Survey (NHIS), 75
National Population Health Survey, 117, 209
National Survey of Children's Health (NSCH), 75, 76
National Survey on Drug Use and Health (NSDUH), 46, 61, 106, 157
Negative deficit-based approach, 240
Neotenous features, 8
Nondiscriminatory procedures, 227
Non-Substance-Related Mental Disorder, 46
Not in Education, Employment nor Training (NEETs), 196
Nuclear family, 95

O

Occupational categories, 190
Occupational health and safety, 191–193, 196
Oft-cited figures, 221
Opioid-related disorders, 49–51
Opioids, 116
Opioid use, 49–51
Organisation for Economic Co-operation and Development (OECD), 153, 178, 217
Oxycodone, 50

P

Parental divorce, 222
Parenthood, 118
Paternal postpartum depression, 118–120
Pathological gambling, 45, 51
Personality disorders, 33
Personality functioning, 160
Pharmaceuticalization, 89
Poor mental health, 185
Positive mental health consequences, 190
Postsecondary education, 196
Postsecondary institutions, 154, 169
Post-traumatic stress disorder (PTSD), 27, 30, 33, 192
Potential mental health benefits, 194
Powerlessness, 45
Precarious employment, 187, 188, 197
Precarious/unskilled employment, 193
Primary education, 159
    ADHD, 160
    childhood educators, 161
    disruptive behaviors, 160
    elevated rates, 160
    gender gaps, 160
    gender stereotypes, 160
    marginalized boys, 161
    mastering basic reading skills, 159
    school culture, 161
Pro-social communities, 225
Protestantism, 36
Psychiatric industry, 88, 89
Psychological distress, 57, 197, 207, 210, 213, 214
Psychological resiliency, 238
Psychophysiological addictive qualities, 192
Psychosocial experience, 213
Psychosocial factors, 119
Psychosocial impact, 80
Psychosocial interventions, 139
Psychosocial job stress, 188
Public health approach, 2
Public health intervention, 227

R

Rape culture, 166, 169
Reasons for living, 35
Reform, 243
Relationship dissolution, 212
Residential schools, 26
Risk of suicide, 24, 32, 34
Risky occupations, 239, 240
Rural and remote regions, 25

S

School diplomas and certificates, 153
School leavers categories, 154
Secondary education, 159
    average misbehavior, 162
    dropout rates, 163
    extracurricular activity, 164
    GCSE, 161, 162
    international survey, 162
    males and females, 162
    OECD, 161
    policy and societal discussion, 162
    preponderance, 163
    pro-social behavior, 164
    school dropout, 163
    statistics, 163
    teacher–pupil engagement, 164
    traditional boyhood pursuits, 164
    US *Condition of Education* report, 162
    US figures, 161
    US statistics, 162
Seduction community, 220, 225
Self-medication, 192

Self-sacrifice, 239
Service-based economy, 163
Severe injury, 192
Sex addiction, 46
Sex steroids, 87
Sexual paranoia, 241
Shifting economy, 196
Single-father motherless households
  ADHD diagnosis, 223
  children at risk, 225
  delinquency, 223
  incarceration ratio, 222
  OR, 223
  psychosocial outcomes, 223
  psychosocial status of children, 222
  subanalysis, 223
Single-jurisdiction surveys, 215
Single-mother household, 220
Single never-married men, 217
Single-occupancy households, 220
Single parent household, 226
Singlism, 215
Smartphone addiction, 46
Social alienation, 35, 216
Social and demographic trends, 217
Social and emotional learning programs, 169
Social capital, 167
Social connection, 35–37
Social context, 3
Social control, 95, 96
Social determinants, 2, 3
Social integration, 35–37, 216
Social interaction, 32, 213
Social media, 241
Social prescribing, 143
Social Readjustment Rating Scale, 207
Social sciences, 2
Social support, 32, 36, 236
Social transformations, 236
Social trends, 4
Social work, 242
Sociocultural determinants
  acute and chronic stress, 236
  deficit-based approach, 237
  goal achievement, 236
  occupation, 235
  social discourse, 237
  social transformations, 236
  traditional masculinity, 237
Socioeconomic changes, 194
Socioeconomic conditions, 196
Socioeconomic groups, 131
Socio-economic macro-environment, 30

Socioeconomic shift, 195
Socioeconomic status (SES), 113, 186, 220
Special education, 159
Stakeholders, 243
STEM fields, 243
Stereotypes, 215, 216, 226, 242, 244
Stigmas, 216
Stolen generation, 26
Strategy and monitoring progress, 243
Stratified subanalysis, 181
Strengths and Difficulties Questionnaire
    (SDQ), 75
Strengths and Weaknesses of ADHD-
    Symptoms and Normal Behaviour
    instrument (SWAN), 75
Strengths-based approach
  clinical interaction, 240
  outcomes, 240
  positive, 240
Strengths-based model, 242
Stressful experience, 214
Stressful transitional period, 212
Subcultures/communities, 217
Substance abuse, 46, 47, 220
Substance Abuse and Mental Health Services
    Administration 2019, 128
Substance use, 33–35
Substance use disorder (SUD), 34, 35, 46, 47,
    54, 129, 156, 157, 183–185, 241
  and addictions, 59–61
  treatments, 61, 62
Substance-Related and Addictive
    Disorders, 46
Suicide, 155, 156
  analogous age-adjusted odds ratio, 182
  blue-collar occupations, 182
  Global Financial Crisis, 182
  higher rate, 181
  high-status occupations, 181
  low-status occupations, 181
  meta-analysis, 181
  pooled relative risk, 181
  unemployment, 181, 182
Suicide mortality rate, 32
Suicide rates, 24
Suicide: A Study in Sociology' (book), 36
Syrian refugee resettlement program, 6
Systematic review, 181

T

Teacher-training programs, 169
Temporariness, 188

Tertiary education, 153, 155, 195
    demographics, 165
    gender differential, 165
    health care, 166
    male engagement, 166
    male underrepresentation, 165
    postsecondary campuses, 166
    postsecondary enrollment, 165
    preponderance, 165
    statistics, 164
    US *Condition of Education* report, 165
    US Department of Education, 165
    villain dichotomy, 166
Therapeutic approach, 237
Three longitudinal studies, 189
Toxic masculinity, 34, 166, 169, 235, 237, 241
Traditional boyhood pursuits, 169
Traditional jurisdictions/subcultures, 214
Traditional masculinity
    APA, 237, 238
    CBT, 238
    clinicians and services, 239
    harm mental health, 238
    ideology, 237
    influence mental health, 237
    men's mental health, 237
    mental health issues, 239
    pathologization, 237
    psychosocial variables, 238

U

UK National Institute for Health Care Excellence (NICE), 82
Underachievement, 168
Underrepresentation, 168
Unemployed females, 184
Unemployed nonmanual workers, 185
Unemployment, 28, 29, 37
    criminality and antisocial behavior, 197
    depression and anxiety, 185, 186
    disintegration, 179
    financial implications, 183
    job loss, 179
    meta-analysis, 180
    nefarious consequences, 197
    negative mental health effects, 180
    positive secondary benefits, 179
    psychological distress, 180
    psychological problems, 180
    relevant reviews, 180
    SUD, 183–185
    suicide, 181–183
Unemployment rates, 195
University administrators, 169
Unmanageability, 45
Unmarried and divorced men, 227
Unmarried men, 214
Unmarried women, 212
Unplanned biographical disruption, 213
US Bureau of Labor Statistics, 178, 190, 191, 195, 196
US Centers for Disease Control and Prevention (CDC), 12, 23
US *Condition of Education* report, 160, 163
US Epidemiological Catchment Area study, 57
US Food and Drug Administration (FDA), 82
US National Ambulatory Medical Care Survey, 89
US National Epidemiologic Survey on Alcohol and Related Conditions (NESARC), 49, 52, 113
US National Health Interview Survey, 107
US National Longitudinal Mortality Study, 211
US National Longitudinal Survey of Youth, 222
US Substance Abuse and Mental Health Services Administration (SAMHSA), 46

V

Victim-blaming, 2, 3, 34, 239
Victim-blaming deficit-based approach, 239
Vitamins, 177

W

Western jurisdictions, 217
White House Gender Policy Council, 243
Women's health, 9
Workplace injuries, 192
Workplace issues, 186
Workplace psychological demands, 189
Workplace stigma, 187, 193, 194
World Health Organization (WHO), 3, 23, 46